Advanced Concepts in Endocarditis - 2021

Edited by Michael S. Firstenberg and Umashankar Lakshmanadoss

Published in London, United Kingdom

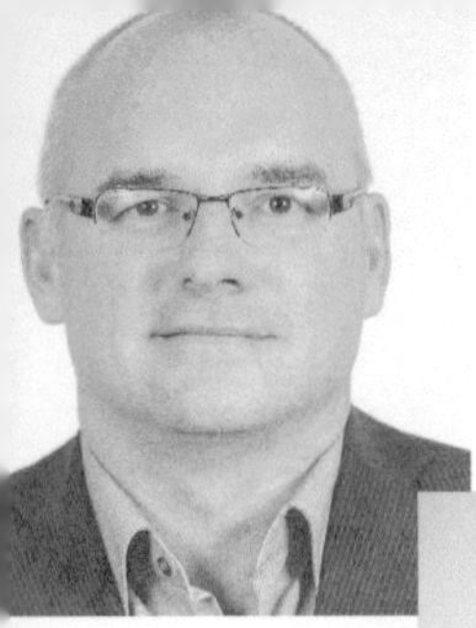
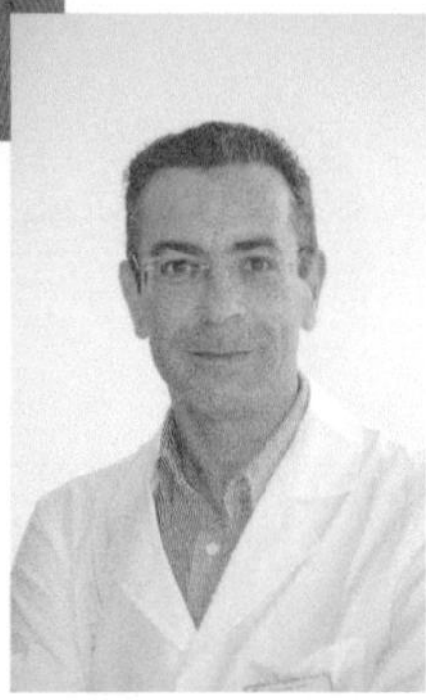
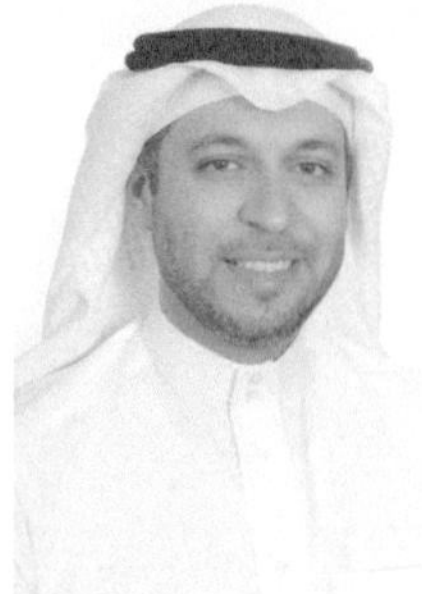
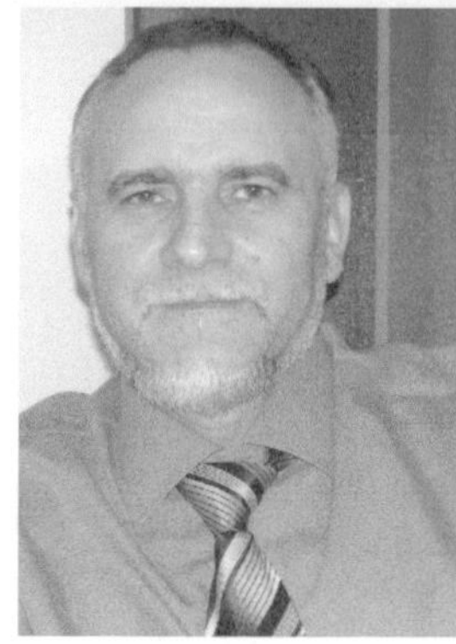
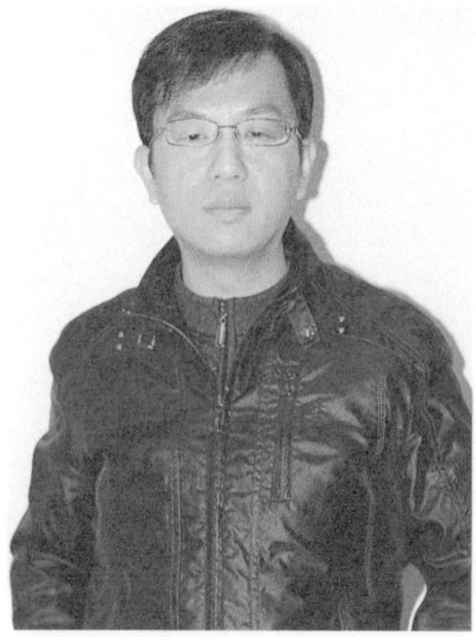
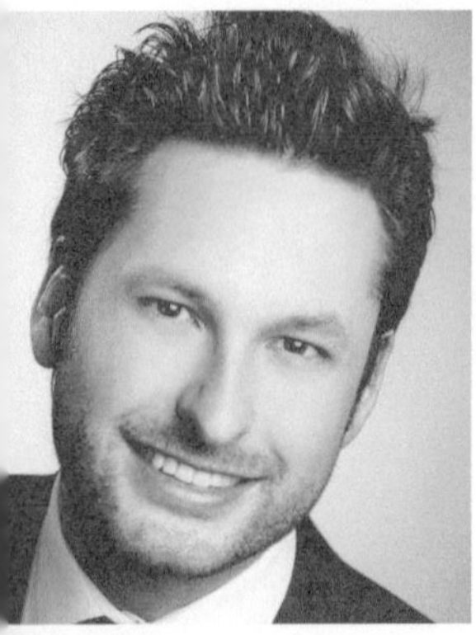
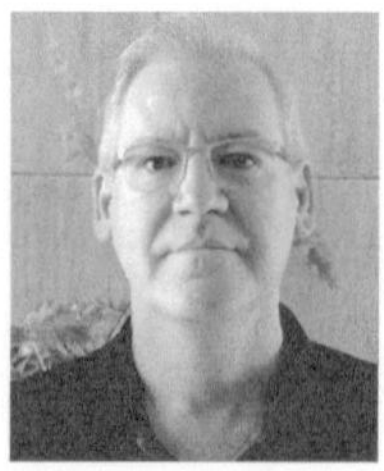

IntechOpen

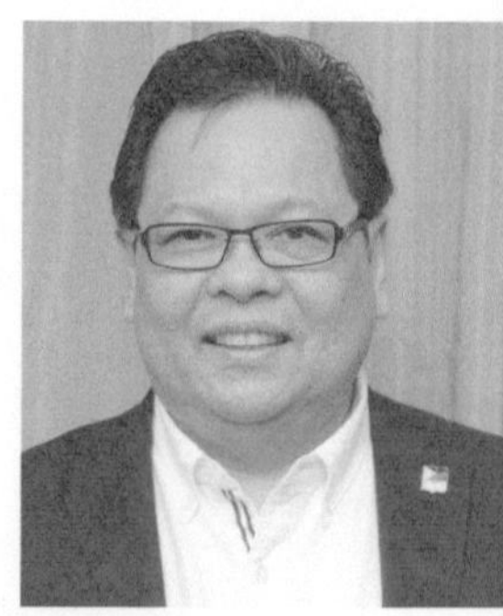
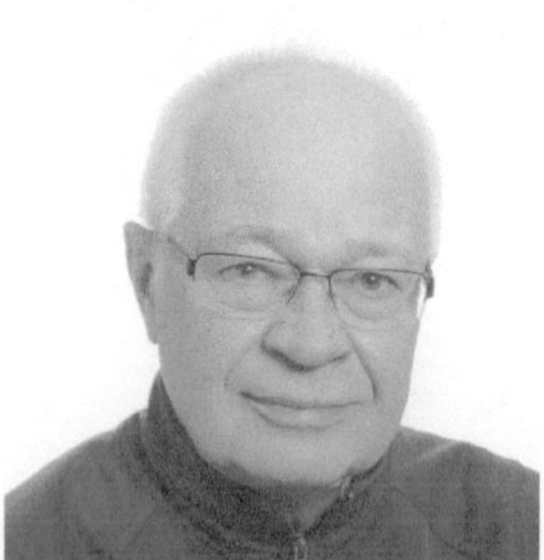
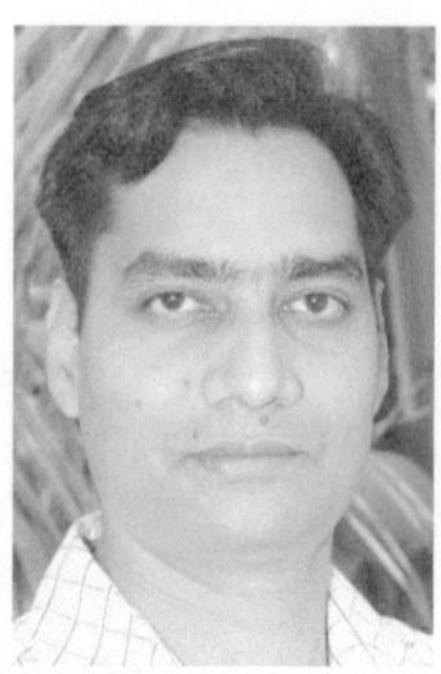
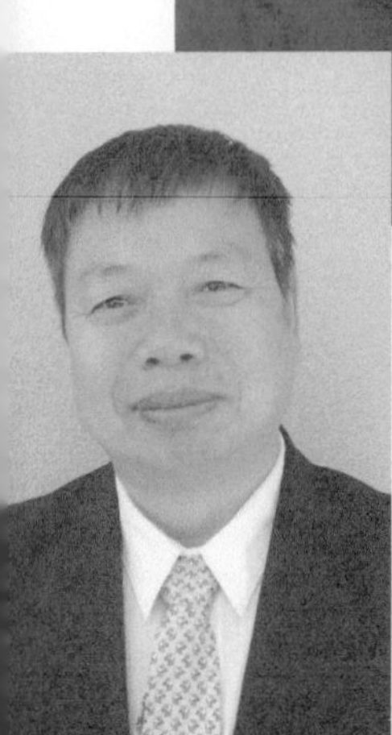
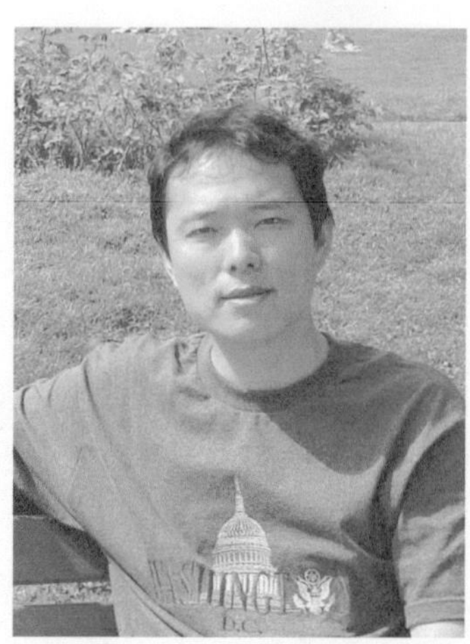
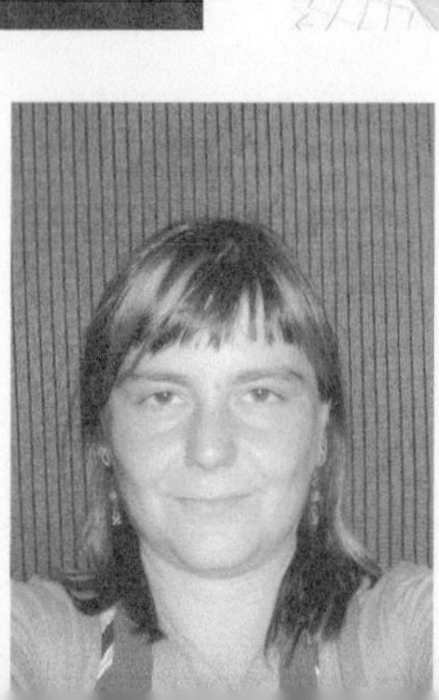

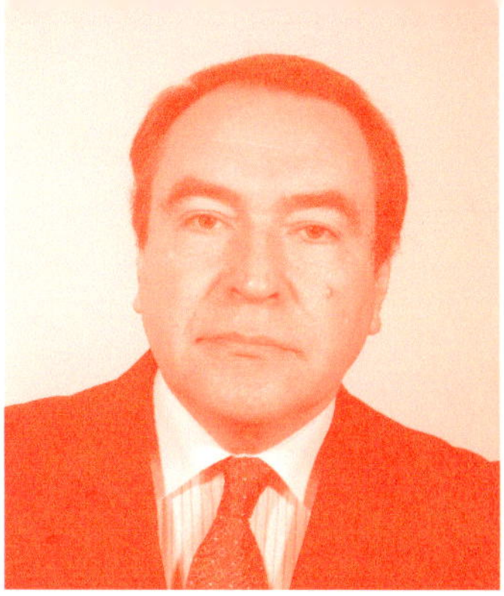
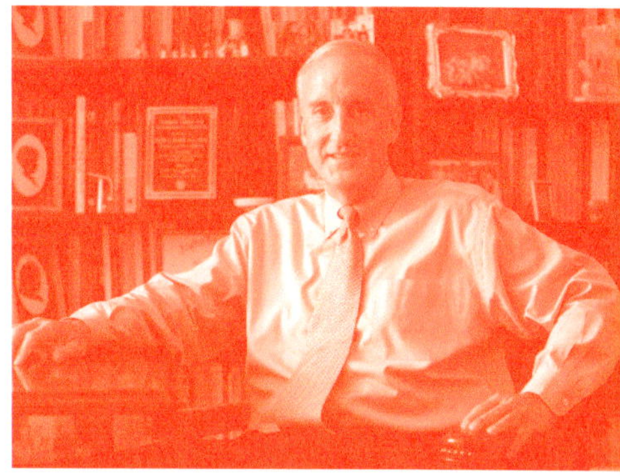
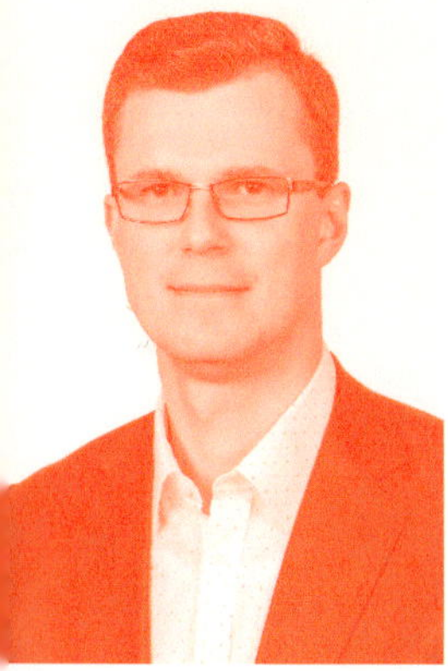
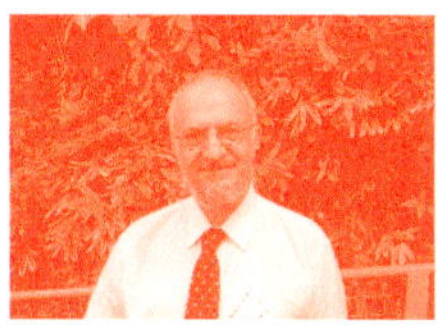
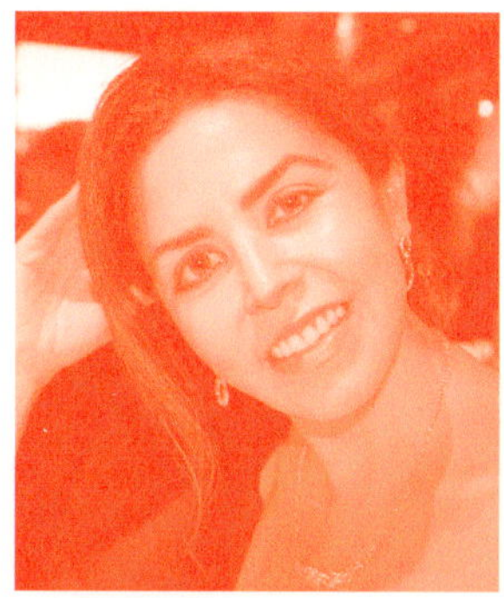

Supporting open minds since 2005

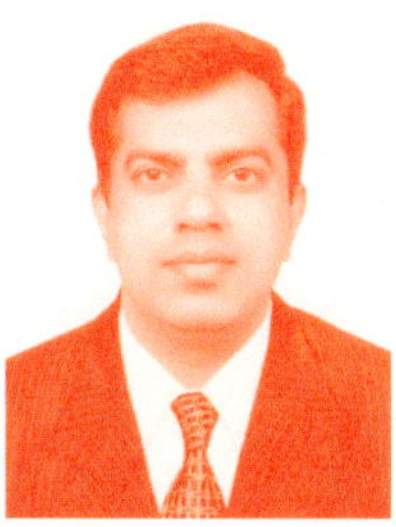
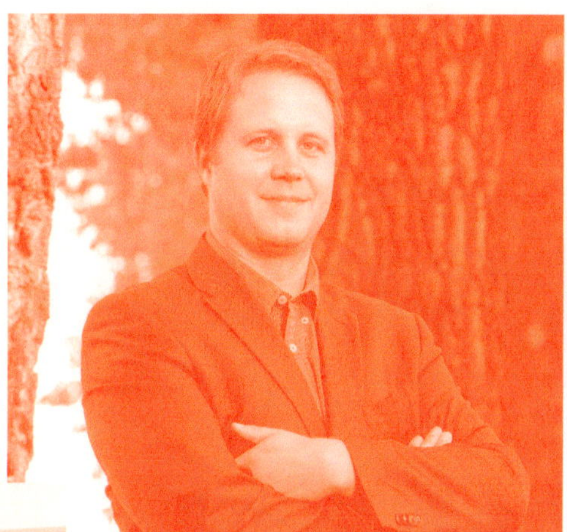
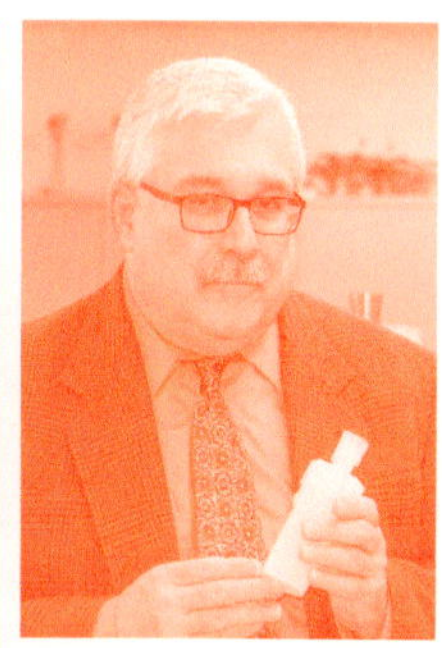
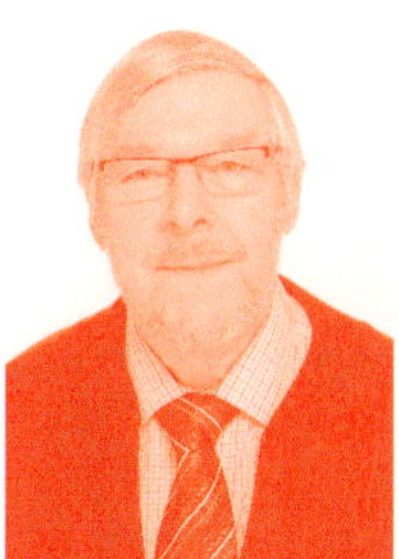
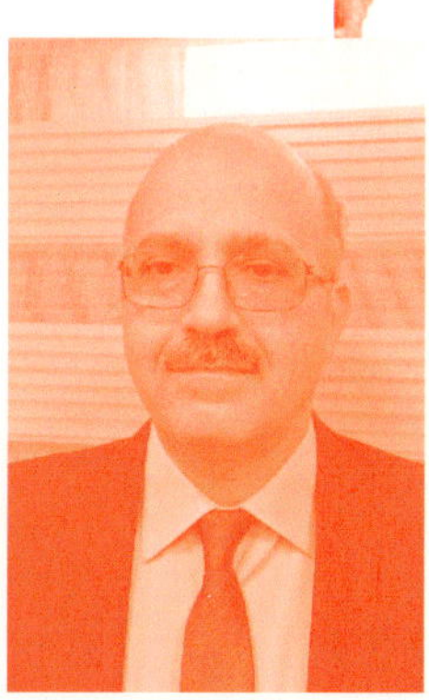
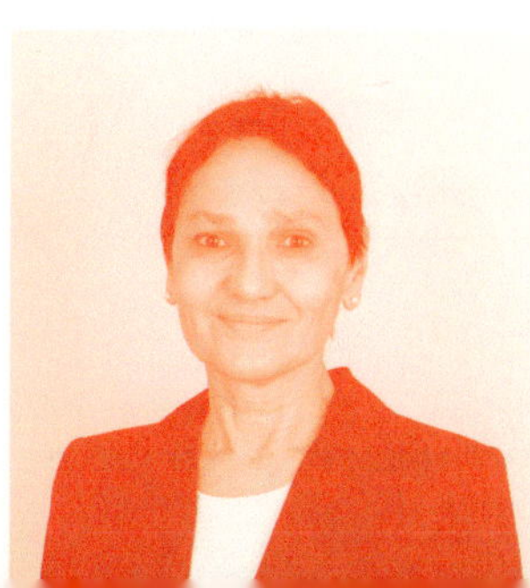
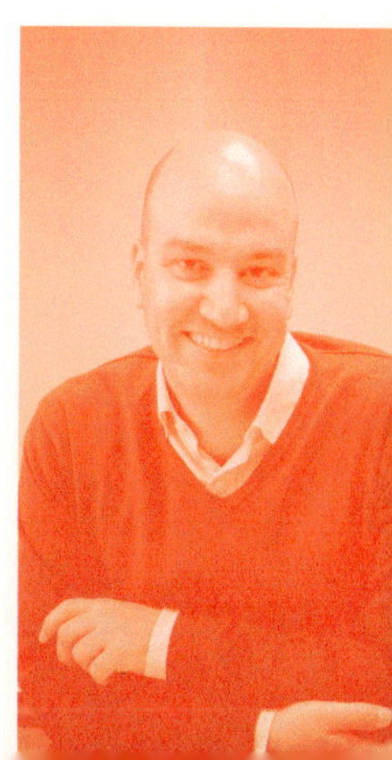

Advanced Concepts in Endocarditis - 2021
http://dx.doi.org/10.5772/intechopen.87377
Edited by Michael S. Firstenberg and Umashankar Lakshmanadoss

---

Contributors
Theodoros Ntoskas, Changbaig Hyun, Sang-Il Suh, Ran Choi, Ta-Li Lu, Madhavi Latha Routhu, Krishna Gudikandula, Eric J. Stöhr, T. Jake Samuel, Mark Joseph, Vira I. Ayzenbart, Sameh M. M. Said, Amparo Benedicto, Lourdes Dominguez, José A. Oteo, Lara García-Álvarez, Michael S. Firstenberg

First published in London, United Kingdom, 2021 by IntechOpen
IntechOpen is the global imprint of INTECHOPEN LIMITED, registered in England and Wales, registration number: 11086078, 5 Princes Gate Court, London, SW7 2QJ, United Kingdom
Printed in Croatia

British Library Cataloguing-in-Publication Data
A catalogue record for this book is available from the British Library

Additional hard and PDF copies can be obtained from orders@intechopen.com

Advanced Concepts in Endocarditis - 2021
Edited by Michael S. Firstenberg and Umashankar Lakshmanadoss
p. cm.
Print ISBN 978-1-83968-479-1
Online ISBN 978-1-83968-480-7
eBook (PDF) ISBN 978-1-83968-481-4

For EU product safety concerns:
IN TECH d.o.o., Prolaz Marije Krucifikse Kozulić 3, 51000 Rijeka, Croatia, info@intechopen.com or visit our website at intechopen.com.

Meet the editor

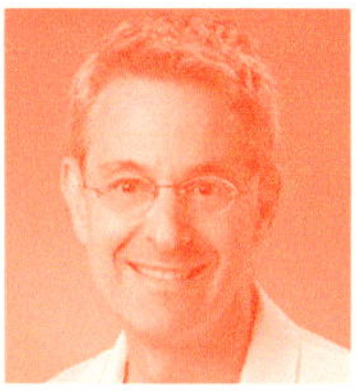

Dr. Michael S. Firstenberg is a thoracic surgeon at the St. Elizabeth Medical Center (Ascension) in Appleton, Wisconsin. He attended Case Western Reserve University Medical School, Cleveland, OH, USA, received his general surgery training at University Hospitals in Cleveland, and completed thoracic surgery fellowships at The Ohio State University and The Cleveland Clinic. He is an active member of the Society of Thoracic Surgeons (STS), American Association of Thoracic Surgeons (AATS), the American College of Cardiology (ACC), and the American College of Academic International Medicine (ACAIM), for which he served as president in 2021–2022. He has authored more than 250 peer-reviewed manuscripts, abstracts, and book chapters and has edited several textbooks and lectured worldwide on topics ranging from medical leadership, COVID-19, endocarditis, and extra-corporeal membrane oxygenation (ECMO).

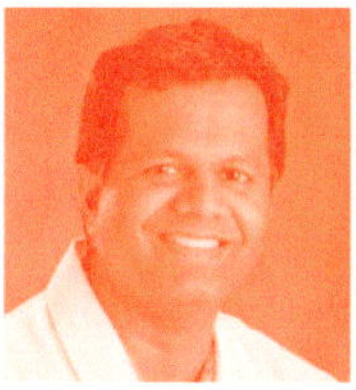

Dr. Umashankar Lakshmanadoss completed his training at the University of Rochester, NY, USA. He served as the director of inpatient medical consult service at Johns Hopkins University School of Medicine, Baltimore, MD, USA, and then joined the Division of Cardiovascular Medicine at Guthrie Clinic, Sayre, PA, USA. Then he pursued training in cardiac electrophysiology at William Beaumont School of Medicine and continued advanced cardiac electrophysiology training at Mayo Clinic, Rochester, MN. He served as an assistant professor of medicine in the Division of Cardiology, Louisiana State University, Shreveport, LA, where he also serves as the director of the complex arrhythmia ablation program. His research interest is in the field of cardiac electrophysiology. Currently, he is the director of cardiac electrophysiology at Mercy Health, Cincinnati, OH, USA.

Contents

Preface

The diagnosis of endocarditis has evolved substantially over the years, and there are many reasons for this. Advances in medical imaging technologies, including echocardiography, computed tomography (CT), and magnetic resonance imaging (MRI) combined with greater utilization of these modalities for the serial diagnosis and management of patients have allowed for improved diagnosis and understanding of various disease conditions. In addition, greater awareness of the problem, especially some of the contributing risk factors such as implantable cardiac devices, intravenous drug/substance abuse, and more advanced chronically ill and immunosuppressed patients, has contributed to a significant increase in the overall incidence of infections involving heart valves and other cardiac structures.

While the diagnosis of endocarditis has remained somewhat consistent over the years, the tools used to evaluate and manage patients have become more widely available, more accurate, and more precise. Because of the increased utilization of advanced imaging technologies on patients at all stages of life, many more patients are being diagnosed with potential infectious complications of their cardiac structures. This has resulted in a growing incidence of unusual, complex, and poorly understood problems, all of which are discussed in this book.

It is also becoming clear that the global increase in substance abuse, especially intravenous drugs and the use of 'dirty' needles or 'contaminated' drugs, has also increased the incidence of infectious problems. While the ethical implications of managing patients with long-standing substance abuse have been previously discussed, various chapters in this book address some of the practical aspects of management of infectious complications associated with 'right-sided problems. Historically, the established international guidelines have focused on the management of 'left-sided disease, namely, involving the aortic and/or mitral valves. However, with the increased incidence of 'right-sided pathology, mainly the tricuspid valve and less commonly the pulmonic valve, the technical aspects of management continued to evolve. Likewise, decision-making regarding indications, medical therapy, and goals of care continue to evolve and become incorporated into professional society guidelines.

With the growing understanding of the incidence, risk factors, management, and overall pathophysiology of endocarditis, there is also the increasing recognition of a potential impact on a broader range of the patient population. For example, with advanced in-cancer therapies and the potential impact on the heart, there is also growing interest in the potential role that oncologic treatment has on the heart, either as a primary impact or a secondary process, such as an increased risk for structural abnormalities including infectious endocarditis, and the ability to distinguish between normal, abnormal, and abnormal from infectious complications versus non-infectious complications. Chapters in this text lend some insights and guidance into these evolving multi-disciplinary areas of cardio-oncologic care.

While the topic of endocarditis is extensive and a comprehensive review is far beyond the scope of a single project, it is the goal of this text to highlight some evolving areas in both the diagnosis and management of infectious complications. Even though the focus is on the pathophysiology of endocarditis, it is also important to recognize that the same advanced diagnostic tools that are being used to identify various pathologic states are also being more widely utilized to better help understand the natural history and evolution from normal structure and function to a pathologic disease state. In other words, a primary goal of this text is to provide some greater insights into the rapidly evolving themes regarding the diagnosis and management of endocarditis with the recognition that to understand abnormal appropriately, we also must be proficient in our understanding of normal.

The editors greatly appreciate the authors for their hard work and thoughtful contributions.

Michael S. Firstenberg
St. Elizabeth Medical Center,
Appleton, Wisconsin, USA

Umashankar Lakshmanadoss MD, FACC, FHRS, CCCDS
Mercy Heart Institute,
Cincinnati, OH, USA

Chapter 1

Introductory Chapter: Endocarditis

Michael S. Firstenberg

1. Introduction

Endocarditis a very complex and diverse set of problems and can include infectious and non-infectious diseases of the heart. The spectrum of problems includes vegetations on valves, fistulas and abscess cavities, and infections that develop on prosthetic materials such as pacemaker and defibrillator leads, prosthetic valves, intra-cardiac catheters, heart pumps, and any other type of intra-cardiac foreign material. The diagnosis and management of these problems can be quite challenging and will typically require an integrated multi-disciplinary team. Nevertheless, with advances in the therapies that are being offered to older and sicker patients, offset by advances in both the medical and surgical management of infectious cardiac problems, the number of cases continue to grow with still major risks for morbidity and mortality. In addition, the global concerns for substance abuse and the risks for the use of contaminated needles has led to a significant increase in associated infectious complications. Without a doubt, endocarditis in the setting of substance abuse is not only a significant medical and surgical problem – but a difficult social problem as well. The financial and ethical implications of endocarditis further highlight the emphasis of a team-based approach to the diagnosis and management.

Unfortunately, even minor invasive procedures have been shown to increase to risk of infections of native or prosthetic valves [1]. Typically, endocarditis was associated with blood-stream infections in the setting of dental procedures, but it is becoming more recognized that even minor procedures, such as gastrointestinal endoscopy, can increase risk for cardiac infections and might prompt a broader reevaluation of the role of prophylactic antibiotics prior to such procedures. Evidence, especially in higher-risk patients such as those with bicuspid aortic valves and mitral valve prolapse, is suggesting that the risk for bloodstream infection might be greater than historically believed [2].

The growing incidence of endocarditis also parallels the growing social problems of modern society as is seen in the evolving epidemiology of patients presenting with infections of their heart, heart valves, and intra-cardiac devices and structures. As mentioned, the global drug abuse epidemic – combined with the increasing utilization of cardiac procedures in older and sicker patients with advanced co-morbidities, reflects the need for a more wide-spread recognition of this problem. Fortunately, advances in diagnostic –especially imaging technology and microbiology serology testing – and surgical techniques can improve outcomes in those who present with even advanced disease. As such, the goal of this book is to emphasize and review some of the evolving concepts in the diagnosis, presentation, epidemiology, and management options of endocarditis.

2. Epidemiology

As discussed above, the areas of greatest focus are currently the implications of the global intravenous drug abuse (IVDA) epidemic and the growing utilization of cardiac implantable devices (CID). Both of these very different set of problems has each contributed to a substantial increase in the incidence of endocarditis and, particularly, involving right-sided cardiac structures such as the tricuspid valve. While there is extensive literature and guidelines for the diagnosis and management of left-sided disease (i.e. aortic and/or mitral valves), the literature for the diagnosis and treatment of right-sided disease is still evolving and will reviewed in several of the chapters of this text. It is not just the medical difficulties in the management of IVDA associated endocarditis that continues to be a problem, but the social and ethical implications for re-infections in patients who continue to abuse drugs or fail to pursue appropriate definitive therapy [3, 4]. The recognition of this growing problem is only slowly being better understood [5]. In addition, as mentioned, with the growing utilization of advanced cardiac therapies and implants, there is also a growing risk and incidence of device-related infectious complications [6, 7]. Unfortunately, the increasing use of such devices is expanding at a rate that is exceeding the healthcare systems ability to better understand how to prevent, diagnosis, and treat such device related infections [8–10]. However, with the development and expansion of "Heart Team" to better guide therapies and management, there exist increasing opportunities to improve outcomes by incorporating a team-based approach to the management of these very difficult problems.

3. Diagnosis

Positive blood cultures are the *sine quo non* in establishing a diagnosis of endocarditis. In addition, the original Dukes Criteria has been used for many years to further help make the diagnosis [11]. Advances in ultrasound imaging has shown to be extremely useful in the management of patients and guiding therapy [12]. Transthoracic and transesophageal imaging are considered first-line tests to evaluate for suspected endocarditis. Current major international society guidelines and appropriateness criteria support their liberal use [2, 12] – the role of other modalities, such as 3D echocardiography, computed tomography (CT), magnetic resonance imaging, and positron-emission tomography (PET) continues to expand [13, 14]. Nevertheless, such diagnostic tools should be readily available and aggressively used, including non-cardiac imaging of the neuro-axis and body structures, to ensure the scope of what is typically a systemic problem is completely defined. Furthermore, any change in the clinical picture or concerns for disease progression or failure of medical therapies should prompt a timely reassessment with repeat imaging.

4. Therapy

Without a doubt the cornerstone to early managed is focused on targeted antibiotic therapies, diagnosis of the primary problem, evaluation for secondary complications (such as embolic complications, like stroke), and engagement of a multi-disciplinary team of physicians and healthcare providers, who, by definition have both an interest and expertise in endocarditis to help define a treatment plan. As with any treatment plan, the recipe for success must consider if and when surgery should be performed (and which operation – not an easy decision process) and how some of the contributing co-morbidities can be attenuated to minimize the risks for recurrence. While it is easy to focus on the initial diagnosis and managed, often an index hospitalization, long-term success requires close follow-up to monitor for compliance to optimize the opportunity an overall successful treatment plan. Because of the challenges of many of the socio-economic problems that patients with endocarditis often face, and are addressed in some of the chapters of this text, full engagement by the entire healthcare team will need to make sure that any and all obstacles to treatment success are removed, if possible. An extensive medical and surgical plan that does not consider the socio-economic variables that are often unique to each patient are probably at risk for treatment failure.

One of the most important decisions in the management of endocarditis is determining the role of surgery – and not just if surgery should be performed, but when, what operation, choices of valves, risks for complications, barriers to follow-up (i.e. need for life-long anticoagulation if mechanical valves are used), and maybe even where and by whom. Such decision making cannot and should not be performed in the vacuum of specific guidelines and indications for surgery but also must consider the entire evolving clinical picture. Regardless of the direction of the care plan, recognition of the impact on timing of therapies is of critical importance. As with most medical problems, delays in therapy might make the problem worse and hence require not just a broad understanding of the evolving literature regarding the timing of surgery, but the importance of timely evaluation of problems, regardless of how trivial they may appear and constant re-assessment of the treatment plan to ensure the original plan is working as planned as does not need to be revised [15–18].

A common theme in many of these chapters is the decision-making process and role for surgery. A point that requires further emphasis is the role for early surgery and how this concept needs to cage every aspect of a larger treatment plan, specifically [19]:

1. Early surgery is recommended in patients with highly-resistant organisms and, in particular, fungal infections.

2. Worsening heart failure (especially acute) due to valvular dysfunction.

3. New or worsening cardiac complications – such as root abscesses, fistulas, heart block, and evidence of new/worsening annular involvement.

4. Surgery is indicated with failure of medical therapy, such as persistent bacteremia or septic symptoms (fever, tachycardia) greater than 5–7 days in the absence of another causes in the setting of targeted antibiotic management.

5. Growing vegetations despite appropriate antibiotic therapy – especially with evidence of recurrent embolic complications.

6. Large and/or mobile vegetations (>1 cm) and/or with severe valve regurgitation – even in the absence of heart failure signs and symptoms.

Unfortunately, such decision-making and indications often mandates surgery in less than optimal conditions – such as patients who are still actively infected, have sustained recent systemic or cerebral embolic complications, or are risk for long-term reinfection due to compliance or concerns of co-existing and incompletely addressed or defined comorbidities. Such is the realities of this disease process and all providers must recognize that sometimes earlier intervention, even if in less-than-ideal surgical conditions, might be ultimately better for the patient in the long run.

Similar considerations are used to guide the management of prosthetic valve endocarditis [20]. Despite the challenges of re-operative surgery in a "septic" patient, it must be appreciated that medical therapies alone are rarely successful, the best opportunity for a cure often requires complete removal of all prosthetic material and replacement.

5. Social implications

The pandemic of intravenous drug abuse has resulted in a substantial increase in the incidence of endocarditis. There is at least a twofold increase in the number of heroin users from 2006 to 2013 [21]. The medical, social, and economic implications are obviously substantial. The role of infected needles, infected drugs, skin contamination, or some combination all contribute to the risk for endocarditis. Acute infections are further challenged by other substantial comorbidities, such as untreated Hepatitis B/C and the Human Immunodeficiency Virus (HIV) [22]. As a consequence of long-standing narcotic use/abuse, infected patients will often chronic pain syndromes and drug tolerance that can make symptom management difficult. In addition, mental health and personality disorders also challenge how these patients are treated – the mental and emotional fatigue placed upon the healthcare team can be substantial and might be used to influence the decision-making process for an individual patient. It is critical to consider all of these co-variates in the context of decision-making, need for compliance, and potential long-term therapy implications. For example, while replacement with biologic valves may predispose to early structural degeneration and need for additional surgery, their use might be a better longer-term strategy than subjecting a potentially non-compliant patient with untreated Hepatitis to life-long anticoagulation. In other words, even if the acute infectious problem is "cured", many of the decisions regarding the management of endocarditis – including the re-infection prevention opportunities – reflect that endocarditis can often be viewed as a life-long problem [23]. The ethical considerations of both acute and chronic disease management, as discussed in this chapter on the ethics of recurrent drug use/abuse, clearly demonstrates that long-term success often is as much a function of the overall team approach to the problems (rarely is endocarditis a singular problem) including the contributing factors, such as substance abuse. The tragic reality, however, is that while the ethics of the social approach to endocarditis often plays a substantial role in the management of individual patients, the foundation for such biases might be inherently flawed. Furthermore, there must be an understanding that despite everything being "done right" many patients, as a function of incurable comorbidities, much like complications of advanced cancers, patients might still die with and from endocarditis.

6. Conclusions

Improvements in diagnostic tools and an increasing understanding of the scope of associated problems have led to an increase in the recognition and management complexity of infectious endocarditis. Challenging social problems, advanced co-morbidities, and complex infections emphasize the role for early and aggressive management by a well-integrated and comprehensive multi-disciplinary team.

Hopefully, while each chapter in this text will stand on its own, taken together, the goal of this project is to help emphasize the importance of collaborative Team work and consideration for all of the contributing co-morbidities, and a comprehensive plan are critical to the short and long-term treatment successes [24, 25].

It cannot be emphasized enough that the goal of this volume is to lend valuable perspectives into some of the rapidly evolving topics and challenges surrounding the treatment of endocarditis – including management of complications, role and time of surgery, and the holistic approach to what often evolves into a life-long problem. Hopefully, with a greater understanding and emphasis on Teamwork, improvements in prevention, diagnosis, and treatment will result in better outcomes for all.

Author details

Michael S. Firstenberg
Ascension NE Wisconsin–St. Elizabeth Campus, Appleton, Wisconsin, United States

*Address all correspondence to: msfirst@gmail.com

References

[1] Janszky I, Gémes K, Ahnve S, Asgeirsson H, Möller J. Invasive Procedures Associated With the Development of Infective Endocarditis. Journal of the American College of Cardiology. 2018 Jun 19;71(24): 2744-2752.

[2] Zegri-Reiriz I, de Alarcón A, Muñoz P, Sellés MM, González-Ramallo V, Miro JM, Falces C, Rico CG, Urkola XK, Lepe JA, Alvarez RR. Infective Endocarditis in Patients With Bicuspid Aortic Valve or Mitral Valve Prolapse. Journal of the American College of Cardiology. 2018 Jun 11;71(24):2731-2740.

[3] Sousa, C., Botelho, C., Rodrigues, D., Azeredo, J. and Oliveira, R., 2012. Infective endocarditis in intravenous drug abusers: an update. European journal of clinical microbiology & infectious diseases, *31*(11), pp.2905-2910.

[4] Habib, G., Lancellotti, P., Antunes, M.J., Bongiorni, M.G., Casalta, J.P., Del Zotti, F., Dulgheru, R., El Khoury, G., Erba, P.A., Iung, B. and Miro, J.M., 2015. 2015 ESC Guidelines for the management of infective endocarditis. *European heart journal*, p.ehv319.

[5] Njoroge LW, Al-Kindi SG, Koromia GA, ElAmm CA, Oliveira GH. Changes in the Association of Rising Infective Endocarditis With Mortality in People Who Inject Drugs. JAMA cardiology. 2018 Jun 20.

[6] Latib, A., Naim, C., De Bonis, M., Sinning, J.M., Maisano, F., Barbanti, M., Parolari, A., Lorusso, R., Testa, L., Dato, G.M.A. and Miceli, A., 2014. TAVR-associated prosthetic valve infective endocarditis: results of a large, multicenter registry. *Journal of the American College of Cardiology*, *64*(20), pp.2176-2178.

[7] Salaun E, Sportouch L, Barral PA, Hubert S, Lavoute C, Casalta AC, Pradier J, Ouk D, Casalta JP, Lambert M, Gouriet F. Diagnosis of Infective Endocarditis After TAVR: Value of a Multimodality Imaging Approach. JACC. Cardiovascular imaging. 2018 Jan;11(1):143-146.

[8] Thornhill, M.H., Dayer, M.J., Jones, S., Prendergast, B., Baddour, L.M. and Lockhart, P.B., 2016. The Effect of Antibiotic Prophylaxis Guidelines on Incidence of Infective Endocarditis. Canadian Journal of Cardiology.

[9] Patanè, S., 2014. Is there a need for bacterial endocarditis prophylaxis in patients undergoing gastrointestinal endoscopy?. Journal of cardiovascular translational research, *7*(3), pp.372-374.

[10] Dayer, M.J., Jones, S., Prendergast, B., Baddour, L.M., Lockhart, P.B. and Thornhill, M.H., 2015. Incidence of infective endocarditis in England, 2000-13: a secular trend, interrupted time-series analysis. The Lancet, *385*(9974), pp.1219-1228.

[11] Baddour, L.M., Wilson, W.R., Bayer, A.S., Fowler, V.G., Tleyjeh, I.M., Rybak, M.J., Barsic, B., Lockhart, P.B., Gewitz, M.H., Levison, M.E. and Bolger, A.F., 2015. Infective Endocarditis in Adults: Diagnosis, Antimicrobial Therapy, and Management of Complications A Scientific Statement for Healthcare Professionals From the American Heart Association. Circulation, *132*(15), pp.1435-1486.

[12] Bruun, N.E., Habib, G., Thuny, F. and Sogaard, P., 2014. Cardiac imaging in infectious endocarditis. European heart journal, *35*(10), pp.624-632.

[13] Habets, J., Tanis, W., Reitsma, J.B., van den Brink, R.B., Willem, P.T.M., Chamuleau, S.A. and Budde, R.P., 2015. Are novel non-invasive imaging techniques needed in patients with suspected prosthetic heart valve endocarditis? A systematic review and meta-analysis. European radiology, *25*(7), pp.2125-2133.

[14] Mahmood M, Kendi AT, Ajmal S, Farid S, O'Horo JC, Chareonthaitawee P, Baddour LM, Sohail MR. Meta-analysis of 18F-FDG PET/CT in the diagnosis of infective endocarditis. Journal of Nuclear Cardiology. 2017 Oct 30:1-4.

[15] Yanagawa B, Pettersson GB, Habib G, Ruel M, Saposnik G, Latter DA, Verma S. Surgical management of infective endocarditis complicated by embolic stroke: practical recommendations for clinicians. Circulation. 2016 Oct 25;134(17):1280-1292.

[16] Aranki, S.F., Santini, F., Adams, D.H., Rizzo, R.J., Couper, G.S., Kinchla, N.M., Gildea, J.S., Collins Jr, J.J. and Cohn, L.H., 1994. Aortic valve endocarditis. Determinants of early survival and late morbidity. Circulation, *90*(5 Pt 2), pp.II175-II182.

[17] Kang, D.H., Kim, Y.J., Kim, S.H., Sun, B.J., Kim, D.H., Yun, S.C., Song, J.M., Choo, S.J., Chung, C.H., Song, J.K. and Lee, J.W., 2012. Early surgery versus conventional treatment for infective endocarditis. New England Journal of Medicine, *366*(26), pp.2466-2473.

[18] Erbel, R.A., 2014. The New Strategy in Infective Endocarditis: Early Surgery Based on Early Diagnosis: Are We Too Late, When Early Surgery is Best?. *Circulation*, pp.CIRCULATIONAHA-114.

[19] Firstenberg MS (November 9th 2016). Introductory Chapter: Endocarditis - A Diagnostic and Therapeutic Challenge, Contemporary Challenges in Endocarditis Michael S. Firstenberg, IntechOpen, DOI: 10.5772/66406. Available from: https://www.intechopen.com/books/contemporary-challenges-in-endocarditis/introductory-chapter-endocarditis-a-diagnostic-and-therapeutic-challenge

[20] Perrotta, S., Jeppsson, A., Fröjd, V. and Svensson, G., 2016. Surgical treatment of aortic prosthetic valve endocarditis: a 20-year single-center experience. The Annals of thoracic surgery, *101*(4), pp.1426-1432.

[21] Wurcel, A.G., Anderson, J.E., Chui, K.K., Skinner, S., Knox, T.A., Snydman, D.R. and Stopka, T.J., 2016, May. Increasing Infectious Endocarditis Admissions Among Young People Who Inject Drugs. In *Open Forum Infectious Diseases* (Vol. 3, No. 3, p. ofw157). Oxford University Press.

[22] Gundelly, P., Burgess, D.S., Boulay, J., Caldwell, G. and Thornton, A., 2014, December. 921Prevalence of Hepatitis C Infection and Epidemiology of Infective Endocarditis in Intravenous Drug Users in Central Kentucky. In *Open Forum Infectious Diseases* (Vol. 1, No. suppl 1, pp. S266-S266). Oxford University Press.

[23] Magsino K, Sanjanwala R, Hiebert B, Rothney J, Manji R, Arora R, Shah P. Treatment Outcomes for Right-Sided Endocarditis in Intravenous Drug Users: A Systematic Review and Analysis of Outcomes in a Tertiary Centre. The Thoracic and cardiovascular surgeon. 2018 Jan 19.

[24] Chambers, J., Sandoe, J., Ray, S., Prendergast, B., Taggart, D., Westaby, S., Arden, C., Grothier, L., Wilson, J., Campbell, B. and Gohlke-Bärwolf, C., 2014. The infective endocarditis team: recommendations from an international

working group. Heart, *100*(7), pp.524-527.

[25] Chirillo, F., Scotton, P., Rocco, F., Rigoli, R., Polesel, E. and Olivari, Z., 2013. Management of patients with infective endocarditis by a multidisciplinary team approach: an operative protocol. Journal of Cardiovascular Medicine, *14*(9), pp.659-668.

Chapter 2

Echocardiographic Assessment of Myocardial Deformation during Exercise

Eric J. Stöhr and T. Jake Samuel

Abstract

The human heart is an asymmetrical structure that consists of oblique, circumferential, and transmural fibers, as well as laminae and sheets. Sequential electrical activation of all the muscle fibers ultimately results in a coordinated contraction of the heart muscle also referred to as "deformation." This is immediately followed by myocardial relaxation, when the preceding deformation is reversed, and the ventricles fill with blood. Given the complexity of these repetitive motions, it is not surprising that there is great diversity in the myocardial deformation between different individuals and between distinct populations. Exercise presents a natural challenge to determine the full capacity of an individual's heart, and modern imaging technologies allow for the non-invasive assessment of myocardial deformation during exercise. In this chapter, the most relevant anatomical basis for myocardial deformation is summarized and definitions of the most relevant parameters are provided. Then, the general cardiac responses to exercise are highlighted before the current knowledge on myocardial deformation during exercise is discussed. The literature clearly indicates that the echocardiographic evaluation of myocardial deformation during exercise holds great promise for the identification of sub-clinical disease. Future studies should aim to determine the mechanisms of differential expression of myocardial deformation during exercise in health and disease.

Keywords: exercise, heart, stress testing, diagnostics, imaging, echocardiography, VO_2max, CPET, strain, twist, torsion, untwisting rate, blood pressure, LVAD, heart failure, speckle tracking, hypertension

1. Introduction

In recent years, technological advances in the field of echocardiography have allowed for a faster acquisition of images with an improved spatial and temporal resolution. As part of these advances, the advent of speckle tracking imaging has resulted in an explosion of investigations into myocardial deformation, as evidenced by more than 5000 articles on PubMed, increasing exponentially since 2005 (https://pubmed.ncbi.nlm.nih.gov/?term=speckle+tracking, accessed 7th of May 2020). The past two decades has also seen in a shift in "stress echocardiography" from being dominated by acute drug-based interventions to primarily exercise challenges. Therefore, this chapter focuses on the current knowledge related to myocardial deformation during acute exercise stress. Instead of just summarizing the current literature, a careful selection of articles is presented that is then used to provide the reader with a narrative that highlights important general principles of cardiac physiology, including the responses to exercise. To achieve this aim, first a brief overview of the principles and mechanisms governing myocardial deformation will be provided summarised and the key terminology will be defined. Then, the general role of exercise stress testing will be discussed, before the benefits of obtaining myocardial deformation during exercise in health and disease will be reviewed.

2. Principles of myocardial deformation

During contraction of the heart, deformation of the whole muscle occurs in four quantifiable dimensions. In general, these have been identified as: longitudinal shortening (=longitudinal strain, %), circumferential shortening (circumferential strain, %), radial lengthening (=radial strain, %) and rotation (apical – basal rotation = net twist angle, degrees), as well as the diastolic reversal of all of these indices. In addition, the rate of systolic shortening and diastolic lengthening can be measured, which is referred to as strain rate, twisting rate, and untwisting rate. An important distinction must be made between myocardial deformation and pure "velocities", which do not consider the relative shortening (contraction) or lengthening (relaxation) of heart muscle itself but only consider the linear displacement of single myocardial points. Although myocardial velocities can also be measured, they are not representative of the contraction and relaxation of heart muscle. For these reasons, parameters such as E' ("E prime"), which typically represent myocardial velocities in a single location on the mitral annulus, are not discussed in this chapter.

The conventional categorizations of deformation into strain and twist are logical from a biophysics and bioengineering perspective, since deformation of the heart can indeed be detected in these distinct 2-dimensional echocardiographic imaging planes. However, as will be reviewed in the following section on the anatomy and electrical conductance, the structure of the heart is far from symmetrical and—to achieve the final coordination of all components with each heartbeat—important functional differences in the various regions within the heart are present. These intricate deformational patterns can be conceptually simplified by considering the region-specific deformation in a 2-dimensional plane, allowing for easier evaluation of cardiac mechanics in both the laboratory and the clinic. However, one must consider the 3D deformation of the heart muscle, where the deformation of the four imaging planes occur simultaneously and with many of these aspects anatomically and functionally interwoven. This anatomical complexity is the focus of the next section.

2.1 Anatomy

Historical reviews have often credited Leonardo da Vinci's observations in the 15th century as some of the first to describe the gross anatomy of the heart and his speculations about the resulting function. In his drawings[1], da Vinci refers to the importance of vortices, which necessitate the presence of helical structures and/or motions that were apparent as "clockwise and counterclockwise spirals within the aorta as the outlet of the left ventricle" [1]. More than a century after da Vinci's death, William Harvey published his seminal book *Exercitatio Anatomica De Motu Cordis Et Sanguinis In Animalibus* (An Anatomical Study on the Motion of the Heart and Blood in Living Beings, 1628 [2]), in which he established the circulation—including the anatomy

[1] In 2019, an exhibition across the UK celebrated the drawings by Leonardo da Vinci, including some of his anatomical sketches (https://www.rct.uk/collection/themes/exhibitions/leonardo-da-vinci-a-life-in-drawing/the-queens-gallery-palace-of).

and motion of the heart—as we mostly know it today, thereby also popularizing the previous work by Ibn al-Nafis [3]. In 1669, Richard Lower provided remarkable detail on the anatomy of the heart in his publication of *Tractatus de Corde...* (Treatise on the Heart. ... [4]). Despite these early discoveries, it wasn't until the contributions by McCallum and then Mall in the early twentieth century that there were new advancements in this field [5, 6]. During the second World War, Robb & Robb provided an exceptionally detailed overview of the accumulated knowledge that covered five centuries of discoveries [7]. Then, 27 years later, in 1969, Streeter et al. published the much-cited myocardial fiber distribution of the left ventricle (LV) in dogs, and Greenbaum et al. confirmed the observations in human cadavers [8, 9].

Today, after centuries of observations, there is still debate on the exact origins and arrangements of the heart [10]. However, general consensus exists that the mammalian LV consists of oblique fibers in the endocardium that gradually change into circumferential fibers in the midwall and continue to oblique fibers in the subepicardium, orientated in the opposite direction to those in the endocardium, thus creating what is often referred to as a helical arrangement [11–14]. Noteworthy insight has also been provided by the description of sheets and laminae, which may not only impact the effect of individual myofibres but also the electrical propagation across the myocardium [15, 16]. With regard to the latter, the coordinated sequence of electrical propagation and activation of the LV occurs in a specific apex-to-base and endocardial-to-epicardial order during systole [17]. Due to these different electrical activation times, each part of the heart muscle is activated for different durations, therefore shortening and lengthening velocities (or systolic and diastolic "strain rates") vary significantly in the different regions of the LV and are not associated with the overall heart rate [18]. A significant addition to the longstanding knowledge on oblique and circumferential fibers was provided by Lunkenheimer et al., who provided evidence for the existence of transmural myofibres that may be of fundamental relevance to the regulation of forces associated with normal myocardial contraction and relaxation [19]. Finally, there is important structural diversity on the myocyte level that contributes to the overall elasticity of the cardiomyocyte, as revealed by different isoforms of the giant protein titin, which may influence myocardial deformation in systole and diastole, not least during exercise [20, 21]. Collectively, the current knowledge indicates a non-uniform, complex mesh of diverse cardiac myofibre arrangements which may be grouped in sheets and laminae, influencing the electrical activation sequence of the heterogeneously distributed autonomic nerves in the heart (**Figure 1**, [22]). In comparison to the LV, the macro-structure of the right ventricle (RV) is not cone-shaped but resembles that of a crescent, almost wrapping around the LV. Yet, the underlying micro-structure is similar to the LV, albeit with some key differences. Like the LV, the epicardial and endocardial fibers are arranged helically, but with a smaller range of oblique angles [23]. The main difference to the LV seems to be in the myofiber arrangement of the midwall. Here, "the circumferentially arranged middle fibres are confined to the LV and septum" [8] and "without such beneficial architectural remodeling [...] seem unsuited structurally to sustain a permanent increase in afterload" [23]. It is probably because of the overall crescent shape (that makes echocardiographic image acquisition in any plane other than the longitudinal challenging), and the lack of an obvious torsional motion, that the assessment of right ventricular deformation has largely focused on longitudinal strain.

2.2 Definitions and selection of myocardial deformation parameters

Because of the increasing number of studies focused on myocardial deformation mentioned in the introduction to this chapter, it has been inevitable that some inconsistencies exist regarding the nomenclature in the literature (**Table 1**). Here, a

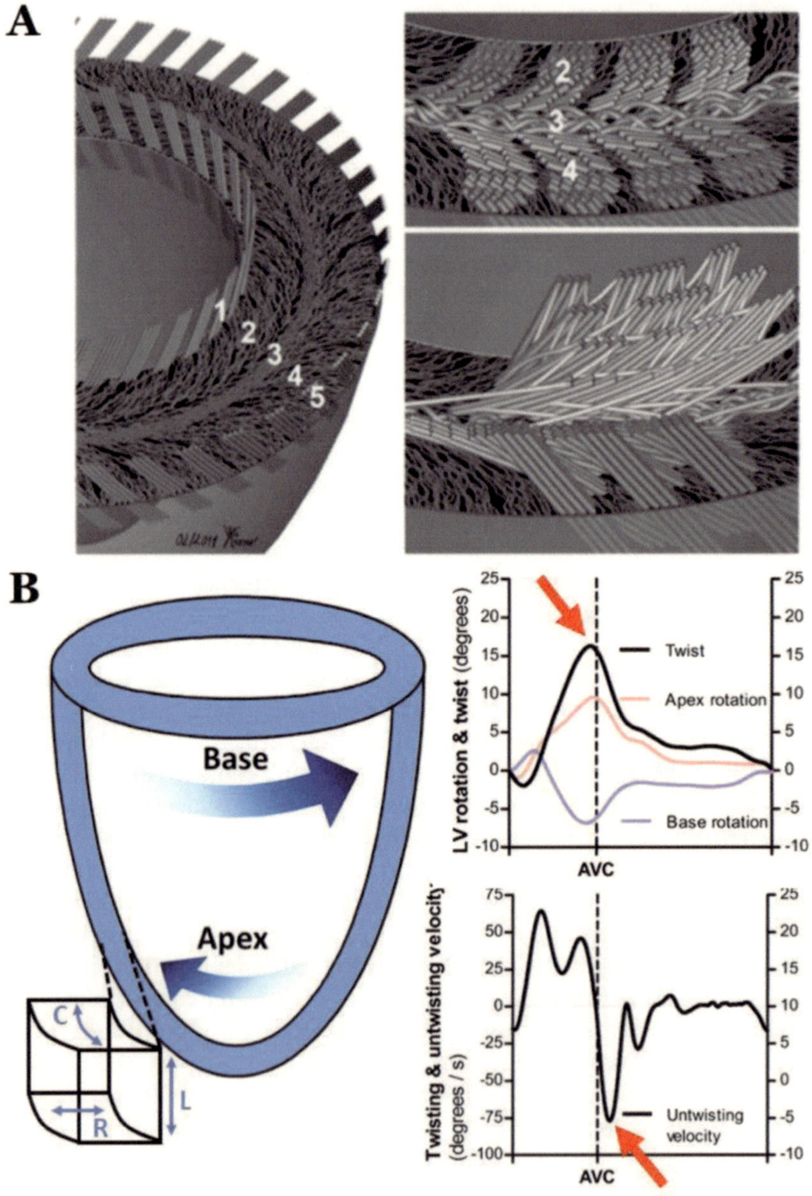

Figure 1.
LV anatomy, strain and twist. (A) Although the detailed anatomy of the heart is still a matter of debate, the most comprehensive, evidence-based model includes a mesh of oblique, circumferential and transmural fibers (1–5). (B) LV strain is typically assessed in three planes, the longitudinal plane (from the apex to the base, L), the circumferential plane, C, and the radial plane (from the endocardium to epicardium, R). Owing to the specific anatomy, contraction of the LV results in a twisting motion around the long-axis, with an opposing rotational movement at the base compared with the apex that is rapidly released in diastole. Resultant twist and twist velocity curves produce a clear signal for peak LV twist and early diastolic untwisting rate (red arrows). Please see further details and the original figures in Refs. [14, 24].

summary of the most common definitions is provided and the reader is also referred to previous review articles for further details on the terminology [24–26].

With regard to the LV, three strain components have been established: longitudinal, circumferential and radial strain [25]. Systolic strain rate was once thought to reflect contractility; however, these hopes have not been sustained. Furthermore, the anatomy of the heart does not support the measurement of radial strain since there are no radial fibers in the LV or RV. Although the transmural fibers may somewhat relate to this type of strain, they maximally constitute ~20% to overall deformation and do not seem to run strictly in the radial direction. Second, the classification of twist or torsion as a "shear strain" or fourth dimension of deformation does not fit the underlying anatomy of the heart either. There is currently no empirical evidence for the existence of a

Parameter (unit)	Description
Circumferential strain (%)	Percentage shortening of the circumference
Global longitudinal strain (%)	Typically, the average strain of multiple walls obtained from different echocardiographic windows (4-chamber, 2-chamber, 3-chamber)
Longitudinal strain (%)	Shortening along the long-axis of the ventricles in a single 2-dimensional imaging plane (for example a 4-chamber view)
Shear strain	The strain resulting from two different normal strains, for example "longitudinal-circumferential shear strain"
Strain (rate) imaging	Generic term that can refer to strain data obtained with either tissue Doppler or speckle tracking echocardiography
Strain rate (/s)	The rate of shortening (strain) or lengthening (strain) of each strain
Tissue Doppler strain (%)	Strain obtained with tissue Doppler echocardiography, which is more angle-dependent than speckle tracking echocardiography
Tissue velocity imaging (%)	Echocardiographic imaging based upon Doppler modality, often synonymous with tissue Doppler strain
Twist (degrees)	Also called the net twist angle, obtained from the net difference in rotation between the left ventricular base and apex. Not to be confused with torsion or rotation, the latter referring to the local angular deformation at the base and apex
Untwisting rate (°/s)	The maximal early diastolic rate of reversal of twist

Table 1.
Deformation parameters.

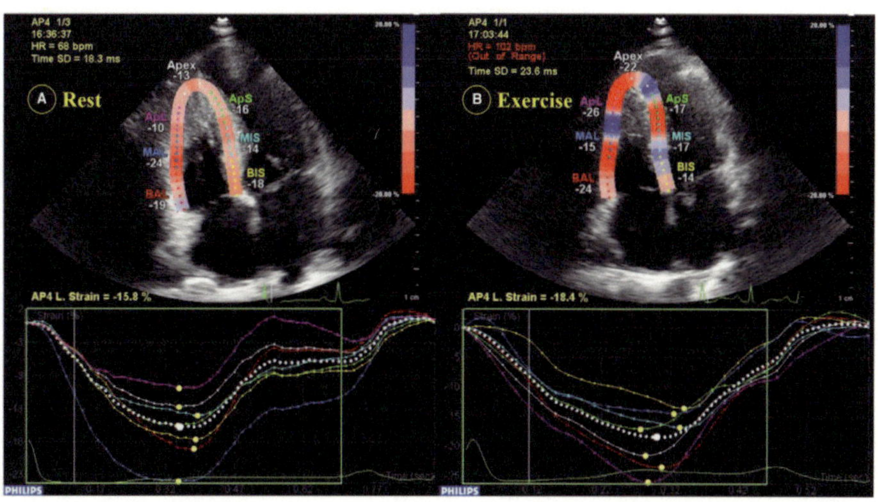

Figure 2.
RV strain. The measurement of RV strain at rest (left) and during exercise (right) in a patient with hypertrophic cardiomyopathy. Because of the anatomical arrangement of the RV, longitudinal strain is the most commonly investigated parameter, although further clarity is required whether to always include or exclude the septum [28]. From a functional perspective, there is strong evidence that the septal deformation is more similar to that of the LV than the RV free wall, as supported by evidence of a shared morphology [29, 30]. Please see further details and the original figure in: Wu et al. [31].

meaningful number of longitudinal fibers that could determine longitudinal deformation of the ventricles. Instead, the oblique fibers that make up most of the fibers within the left ventricular walls are likely responsible for deformation in the longitudinal direction. Consequently, it does not seem appropriate to calculate twist or torsion from the longitudinal and circumferential shear angle, also because this approach does not capture the potential regional differences that exist between the base and apex in both the LV and RV. Despite these drawbacks to the radial and longitudinal parameters, it must be acknowledged that longitudinal strain has become the most established measure as a clinical marker with diagnostic potential [27]. For these reasons, in the context of this chapter, it seems appropriate to ignore LV radial strain but include LV longitudinal and circumferential strain as well as twist and untwisting rate. Since no clear circumferential fibers or twisting motion have been detected in the RV, the focus for that chamber will be exclusively on longitudinal strain **Figure 2**.

3. Echocardiographic assessment of myocardial deformation during exercise

3.1 Why exercise?

Even if all humans were elite athletes, we would spend most of the time in a day in a biological state of rest—or certainly in a state of low physical activity that only constitutes a fraction of the total capacity of our cardiovascular system. Accordingly, the routine clinical practice of examining cardiac function at rest is a good representation of the condition we find ourselves in most of the time. However, when a person requires an echocardiographic examination, it is typically for clinical reasons initiated by the presence of negative symptoms, often presenting as "exertional dyspnea" or angina. If an echocardiographic examination then detects structural and functional abnormalities of the heart that are congruent with the individual's symptoms, the diagnosis of heart disease is likely. However, resting assessment of cardiac function often fails to recapitulate conditions of exertional dyspnea, and thus can sometimes lead to misdiagnosis. Equally, waiting until the emergence of symptoms postpones clinical treatment. For this reason, "stress testing" has been suggested to offer the opportunity of a "window into the future". By taking the person out of their typical state of rest or low physical activity and stressing the full range of their cardiovascular system until maximum effort, underlying abnormalities may be detected that remain otherwise unknown. Examples for the benefit of exercise testing have been presented in relation to "unmasking masked hypertension" [32, 33]. Similarly, in pregnancy it has been proposed that the cardiovascular responses to exercise tests prior to conception may be indicators of the presence or absence of complications during future pregnancies [34–37]. Furthermore, the complex etiology of heart failure has justified detailed exercise testing to identify the most important contributors out of the numerous cardiac or peripheral factors that may be involved in the development and/or the state of heart failure [38–40].

It is now recognized among clinical practitioners that the investigation of myocardial deformation during exercise can provide additive value, since previous research studies have revealed new (and sometimes surprising) insight into the behavior of the heart during exercise. As will be discussed in detail in Section 3.3, these findings have informed our basic understanding of cardiac function and sometimes guided future clinical investigation. Since myocardial function, including parameters of myocardial deformation, are influenced by the general loading state of the heart, any exercise responses must be seen in the context of general cardiovascular responses, as discussed in the next section.

3.2 General cardiovascular responses to exercise

In the context of myocardial deformation, the most relevant cardiovascular and cardiopulmonary responses to a standardized exercise test pertain to stroke volume, cardiac output, end-diastolic volume, blood pressure, arterial resistance, lactate, and maximal oxygen consumption (VO_2max). In healthy individuals, a clear change in these parameters can be expected at the onset of low intensity dynamic exercise that should continue to change linearly up to moderate intensities. Importantly, dynamic exercise tests cause a disproportionate peripheral vasodilation in relation to the increase in cardiac output, and hence total peripheral resistance drops sharply at the onset of exercise and then remains constant across moderate and high exercise intensities [41]. From a diastolic perspective, end-diastolic volume has been shown to increase in some studies while others have not observed any change with exercise. This is not trivial since an acute increase in end-diastolic volume has been associated with an increased stroke volume, an effect also known as the Frank-Starling mechanism [42]. However, the overall contribution of end-diastolic volume to stroke volume is still relatively low because most of the increase in stroke volume has been attributed to the enhanced contractility that reduces the end-systolic volume.

At workloads above moderate intensity, several important physiological changes occur in healthy individuals. Blood lactate concentrations increase exponentially and CO_2 production rises above O_2 consumption, both reflecting the greater contribution of anaerobic metabolic pathways to overall energy utilization and causing a strong stimulus for vasodilation not least in the cerebral circulation. During the highest effort, stroke volume and VO_2 have been reported to plateau and even decrease, but the exact pattern and the underlying mechanisms to this response remain a matter of debate [43]. Fortunately, this does not seem to impact the interpretation of cardiovascular responses to exercise in patients, since the sub-maximal data are currently thought to be of sufficient clinical value to determine whether exercise performance is normal or impaired [44].

One important distinction between the LV and RV responses to exercise is the potential for a "disproportionate load" on the RV [45], which is perhaps explained by both a greater relative rise in pulmonary blood pressure compared with that in the aorta, and differences in RV intrinsic factors such as force development. The differences between the LV and RV responses to exercise highlight the specific impact exercise has on the cardiovascular system. Consequently, determining the true origin of exercise limitations is challenging because many components of the cardiovascular system may be affected. For example, studies have shown that an exaggerated rise in blood pressure during exercise may be associated with negative outcomes, but whether this is caused by the heart or the periphery may be more difficult to determine [46–48]. Even in heart failure, the reduced exercise tolerance has been suggested to be a result of both central and non-cardiac limitations [38–40, 49]. Consequently, assessing myocardial deformation *in relation* to conventional exercise responses is essential for the quantification of the contributions of the heart muscle itself.

3.3 Myocardial deformation during exercise

Whatever myocardial parameter one chooses to examine during exercise, the interpretation of the responses can be tricky. For example, an increase in myocardial deformation with sub-maximal cycle exercise along with a typical drop in arterial resistance and concomitant reductions in end-systolic volume, in the presence of no adverse structural remodeling would be reflective of a "healthy" response. Equally, it is theoretically possible that the absence of a clear increase in myocardial deformation—which could be interpreted to represent myocardial dysfunction—may be a normal response if the increase in blood pressure and peripheral resistance were excessively high (or the exercise test did in fact create a condition of increased afterload). In this case, it is conceivable that the origin of the exercise limitation may not be cardiac despite the attenuated deformation, but perhaps peripheral in nature causing an exercise failure before the cardiac reserve is fully used [39]. Therefore, this section provides an overview of the general trend of myocardial deformation during exercise, but the reader is alerted that a qualitative interpretation must be performed after consideration of the wider physiology. Articles in this section were included if the studies had obtained data with echocardiography during exercise (tissue Doppler and tissue velocity imaging data were mostly excluded because both techniques are angle-dependent and typically represent only data from a single segment within the mitral annulus). Although a promising and exciting alternative to echocardiography, myocardial deformation during exercise obtained using MRI is not the focus of this chapter [50, 51]. Studies were also excluded if they obtained data immediately following exercise effort, as discussed in more detail in the section on methodological considerations. Finally, the avid reader is referred to some excellent review articles that cover more of the literature than this book chapter can accommodate [52–55].

3.3.1 Physiological insight from healthy individuals

The physiology of myocardial deformation during exercise in healthy people is the fundamental basis upon which to interpret the responses in patient populations. Although many clinical research studies also include a healthy control group, sometimes these are matched to the patient groups in their demographics and, therefore, may not represent truly "healthy" individuals. Wherever possible, the data presented here will be from populations purposefully recruited as young healthy reference groups. To date, studies have revealed a variety of new perspectives that may be of great importance for the interpretation of clinical populations.

A decade ago, two studies revealed the strain and twist responses during incremental exercise. First, Doucende et al. showed that left ventricular twist and circumferential strain increased linearly up to moderate exercise intensities, while longitudinal strain increased initially but then plateaued at low exercise efforts [56]. This study also highlighted the interdependence of systolic and diastolic deformation, the role of untwisting rate in LV filling during exercise and the contribution of the LV apex to the overall myocardial response. Second, it was shown that LV twist and untwisting rate increased linearly up to near-maximal efforts, correlating with stroke volume and, thus, perhaps contributing to maximal exercise capacity in humans [57]. The importance of regional LV deformation, at the LV apex, was again highlighted. Several other studies have revealed similar patterns of LV twist during exercise in pre- and postmenopausal women, in athletes and of humans ascending to high altitude [58–62]. Consequently, it is now generally accepted that an increase in LV twist with exercise up to moderate intensities can be expected as a normal response (**Figure 3**). Surprisingly few studies dedicated to healthy individuals have measured LV strain during exercise, but they agree in general that longitudinal strain also increases with exercise [56, 61–64]. Because of the risk of potential confounders, it is not possible to directly compare the response in LV twist and strain obtained in different studies. But in general, it is of great importance to note that the patters of the responses to exercise are not always the same for the two parameters, reminding us that they do not represent the same myocardial deformation. In agreement with the general physiological response to incremental exercise, LV twist increases linearly while longitudinal strain seems to plateau at low exercise efforts. This was more recently confirmed by Williams et al., who reported the same

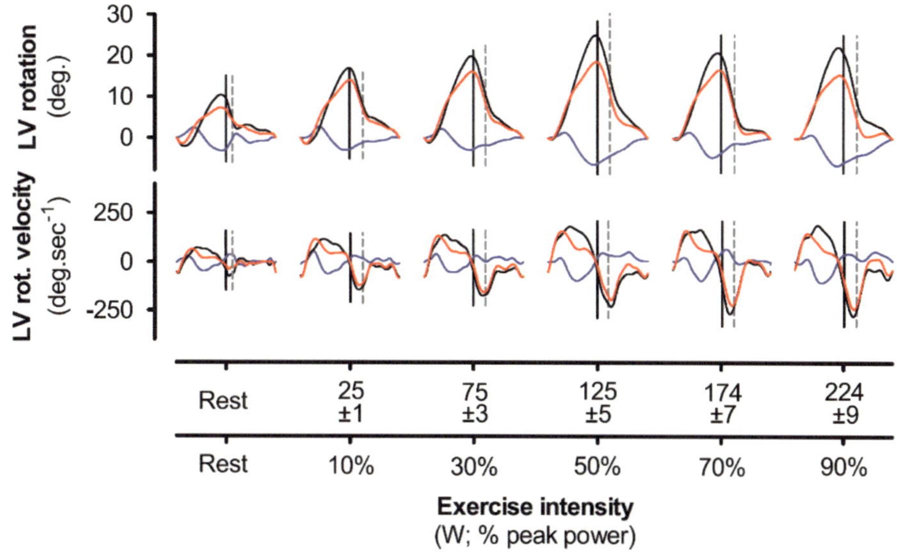

Figure 3.
Myocardial deformation to incremental exercise. LV twist curves during incremental exercise, revealing a linear increase up to 70–80% of maximal individual exercise effort for both peak systolic LV twist (highest value in black lines top row) and peak diastolic untwisting rate (lowest value within black lines bottom row). Red lines represent myocardial deformation at the LV apex, blue lines at the LV base. Black lines are the composite of apical and basal data. Please see further details and the original figure in Ref. [57].

disparity between parameters in young healthy men [62]. Interestingly, in the same study, women seemed to have more of a linear response in longitudinal strain akin to LV twist. The disparity between LV twist and longitudinal strain has also been noted in studies on aging where LV twist consistently increases, but longitudinal strain does not change or decreases. Considering the well-established progression of aortic stiffness with aging [65], longitudinal strain appears to be at odds again with general physiology. Future studies should not only examine the parameters in relation to their sensitivity as a clinical marker but also consider the fit with general physiology.

Studying the acute effects of exercise on myocardial deformation may be influenced by the chronic remodeling that humans have experienced. In this regard, Burns et al. showed that aging seems to be associated with a reduced LV twist reserve during exercise in a population of 60-year old individuals [66]. Similarly, "female aging", as represented by the menopause, seems to impact the myocardial response to exercise, which may be further altered by exercise training [58]. One of the more surprising observations has been that of Cooke et al. who proposed that endurance trained athletes with enlarged "athlete's heart" and a greater stroke volume had a similar systolic LV function, including LV twist, during submaximal exercise compared to untrained humans with smaller stroke volume [67]. Similar to the results presented by Doucende and Williams discussed above [56, 62], this particular exercise response strongly suggests that the mechanical[2] systolic function of the heart may not be strictly associated with its output (stroke volume). Some mathematical calculations support the potentially poor linear association between systolic LV mechanical function and ejection fraction while others suggest a strong relationship [68]. In any case, the previous findings suggest that future investigations into the interaction between systolic deformation and ejection, and diastolic deformation and filling are needed to clarify the current uncertainty. One reason for the existing disagreement between

[2] The term mechanical is most commonly used in the literature on myocardial deformation. However, from a biophysical perspective, it may be more appropriate to refer to "kinematics".

mechanical function and associated hemodynamics may be the technical limitations causing restricted views from a 2D echocardiographic window. In the case of exercise responses, this may be particularly evident at the LV apex, since the apex has been proposed as an important contributor to exercise responses (in particular in diastolic function) [56, 57, 69]. However, in the echocardiographic images relevant for the measurement of global longitudinal strain, the representation of the apical segments is proportionately small and their contribution to longitudinal strain and strain rate may be underestimated compared with short-axis views [18]. Thus, some of the insight provided by myocardial deformation during exercise in healthy people relates to our more general understanding of cardiac function.

Compared with LV strain, RV longitudinal strain seems to be ~10 percentage points higher in healthy young humans at rest, likely reflecting the different anatomy combined with a lower pulmonary resistance compared with the aorta. Most studies reporting RV strain in healthy individuals during exercise have done so by including healthy controls as comparators to cardiac patients. From those studies, some patterns have emerged that suggest a consistently increased RV longitudinal strain during submaximal exercise in healthy individuals [28, 31, 70]. The mechanisms for this are probably similar to those of the LV, where an increased sympathetic state increases contractility while peripheral (pulmonary) vasodilation decreases downstream resistance [71]. However, during intense exercise, it seems that right ventricular myocardial deformation increases perhaps less than the LV, and it has even been shown to *decrease*. Given that both ventricles should produce approximately the same stroke volume under stable conditions, the lower RV strain during exercise is another indicator that the interaction between the mechanical function of the ventricles and the circulation may depend as much on the local arterial resistance as it may depend on the muscular performance (and therefore health) of the ventricles, and thus fitting the long-standing concept of a greater afterload-sensitivity of the RV. Recent studies in advanced heart failure patients who were surgically implanted with left ventricular assist devices (LVAD) may support this, since the mechanical pumps "unload" the LV and shift blood volume to the rest of the circulation, maybe creating "A Different Kind of Stress Test for the RV" [72, 73]. The accurate measurement of pulmonary and aortic resistance beyond the measurement or estimation of blood pressure is certainly going to elucidate the differential exposure and performance of the two ventricles [74]. At present, it seems that exercise does indeed cause a greater afterload challenge for the RV compared with the LV. In fact, it is worth noting that the exercise modalities used in the studies presented so far in this section have mostly employed "dynamic" exercise (see Section 3.4). In this context, it is essential to point out that this type of exercise increases sympathetic activation of the myocardium and reduces arterial resistance compared with the resting state, therefore creating an environment for the LV (and at low intensities for the RV) that is characterized by reduced afterload. During higher exercise intensities, pulmonary resistance can increase during dynamic exercise and create an augmented afterload challenge [45]. Strength exercise, also called resistance exercise, and isometric handgrip exercise are two other modalities that can provide an afterload challenge for the LV [75]. Interestingly, studies employing these exercise modalities in a number of different populations have consistently shown that the reduced systolic deformation is in part compensated for by an increase in heart rate, but can also be uncoupled from diastolic function [76–79]. Given that resistance exercise produces a very different challenge to dynamic exercise, and that strength training is an important addition to rehabilitation, future research should consider incorporating responses during high resistive efforts [80, 81].

3.3.2 Exercise responses in patients with cardiovascular disease

In a seminal study, Notomi et al. provided mechanistic insight into the complex interdependence between systolic and diastolic function in hypertrophic cardiomyopathy [20]. Although the study used Tissue Doppler Imaging, it is a landmark study that has provided new insight and has popularized the use of exercise testing for both basic science and new insight into cardiac performance in patients. The study revealed that LV twist during exercise was significantly reduced in patients with hypertrophic cardiomyopathy. Similarly, two other studies concluded that systolic deformation reserve is reduced in patients with hypertrophic cardiomyopathy [82, 83]. However, one challenge in patient populations is that the change in heart rate is often different compared with control groups, and therefore it is possible that the groups experienced different physiological stimuli. This is a recurring problem in exercise studies that currently reduces the confidence in some conclusions. Equally, sometimes the matching of the change in heart rate between groups may lead to unequal workloads or changes in blood pressure, highlighting again the need to interpret myocardial deformation during exercise in the context of general physiological responses. Notwithstanding, the overall trend is that LV myocardial deformation in patients is reduced in response to an acute exercise challenge, including in cardiac amyloidosis, hypertension, cancer, coronary artery disease, as well as in patients with valve disease before and after surgical correction [84–89]. Some subtle observations, however, are worthy of discussion. For example, in patients with microvascular angina, only the subendocardial strain was reduced, and diastolic function during exercise was more severely affected than systolic reserve [90]. Similarly, myocardial regions can respond differently during exercise in coronary artery disease patients, as shown by differential basal vs. apical rotational mechanics [89]. In an elegant study in patients with hypertrophic cardiomyopathy, Soullier et al. showed that there was significant heterogeneity in the response of the different deformation parameters to exercise, and that resting twist was even increased in patients while diastolic untwisting rate was less affected [83]. In patients with a prior heart transplant, the age of the recipients and donors seem to influence the longitudinal and circumferential strain response to exercise [91, 92]. All these observations highlight the very subtle changes that can occur between parameters, and between systolic and diastolic function. To determine the full significance of such differences should be the focus of future investigations. Furthermore, it will be essential to relate myocardial deformation more often to parameters like cardiac output, to enable the meaningful interpretation of deformation indices and their contribution to the overall capacity of the heart. When this was done in previous studies, the myocardial deformation during exercise provided a clear advancement of our general understanding of the etiology and/or progression of cardiac disease [93].

Because of the prevalence and importance of pulmonary hypertension, and the exercise limitations of heart failure patients, myocardial deformation of the RV during exercise has received heightened attention [94]. Similar to the LV response, the expected increase in RV myocardial deformation during exercise is generally blunted, not just in pulmonary hypertension but also in tetralogy of Fallot, systemic sclerosis, and hypertrophic cardiomyopathy [31, 95–97]. Most often, there is clear evidence that pulmonary artery pressures increased disproportionately in the groups that had a blunted increase in RV longitudinal strain during exercise. Importantly, these patients often have normal pulmonary artery pressures at rest, which not only emphasizes the diagnostic value of exercise testing, it also highlights the possibility that patients with suspected LV pathology should be tested for the RV myocardial response to exercise.

3.4 Important practical considerations

Any echocardiographic examination consists of two main parts: (1) the acquisition of standardized echocardiographic images, and (2) the analysis of images for the quantification of relevant parameters [98, 99]. When conducting echocardiography during exercise, both parts require modified approaches to ensure that the conclusions drawn remain valid. Here, based upon our extensive practical experience, we present some "take-home-messages" that we consider essential for the echocardiographic assessment of myocardial deformation during exercises.

- Typically, exercise tests are performed in a stepwise (constant intensity for some minutes, then increasing) or incremental (gradually increasing intensity with every second) manner. Because different protocols provoke different physiological responses, the correct protocol must be selected carefully.

- Exercise responses depend on the *relative* workload of an individual. Therefore, exercise intensities should be adjusted to an individual's anticipated capacity and patients' myocardial deformation interpreted in relation to the relative workload [100].

- The individual adjustment of workload increments during the test should also acknowledge fitness, age, sex, medical history, and acute or chronic injuries.

- For the assessment of myocardial deformation during exercise, running or cycling modalities are the most common. For the reason of improved image quality and because it is relatively safe/feasible, the preferred choice for exercise echocardiography may be supine cycling.

- While it is generally accepted that gentle end-expiratory breath holds can be performed to obtain images, it is preferable to obtain echocardiographic cine loops during free breathing and average some cardiac cycles during inspiration and expiration.

- It is important to distinguish between the physiological demands of different exercise modalities, categorized as: dynamic, static, and impact [101]. Consequently, certain types of exercise can be considered more as an "afterload challenge" than others, and the responses of myocardial deformation may vary greatly between these types of exercise. In this context, the reader is reminded that exercise training interventions for health will need to consider the same complexities, as evidenced by the potential for differential effects of moderate continuous exercise training *versus* high-intensity interval training in some cardiac patients [102].

- One concern with regard to exercise testing is the risk of triggering adverse events. Although this will depend on the specific individual being tested and must be decided by qualified personnel on a case-by-case basis, as evidenced by a comprehensive study performed by Rognmo et al. [103], the overall risk for serious adverse events seems to be relatively low. Particular health and safety precautions should be taken in patients with overt or suspected arrhythmia and the decision "not allowed to perform an exercise test" may have to be taken.

- Standardization of echocardiographic data acquisition during exercise is absolutely necessary. Sonographers should minimize the sector width and depth, maximize imaging frame rates, only use one focal point and position this in the optimal location, and optimize the overall image to maximize the visibility of the endocardial border for speckle tracking analysis. Although 3D echocardiography may solve some of the limitations of 2D echocardiography, at present the frame rates are too low to obtain the necessary temporal resolution for quantification of myocardial deformation during exercise, although this is expected to change in the near future.

- During exercise, when respiration and heart are increased, the quick location of the optimal echocardiographic window is necessary. Marking up the location on the chest after the resting assessment serves as a "quick help" during exercise. The sonographer must, however, still optimize the image and perhaps move the transducer slightly during exercise.

- Since heart rate increases during exercise but imaging frame rates are already maximized, the effective frame rate (data points per cardiac cycle) decreases. Although this cannot be fully corrected, it seems advisable to perform cubic spline interpolation to attenuate some of these limitations [104]. Note that cubic spline interpolation will not only add points in time (for example for the more confident assessment of dyssynchrony), it also slightly adjusts the peak values.

- Data acquisition immediately following exercise is not the same as "during" exercise. With the cessation of exercise, especially after a strenuous effort with strong muscular contractions, instant changes in whole-body hemodynamics set in [105]. Hence, these data do not reflect an exercise challenge but a "exercise recovery" state.

- For the acquisition of LV twist, apical data must be obtained by moving the transducer close to the point of obtaining a 4-chamber view, otherwise severely misrepresentative data will be collected [24].

4. Summary and conclusions

The assessment of LV and RV myocardial deformation during exercise is feasible and has contributed unique insight into cardiac physiology in health and disease. Inherent methodological challenges require appropriate training and a careful approach to image acquisition, analysis and interpretation. However, ongoing technological advancements and an increasing knowledge suggest that the echocardiographic assessment of myocardial deformation during exercise will play an ever-increasing role in future research and the clinical examination of the cardiac patient.

Acknowledgements

The authors express their sincere gratitude to the publisher, IntechOpen, for their very kind and generous financial support of this chapter.

Author details

Eric J. Stöhr[1,2]* and T. Jake Samuel[3]

1 School of Sport and Health Sciences, Cardiff Metropolitan University, Cardiff, UK

2 Division of Cardiology, Advanced Heart Failure Program, Columbia University Irving Medical Center, New York City, USA

3 Department of Kinesiology, University of Texas at Arlington, Texas, USA

*Address all correspondence to: estohr@cardiffmet.ac.uk; ejs2212@cumc.columbia.edu

References

[1] Buckberg GD. Basic science review: The helix and the heart. The Journal of Thoracic and Cardiovascular Surgery. 2002;**124**(5):863-883

[2] Harvey W, Whitteridge G. Anatomical Disputation Concerning the Movement of the Heart and Blood in Living Creatures. Oxford: Blackwell; 1976

[3] Loukas M, Lam R, Tubbs RS, Shoja MM, Apaydin N. Ibn al-Nafis (1210-1288): The first description of the pulmonary circulation. The American Surgeon. 2008;**74**(5):440-442

[4] Grant RP. Notes on the muscular architecture of the left ventricle. Circulation. 1965;**32**:301-308

[5] Mall P. On the muscular architecture of the ventricles of the human heart. The American Journal of Anatomy. 1911;**11**(3):211-260

[6] Mac Callum JB. On the Muscular Architecture and Growth of the Ventricles of the Heart. Welch Festschrift, Johns Hopkins Hospital Reports1900. p. 9

[7] Robb JS, Robb RC. The normal heart—anatomy and physiology of the structural units. American Heart Journal. 1942;**23**(4):455-467

[8] Greenbaum RA, Ho SY, Gibson DG, Becker AE, Anderson RH. Left ventricular fibre architecture in man. British Heart Journal. 1981;**45**(3): 248-263

[9] Streeter DD Jr, Spotnitz HM, Patel DP, Ross J Jr, Sonnenblick EH. Fiber orientation in the canine left ventricle during diastole and systole. Circulation Research. 1969;**24**(3): 339-347

[10] Lunkenheimer PP, Redmann K, Niederer P, Schmid P, Smerup M, Stypmann J, et al. Models versus established knowledge in describing the functional morphology of the ventricular myocardium. Heart Failure Clinics. 2008;**4**(3):273-288

[11] Harrington KB, Rodriguez F, Cheng A, Langer F, Ashikaga H, Daughters GT, et al. Direct measurement of transmural laminar architecture in the anterolateral wall of the ovine left ventricle: New implications for wall thickening mechanics. American Journal of Physiology. Heart and Circulatory Physiology. 2005;**288**(3):H1324-H1330

[12] Hsu EW, Muzikant AL, Matulevicius SA, Penland RC, Henriquez CS. Magnetic resonance myocardial fiber-orientation mapping with direct histological correlation. The American Journal of Physiology. 1998;**274**(5 Pt 2):H1627-H1634

[13] Poveda F, Marti E, Gil D, Carreras F, Ballester M. Helical structure of ventricular anatomy by diffusion tensor cardiac MR tractography. JACC: Cardiovascular Imaging. 2012;**5**(7):754-755

[14] Lunkenheimer PP, Niederer P, Sanchez-Quintana D, Murillo M, Smerup M. Models of ventricular structure and function reviewed for clinical cardiologists. Journal of Cardiovascular Translational Research. 2013;**6**(2):176-186

[15] Hooks DA, Trew ML, Caldwell BJ, Sands GB, LeGrice IJ, Smaill BH. Laminar arrangement of ventricular myocytes influences electrical behavior of the heart. Circulation Research. 2007;**101**(10):e103-e112

[16] LeGrice IJ, Smaill BH, Chai LZ, Edgar SG, Gavin JB, Hunter PJ. Laminar structure of the heart: Ventricular

myocyte arrangement and connective tissue architecture in the dog. The American Journal of Physiology. 1995;**269**(2 Pt 2):H571-H582

[17] Sengupta PP, Khandheria BK, Korinek J, Wang J, Jahangir A, Seward JB, et al. Apex-to-base dispersion in regional timing of left ventricular shortening and lengthening. Journal of the American College of Cardiology. 2006;**47**(1):163-172

[18] Stöhr EJ, Stembridge M, Esformes JI. *In vivo* human cardiac shortening and lengthening velocity is region-dependent and not coupled with heart rate: 'longitudinal' strain rate markedly underestimates apical contribution. Experimental Physiology. 2015;**100**(5):507-518

[19] Lunkenheimer PP, Redmann K, Florek J, Fassnacht U, Cryer CW, Wubbeling F, et al. The forces generated within the musculature of the left ventricular wall. Heart. 2004;**90**(2):200-207

[20] Notomi Y, Martin-Miklovic MG, Oryszak SJ, Shiota T, Deserranno D, Popovic ZB, et al. Enhanced ventricular untwisting during exercise: A mechanistic manifestation of elastic recoil described by Doppler tissue imaging. Circulation. 2006;**113**(21):2524-2533

[21] Najafi A, van de Locht M, Schuldt M, Schonleitner P, van Willigenburg M, Bollen I, et al. End-diastolic force pre-activates cardiomyocytes and determines contractile force: Role of titin and calcium. The Journal of Physiology. 2019;**597**(17):4521-4531

[22] Kawano H, Okada R, Yano K. Histological study on the distribution of autonomic nerves in the human heart. Heart and Vessels. 2003;**18**(1):32-39

[23] Nielsen E, Smerup M, Agger P, Frandsen J, Ringgard S, Pedersen M, et al. Normal right ventricular three-dimensional architecture, as assessed with diffusion tensor magnetic resonance imaging, is preserved during experimentally induced right ventricular hypertrophy. Anatomical Record. 2009;**292**(5):640-651

[24] Stöhr EJ, Shave RE, Baggish AL, Weiner RB. Left ventricular twist mechanics in the context of normal physiology and cardiovascular disease: A review of studies using speckle tracking echocardiography. American Journal of Physiology. Heart and Circulatory Physiology. 2016;**311**(3):H633-H644

[25] D'Hooge J, Heimdal A, Jamal F, Kukulski T, Bijnens B, Rademakers F, et al. Regional strain and strain rate measurements by cardiac ultrasound: Principles, implementation and limitations. European Journal of Echocardiography. 2000;**1**(3):154-170

[26] Pastore MC, De Carli G, Mandoli GE, D'Ascenzi F, Focardi M, Contorni F, et al. The prognostic role of speckle tracking echocardiography in clinical practice: Evidence and reference values from the literature. Heart Failure Reviews. 2020

[27] Marwick TH, Shah SJ, Thomas JD. Myocardial strain in the assessment of patients with heart failure: A review. JAMA Cardiology. 2019;**4**(3):287-294

[28] Sanz-de la Garza M, Giraldeau G, Marin J, Imre Sarvari S, Guasch E, Gabrielli L, et al.: Should the septum be included in the assessment of right ventricular longitudinal strain? An ultrasound two-dimensional speckle-tracking stress study. The International Journal of Cardiovascular Imaging. 2019; 35 (10): 1853-1860

[29] Addetia K, Takeuchi M, Maffessanti F, Nagata Y, Hamilton J, Mor-Avi V, et al. Simultaneous

longitudinal strain in all 4 cardiac chambers: A novel method for comprehensive functional assessment of the heart. Circulation. Cardiovascular Imaging. 2016;**9**(3):e003895

[30] Hristov N, Liakopoulos OJ, Buckberg GD, Trummer G. Septal structure and function relationships parallel the left ventricular free wall ascending and descending segments of the helical heart. European Journal of Cardio-Thoracic Surgery. 2006;**29**(Suppl 1):S115-S125

[31] Wu XP, Li YD, Wang YD, Zhang M, Zhu WW, Cai QZ, et al. Impaired right ventricular mechanics at rest and during exercise are associated with exercise capacity in patients with hypertrophic cardiomyopathy. Journal of the American Heart Association. 2019;**8**(5):e011269

[32] Peacock J, Diaz KM, Viera AJ, Schwartz JE, Shimbo D. Unmasking masked hypertension: Prevalence, clinical implications, diagnosis, correlates and future directions. Journal of Human Hypertension. 2014;**28**(9):521-528

[33] Schultz MG, Hare JL, Marwick TH, Stowasser M, Sharman JE. Masked hypertension is "unmasked" by low-intensity exercise blood pressure. Blood Pressure. 2011;**20**(5):284-289

[34] Meah VL, Backx K, Davenport MH. International working group on maternal H: Functional hemodynamic testing in pregnancy: Recommendations of the international working group on maternal hemodynamics. Ultrasound in Obstetrics & Gynecology. 2018;**51**(3):331-340

[35] Meah VL, Cockcroft JR, Stöhr EJ. Maternal cardiac twist pre-pregnancy: Potential as a novel marker of pre-eclampsia. Fetal and Maternal Medicine Review. 2013;**24**(4):289-295

[36] Man J, Foo L, Masini G, McEniery CM, Wilkinson IB, Bennett P, et al. Pre-pregnancy exercise stress testing is related to normal physiological adaptation from pre-pregnancy to mid-pregnancy. Ultrasound in Obstetrics & Gynecology. 2017;**50**(Suppl 1):48-153

[37] Bijl RC, Cornette JMJ, van den Bosch AE, Duvekot JJ, Molinger J, Willemsen SP, et al. Study protocol for a prospective cohort study to investigate hemodynamic adaptation to pregnancy and placenta-related outcome: The HAPPO study. BMJ Open. 2019;**9**(11):e033083

[38] Pieske B, Tschope C, de Boer RA, Fraser AG, Anker SD, Donal E, et al. How to diagnose heart failure with preserved ejection fraction: The HFA-PEFF diagnostic algorithm: A consensus recommendation from the heart failure association (HFA) of the European Society of Cardiology (ESC). European Heart Journal. 2019;**40**(40):3297-3317

[39] Tucker WJ, Haykowsky MJ, Seo Y, Stehling E, Forman DE. Impaired exercise tolerance in heart failure: Role of skeletal muscle morphology and function. Current Heart Failure Reports. 2018;**15**(6):323-331

[40] Dhakal BP, Malhotra R, Murphy RM, Pappagianopoulos PP, Baggish AL, Weiner RB, et al. Mechanisms of exercise intolerance in heart failure with preserved ejection fraction: The role of abnormal peripheral oxygen extraction. Circulation. Heart Failure. 2015;**8**(2):286-294

[41] González-Alonso J, Calbet JA. Reductions in systemic and skeletal muscle blood flow and oxygen delivery limit maximal aerobic capacity in humans. Circulation. 2003;**107**(6):824-830

[42] Helmes M, Lim CC, Liao R, Bharti A, Cui L, Sawyer DB. Titin determines the Frank-Starling relation

in early diastole. The Journal of General Physiology. 2003;**121**(2):97-110

[43] Gonzalez-Alonso J. Point: Stroke volume does/does not decline during exercise at maximal effort in healthy individuals. Journal of Applied Physiology. 2008;**104**(1):275-276; discussion 9-80

[44] Guazzi M, Bandera F, Ozemek C, Systrom D, Arena R. Cardiopulmonary exercise testing: What is its value? Journal of the American College of Cardiology. 2017;**70**(13):1618-1636

[45] La Gerche A, Heidbuchel H, Burns AT, Mooney DJ, Taylor AJ, Pfluger HB, et al. Disproportionate exercise load and remodeling of the athlete's right ventricle. Medicine and Science in Sports and Exercise. 2011;**43**(6):974-981

[46] Schultz MG, Otahal P, Picone DS, Sharman JE. Clinical relevance of exaggerated exercise blood pressure. Journal of the American College of Cardiology. 2015;**66**(16):1843-1845

[47] Park C, Fraser A, Howe LD, Jones S, Davey Smith G, Lawlor DA, et al. Elevated blood pressure in adolescence is attributable to a combination of elevated cardiac output and total peripheral resistance. Hypertension. 2018;**72**(5):1103-1108

[48] Falkner B. Cardiac output versus total peripheral resistance. Hypertension. 2018;**72**(5):1093-1094

[49] Morris RI, Sobotka PA, Balmforth PK, Stöhr EJ, McDonnell BJ, Spencer D, et al. Iliocaval venous obstruction, cardiac preload reserve and exercise limitation. Journal of Cardiovascular Translational Research. 2020

[50] La Gerche A, Claessen G, Van de Bruaene A, Pattyn N, Van Cleemput J, Gewillig M, et al. Cardiac MRI: A new gold standard for ventricular volume quantification during high-intensity exercise. Circulation. Cardiovascular Imaging. 2013;**6**(2):329-338

[51] Beaudry RI, Samuel TJ, Wang J, Tucker WJ, Haykowsky MJ, Nelson MD. Exercise cardiac magnetic resonance imaging: A feasibility study and meta-analysis. American Journal of Physiology. Regulatory, Integrative and Comparative Physiology. 2018;**315**(4):R638-RR45

[52] Celutkiene J, Plymen CM, Flachskampf FA, de Boer RA, Grapsa J, Manka R, et al. Innovative imaging methods in heart failure: A shifting paradigm in cardiac assessment. Position statement on behalf of the heart failure Association of the European Society of cardiology. European Journal of Heart Failure. 2018;**20**(12):1615-1633

[53] Crowe T, Jayasekera G, Peacock AJ. Non-invasive imaging of global and regional cardiac function in pulmonary hypertension. Pulmonary Circulation. 2018;**8**(1):2045893217742000

[54] Donal E, Lund LH, Oger E, Reynaud A, Schnell F, Persson H, et al. Value of exercise echocardiography in heart failure with preserved ejection fraction: A substudy from the KaRen study. European Heart Journal Cardiovascular Imaging. 2016;**17**(1):106-113

[55] Gupta DK, Solomon SD. Imaging in heart failure with preserved ejection fraction. Heart Failure Clinics. 2014;**10**(3):419-434

[56] Doucende G, Schuster I, Rupp T, Startun A, Dauzat M, Obert P, et al. Kinetics of left ventricular strains and torsion during incremental exercise in healthy subjects: The key role of torsional mechanics for systolic-diastolic coupling.

Circulation. Cardiovascular Imaging. 2010;**3**(5):586-594

[57] Stöhr EJ, González-Alonso J, Shave R. Left ventricular mechanical limitations to stroke volume in healthy humans during incremental exercise. American Journal of Physiology. Heart and Circulatory Physiology. 2011;**301**(2):H478-H487

[58] Nio AQX, Rogers S, Mynor-Wallis R, Meah VL, Black JM, Stembridge M, et al. The menopause alters aerobic adaptations to high-intensity interval training. Medicine and Science in Sports and Exercise. 2020

[59] Stöhr EJ, McDonnell B, Thompson J, Stone K, Bull T, Houston R, et al. Left ventricular mechanics in humans with high aerobic fitness: Adaptation independent of structural remodelling, arterial haemodynamics and heart rate. The Journal of Physiology. 2012;**590**(9):2107-2119

[60] Stembridge M, Ainslie PN, Hughes M, Stöhr EJ, Cotter J, Tymko M, et al. Impaired myocardial function does not explain reduced left ventricular filling and stroke volume s0at rest or during exercise at high altitude. Journal of Applied Physiology. 2015;**117**:334-343

[61] Vitiello D, Cassirame J, Menetrier A, Rupp T, Schuster I, Reboul C, et al. Depressed systolic function after a prolonged and strenuous exercise. Medicine and Science in Sports and Exercise. 2013;**45**(11):2072-2079

[62] Williams AM,Shave RE, Coulson JM, White H, Rosser-Stanford B, Eves ND. Influence of vagal control on sex-related differences in left ventricular mechanics and hemodynamics. American Journal of Physiology. Heart and Circulatory Physiology. 2018;**315**(3):H687-HH98

[63] Unnithan VB, Rowland TW, George K, Lord R, Oxborough D. Left ventricular function during exercise in trained pre-adolescent soccer players. Scandinavian Journal of Medicine & Science in Sports. 2018;**28**(11):2330-2338

[64] von Scheidt F, Kiesler V, Kaestner M, Bride P, Kramer J, Apitz C. Left ventricular strain and strain rate during submaximal semisupine bicycle exercise stress echocardiography in healthy adolescents and young adults: Systematic protocol and reference values. Journal of the American Society of Echocardiography. 2020

[65] McEniery CM, Yasmin, Hall IR, Qasem A, Wilkinson IB, Cockcroft JR. Normal vascular aging: Differential effects on wave reflection and aortic pulse wave velocity: The Anglo-Cardiff collaborative trial (ACCT). Journal of the American College of Cardiology. 2005;**46**(9):1753-1760

[66] Burns AT, La Gerche A, Mac Isaac AI, Prior DL. Augmentation of left ventricular torsion with exercise is attenuated with age. Journal of the American Society of Echocardiography. 2008;**21**(4):315-320

[67] Cooke S, Samuel TJ, Cooper SM, Stöhr EJ. Adaptation of myocardial twist in the remodelled athlete's heart is not related to cardiac output. Experimental Physiology. 2018;**103**(11):1456-1468

[68] Lipiec P, Wisniewski J, Kasprzak JD. Should we search for linear correlations between global strain parameters and ejection fraction? European Heart Journal Cardiovascular Imaging. 2014;**15**(11):1301

[69] Stöhr EJ, Gonzalez-Alonso J, Bezodis IN, Shave R. Left ventricular energetics: New insight into the plasticity of regional contributions at rest and during exercise. American Journal of Physiology. Heart and Circulatory Physiology. 2014;**306**(2):H225-H232

[70] Claeys M, Claessen G, Claus P, De Bosscher R, Dausin C, Voigt JU, et al. Right ventricular strain rate during exercise accurately identifies male athletes with right ventricular arrhythmias. European Heart Journal Cardiovascular Imaging. 2020;**21**(3):282-290

[71] Kovacs G, Olschewski A, Berghold A, Olschewski H. Pulmonary vascular resistances during exercise in normal subjects: A systematic review. The European Respiratory Journal. 2012;**39**(2):319-328

[72] Stöhr EJ. Left ventricular assist device therapy - a different kind of stress test for the right ventricle. Med Sci sports Exerc. 2019. In: Symposium Presentation at the 2019 Annual Meeting of the American College of Sports Medicine. p. 48. Available from: https://www.acsm.org/docs/default-source/annual-meeting-documents/acsm-annual-meeting-2019-full-program.pdf?sfvrsn=5f858f5c_12

[73] Houston BA, Kalathiya RJ, Hsu S, Loungani R, Davis ME, Coffin ST, et al. Right ventricular afterload sensitivity dramatically increases after left ventricular assist device implantation: A multi-center hemodynamic analysis. The Journal of Heart and Lung Transplantation. 2016;**35**(7):868-876

[74] Pahuja M, Burkhoff D. Right ventricular afterload sensitivity has been on my mind. Circulation. Heart Failure. 2019;**12**(9):e006345

[75] Samuel TJ, Beaudry R, Haykowsky MJ, Sarma S, Nelson MD. Diastolic stress testing: Similarities and differences between isometric handgrip and cycle echocardiography. Journal of Applied Physiology. 2018;**125**(2):529-535

[76] Balmain B, Stewart GM, Yamada A, Chan J, Haseler LJ, Sabapathy S. The impact of an experimentally induced increase in arterial blood pressure on left ventricular twist mechanics. Experimental Physiology. 2016;**101**(1):124-134

[77] Weiner RB, Weyman AE, Kim JH, Wang TJ, Picard MH, Baggish AL. The impact of isometric handgrip testing on left ventricular twist mechanics. The Journal of Physiology. 2012;**590**(20):5141-5150

[78] Meah VL, Shave R, Backx K, Stöhr EJ. Cardiovascular responses to increased pressure during healthy pregnancy. Artery Research. 2019;**20**:109-110

[79] Stöhr EJ, Stembridge M, Shave R, Samuel TJ, Stone K, Esformes JI. Systolic and diastolic left ventricular mechanics during and after resistance exercise. Medicine and Science in Sports and Exercise. 2017;**49**(10):2025-2031

[80] Bjarnason-Wehrens B. Recommendations for resistance exercise in cardiac rehabilitation: Do they need reconsideration? European Journal of Preventive Cardiology. 2019;**26**(14):1479-1482

[81] Hansen D, Abreu A, Doherty P, Voller H. Dynamic strength training intensity in cardiovascular rehabilitation: Is it time to reconsider clinical practice? A systematic review. European Journal of Preventive Cardiology. 2019;**26**(14):1483-1492

[82] Badran HM, Faheem N, Ibrahim WA, Elnoamany MF, Elsedi M, Yacoub M. Systolic function reserve using two-dimensional strain imaging in hypertrophic cardiomyopathy: Comparison with essential hypertension. Journal of the American Society of Echocardiography. 2013;**26**(12):1397-1406

[83] Soullier C, Obert P, Doucende G, Nottin S, Cade S, Perez-Martin A, et al.

Exercise response in hypertrophic cardiomyopathy: Blunted left ventricular deformational and twisting reserve with altered systolic-diastolic coupling. Circulation. Cardiovascular Imaging. 2012;**5**(3):324-332

[84] Cusma Piccione M, Zito C, Khandheria B, Madaffari A, Oteri A, Falanga G, et al. Cardiovascular maladaptation to exercise in young hypertensive patients. International Journal of Cardiology. 2017;**232**:280-288

[85] Clemmensen TS, Eiskjaer H, Molgaard H, Larsen AH, Soerensen J, Andersen NF, et al. Abnormal coronary flow velocity reserve and decreased myocardial contractile reserve are main factors in relation to physical exercise capacity in cardiac amyloidosis. Journal of the American Society of Echocardiography. 2018;**31**(1):71-78

[86] Kaneko S, Tham EB, Haykowsky MJ, Spavor M, Khoo NS, Mackie AS, et al. Impaired left ventricular reserve in childhood cancer survivors treated with anthracycline therapy. Pediatric Blood & Cancer. 2016;**63**(6):1086-1090

[87] Kearney MC, Gallop-Evans E, Cockcroft JR, Stohr EJ, Lee E, Backx K, et al. Cardiac dysfunction in cancer survivors unmasked during exercise. European Journal of Clinical Investigation. 2017;**47**(3):213-220

[88] Magne J, Mahjoub H, Dulgheru R, Pibarot P, Pierard LA, Lancellotti P. Left ventricular contractile reserve in asymptomatic primary mitral regurgitation. European Heart Journal. 2014;**35**(24):1608-1616

[89] Peteiro J, Bouzas-Mosquera A, Broullon J, Sanchez-Fernandez G, Barbeito C, Perez-Cebey L, et al. Left ventricular torsion and circumferential strain responses to exercise in patients with ischemic coronary artery disease. The International Journal of Cardiovascular Imaging. 2017;**33**(1):57-67

[90] Cadeddu C, Nocco S, Deidda M, Pau F, Colonna P, Mercuro G. Altered transmural contractility in postmenopausal women affected by cardiac syndrome X. Journal of the American Society of Echocardiography. 2014;**27**(2):208-214

[91] Cifra B, Dragulescu A, Brun H, Slorach C, Friedberg MK, Manlhiot C, et al. Left ventricular myocardial response to exercise in children after heart transplant. The Journal of Heart and Lung Transplantation. 2014;**33**(12):1241-1247

[92] Esch BT, Scott JM, Warburton DE, Thompson R, Taylor D, Cheng Baron J, et al. Left ventricular torsion and untwisting during exercise in heart transplant recipients. The Journal of Physiology. 2009;**587**(Pt 10):2375-2386

[93] Pugliese NR, Fabiani I, Santini C, Rovai I, Pedrinelli R, Natali A, et al. Value of combined cardiopulmonary and echocardiography stress test to characterize the haemodynamic and metabolic responses of patients with heart failure and mid-range ejection fraction. European Heart Journal Cardiovascular Imaging. 2019;**20**(7):828-836

[94] Taylor BJ, Shapiro BP, Johnson BD. Exercise intolerance in heart failure: The important role of pulmonary hypertension. Experimental Physiology. 2020

[95] Bhatt SM, Wang Y, Elci OU, Goldmuntz E, McBride M, Paridon S, et al. Right ventricular contractile reserve is impaired in children and adolescents with repaired tetralogy of Fallot: An exercise strain imaging study. Journal of the American Society of Echocardiography. 2019;**32**(1):135-144

[96] Chia EM, Lau EM, Xuan W, Celermajer DS, Thomas L. Exercise testing can unmask right ventricular

dysfunction in systemic sclerosis patients with normal resting pulmonary artery pressure. International Journal of Cardiology. 2016;**204**:179-186

[97] Bourji KI, Hassoun PM. Right ventricle dysfunction in pulmonary hypertension: Mechanisms and modes of detection. Current Opinion in Pulmonary Medicine. 2015;**21**(5):446-453

[98] Lang RM, Badano LP, Mor-Avi V, Afilalo J, Armstrong A, Ernande L, et al. Recommendations for cardiac chamber quantification by echocardiography in adults: An update from the American Society of Echocardiography and the European Association of Cardiovascular Imaging. Journal of the American Society of Echocardiography. 2015;**28**(1):1-39.e14

[99] Harkness A, Ring L, Augustine DX, Oxborough D, Robinson S, Sharma V, et al. Normal reference intervals for cardiac dimensions and function for use in echocardiographic practice: A guideline from the British Society of Echocardiography. Echo Research and Practice. 2020;**7**(1):G1-G18

[100] Armstrong C, Samuel J, Yarlett A, Cooper SM, Stembridge M, Stöhr EJ. The effects of exercise intensity vs. metabolic state on the variability and magnitude of left ventricular twist mechanics during exercise. PLoS One. 2016;**11**(4):e0154065

[101] Levine BD, Baggish AL, Kovacs RJ, Link MS, Maron MS, Mitchell JH, et al. Eligibility and disqualification recommendations for competitive athletes with cardiovascular abnormalities: Task force 1: Classification of sports: Dynamic, static, and impact: A scientific statement from the American Heart Association and American College of Cardiology. Circulation. 2015;**132**(22):e262-e266

[102] Wisloff U, Stoylen A, Loennechen JP, Bruvold M, Rognmo O, Haram PM, et al. Superior cardiovascular effect of aerobic interval training versus moderate continuous training in heart failure patients: A randomized study. Circulation. 2007;**115**(24):3086-3094

[103] Rognmo O, Moholdt T, Bakken H, Hole T, Molstad P, Myhr NE, et al. Cardiovascular risk of high-versus moderate-intensity aerobic exercise in coronary heart disease patients. Circulation. 2012;**126**(12):1436-1440

[104] Burns AT, La Gerche A, Prior DL, MacIsaac AI.s Reduced and delayed untwisting of the left ventricle in patients with hypertension and left ventricular hypertrophy: A study using two-dimensional speckle tracking imaging. European Heart Journal. 2008;**29**(6):825-826

[105] Laugshlin MH. Cardiovascular response to exercise. The American Journal of Physiology. 1999;**277**(6 Pt 2): S244-S259

Chapter 3

Echocardiographic Features in Canine Myxomatous Mitral Valve Disease: An Animal Model for Human Mitral Valve Prolapse

Sang-Il Suh, Ta-Li Lu, Ran Choi and Changbaig Hyun

Abstract

Myxomatous mitral valve disease (MMVD) is the most common heart disease in dogs and has many similarities to human mitral valve prolapse (MVP). Transthoracic echocardiography is a non-invasive method for making a diagnosis and predicting the progression of heart failure (HF) in dogs and humans with mitral regurgitation (MR). It enables clinicians to detect the mitral valve (MV) lesions, to evaluate MR severity, and to assess its impact on cardiac remodeling, myocardial function, left ventricular (LV) filling pressures, as well as pulmonary arterial pressure. Furthermore, advanced ultrasound technologies such as tissue Doppler imaging (TDI), strain and strain rate imaging, and two-dimensional (2D) speckle tracking echocardiography (STE) provide a better assessment of global and regional myocardial function. Although the severity of MR and HF in dogs with MMVD is being evaluated as similar to human cardiology, the veterinary cardiologists are more focused on the severity of cardiac remodeling and cardiac dysfunction caused by MR, because surgical restoration of defected mitral apparatus is rarely done in dogs. The chapter will review conventional echocardiographic features of MMVD in dogs to provide a better understanding of the similarities and discrepancies between canine MMVD and human MVP to veterinary and human cardiologists and researchers.

Keywords: mitral valve prolapse, myxomatous mitral valve disease, mitral valve insufficiency, heart failure, mitral regurgitation

1. Introduction

Myxomatous mitral valve disease (MMVD) accounts for 75–80% of heart diseases in dogs and is more prevalent in small and elderly dogs [1, 2]. Due to similarities to human mitral valve prolapse (MVP), it gains huge interest in veterinary and human cardiologists. MMVD and MVP are characterized by progressive myxomatous degeneration of atrioventricular valves and subsequent mitral regurgitation (MR) [3], causing left atrial (LA) and left ventricular (LV) volume overload and left-sided congestive heart failure (CHF) [4]. Although there are many similarities in both diseases (e.g. macroscopic and microscopic pathology, strong genetic background, marked effect of age on prevalence and severity, slow progression), discrepancies in these two diseases (e.g. much more prevalent in dogs than in humans, less prone to develop endocarditis in dogs, less prominent systolic clicks in dogs) exist [5].

Although there are many diagnostic methods for MMVD, the standard transthoracic echocardiographic examination is a gold standard test for diagnosis and prognosis of MMVD and MVP in dogs and humans, respectively. The echocardiography is non-invasive and enables the clinicians to detect the mitral valve (MV) lesions, to evaluate MR severity, and to assess its impact on cardiac remodeling, myocardial function, left ventricular filling pressures, as well as pulmonary arterial pressure [6–11]. However, conventional ultrasound imaging modalities such as two-dimensional (2D), M-mode, color Doppler, pulse-wave (PW), and continuous-wave (CW) Doppler echocardiography may not be enough to precisely evaluate the severity of mitral valve diseases and to monitor disease progression. Advanced ultrasound technologies such as tissue Doppler imaging (TDI), strain and strain rate imaging, and two-dimensional speckle tracking echocardiography (STE) gain popularity in veterinary and human cardiologists because these technologies can assess and monitor global and regional myocardial function more precisely [12], although those require more expensive ultrasound machine and training.

Human MVP causing MR is divided into two groups: primary (i.e. structural intrinsic valvular disease) and secondary (i.e. nonstructural functional MR caused by non-mitral valve diseases). Like dogs, causes of primary MR are degenerative diseases on the mitral valve, such as Barlow, fibroelastic degeneration, Marfan, Ehlers-Danlos, and annular calcification, although rheumatic disease and toxic valvulopathy can also cause MR in humans [13]. Severity of MR in humans is graded qualitatively (e.g. mitral valve morphology, color flow MR jet, flow convergence zone, CW signal of MR jets), semi-quantitatively (e.g. vena contracta [VC] width, pulmonary vein flow, mitral inflow, TVI mit/TVI Ao), and quantitatively (effective regurgitant orifice area [EROA], regurgitant volume [R Vol]) [13]. LV and LA size and the systolic pulmonary arterial pressure are also used to determine the severity of CHF caused by MR.

Although the severity MR and CHF in dogs with MMVD are being evaluated as similar to human cardiology, the veterinary cardiologists are more focused on the severity of cardiac remodeling (e.g. LA and LV dilation) and cardiac dysfunction caused by MR, because surgical restoration of defected mitral apparatus is rarely done in dogs. Therefore, the echocardiographic indices related to MR severity (e.g. MV morphology, flow convergence zone) are not routinely assessed in dogs with MMVD.

The chapter reviews conventional echocardiographic indices being used for diagnosis and prognosis of canine MMVD to provide a better understanding of the similarities and discrepancies between canine MMVD and human MVP to veterinary and human cardiologists and researchers.

2. Assessment of MR severity

Echocardiography is a gold standard test in the assessment and management of humans and dogs with MR. Although color flow MR jets and CW signal of MR jets are useful for detecting MR, a more quantitative approach is required for determining the severity of MR in humans and dogs.

2.1 Semi-quantification of MR

Although quantitative assessment of MR (e.g. EROA and R Vol) is being used for grading the severity of MR in humans [13], it is rarely used in canine practice, because it requires more time-consuming interrogation and is often hard to define the location of EROA and flow convergence shape in dogs with MR [14]. Therefore, canine study, especially in practice, focuses more on the semi-quantification of MR (e.g. the maximal ratio of the regurgitant jet area signal to LA area [ARJ/LAA ratio] and vena contracta).

The ARJ/LAA ratio can be easily obtained with the color Doppler imaging (CDI) method and showed good repeatability and reproducibility in dogs [15, 16]. MR can be graded as mild (<30%), moderate (30–70%), or severe (>70%), based on the ARJ/LAA ratio on the CDI study in dogs with MMVD (**Figure 1A**) [15, 16]. Unfortunately, the ARJ/LAA ratio can be affected by many intrinsic factors (e.g. SAP, LA pressure, the spatial orientation of MR jet) and extrinsic factors (e.g. pulse repetition frequency and gain settings) [17]. Several studies found the ARJ/LAA ratio was not closely correlated with the severity of MMVD in dogs, especially in dogs with American College of Veterinary Internal Medicine (ACVIM) B2 and C [18, 19].

The vena contracta is the narrowest width of the MR jet that occurs at or just downstream from the regurgitant orifice and can reflect the severity of MR (obtained from measuring the regurgitant orifice size by the CDI study) (**Figure 1B**) [17]. Although it requires less time-consuming interrogation and is technically easier to obtain, this method is prone to errors, especially in dogs having dynamic regurgitant orifices [14]. Several studies found the VC and VC-derived variables were closely correlated with the severity of MR and survival time in dogs with MMVD [20–22]. One study found the mean (±SD) diameter of the mitral regurgitation vena contracta in a right parasternal long-axis (RPLx) view (VC_R:Ao) and a left apical four-chamber view (VC_L:Ao) indexed to aortic diameter were 0.21 ± 0.14 and 0.24 ± 0.12, respectively, in dogs with MMVD [21]. Furthermore, the VC_L:Ao > 0.24 was closely correlated with survival time (hazard ratio 4.87) [21].

2.2 Quantification of MR

The measurement of the flow convergence area by proximal isovelocity surface area (PISA) is a gold standard method to quantify the MR jet in humans [13]. Although one study found the PISA method was repeatable and reproducible in awake dogs [16], it is more time-consuming and requires several precautions to obtain the optimal acquisition of the flow convergence images in dogs with MMVD [14]. The regurgitation fraction (RF) obtained by the PISA can be used for

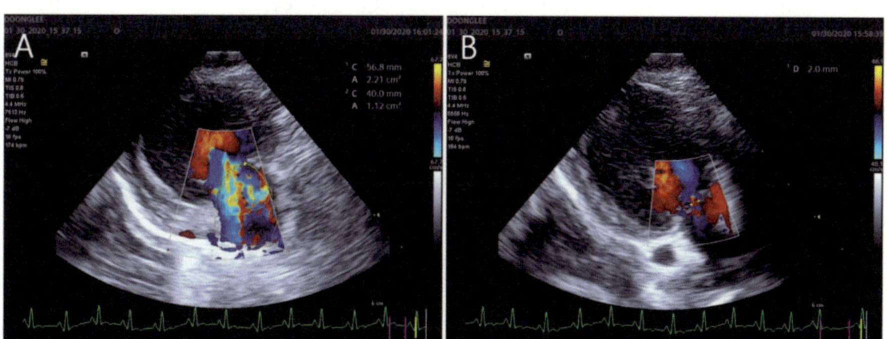

Figure 1.
(A) Semi-quantification of mitral regurgitation (MR). The maximal ratio of the regurgitant jet area signal to the left atrial area (ARJ/LAA ratio) was obtained from a left apical four-chamber view. The ARJ (1.12 cm²)/ LAA (2.12 cm²) of this case was 53%, indicating moderate MR. (B) the vena contracta diameter from a left apical four-chamber view (VC_L) was measured as the diameter of the narrowest point of the mitral regurgitation jet, downstream of the region of proximal flow convergence.

determining the severity of MR in dogs (e.g. mild if <30%, moderate if 30–75%, and severe if >75% of RF). Several studies found the RF was closely correlated with the severity of MMVD and other echocardiographic variables (e.g. LA/Ao and systolic PA pressure) [16, 23, 24]. However, one study found the MR quantification of the PISA method showed a wide range of RF (~33% asymptomatic MMVD dogs had moderate to severe RF) and thus is not routinely done in canine practice [16].

3. Assessment of left heart remodeling

Chronic and hemodynamically significant MR can cause LA and LV volume overload, leading to subsequent LA and LV enlargement. The severity of LA and LV remodeling can be assessed by LA to aortic root ratio (LA/Ao), indexed LA diameter (iLA), LV end-diastolic internal dimension to aortic root ratio (LVID/Ao), and normalized LV end-diastolic internal dimension (nLVID).

3.1 LA assessment

Estimation of LA diameter is one of the best predictors of outcome in dogs with MMVD [25, 26]. It also enables to make a decision for the initiation of medication in dogs with preclinical MMVD (ACVIM B1 and B2) and to estimate the risk for development of left-sided CHF [27, 28]. Hemodynamically significant chronic MR generally induces LA volume overload and thus leads to increase in LA volume [29].

In dogs with MMVD, MR causes LA and LV dilation, and thus the assessments of LA and LV chamber dimensions enable clinicians to predict the progression of MMVD and risk of CHF [27, 30–33]. One study evaluated the linear dimensions of the LA, LV, and Ao from the right parasternal long-axis view in dogs with MMVD and found that the mean (standard deviation; SD) for LA/LV, LV/Ao, and LA/Ao in dogs with MMVD were 1.1 (±0.09), 2.7 (±0.5), and 3.0 (±0.5), respectively, compared with 1.0 (±0.05), 2.1 (±0.2), and 2.1 (±0.1), respectively, in healthy control dogs [34]. This study showed good applicability and repeatability of the LA/LV, LV/Ao, and LA/Ao for assessing LV and LA enlargement in dogs with MMVD [34].

Conventional echocardiographic marker assessing LA enlargement is LA/Ao at the aortic root level of LV short-axis plane (**Figure 2A** and **B**). The degree of LA dilation is closely related to the progression of CHF and survival time in both symptomatic and asymptomatic dogs with MMVD [23, 25, 35]. One study enrolled in 558 dogs with MMVD found LA/Ao > 1.7 was the only significant prognostic index among echocardiographic indices [25]. Although the LA/Ao is a major echocardiographic index for determining the degree of LA dilation, the method for measuring the diameter of Ao is not standardized. The first method assessing LA size [36] was as follows: step 1 measures the internal short-axis diameter of the Ao along the commissure between the noncoronary and right coronary aortic valve cusps on the first frame after aortic valve closure and step 2 measures the internal short-axis diameter of the LA in the same frame in a line extending from and parallel to the commissure between the noncoronary and left coronary aortic valve cusps to the distant margin of the left atrium (**Figure 2A**). However, many other studies used a different way of measurement (the second method), i.e. measuring the internal short-axis diameter of the Ao along the commissure between the noncoronary and left coronary aortic valve cusps on the first frame after aortic valve closure (**Figure 2B**). Our study found the Ao diameters measured by the first method were longer than those measured by the second method. Therefore, the LA/Ao measured by the first method was smaller [37]. Because the LA/Ao is a major echocardiographic index for selecting MMVD study groups for drug trials and clinical trials, the standardization of measurement of Ao diameter is required in the future study.

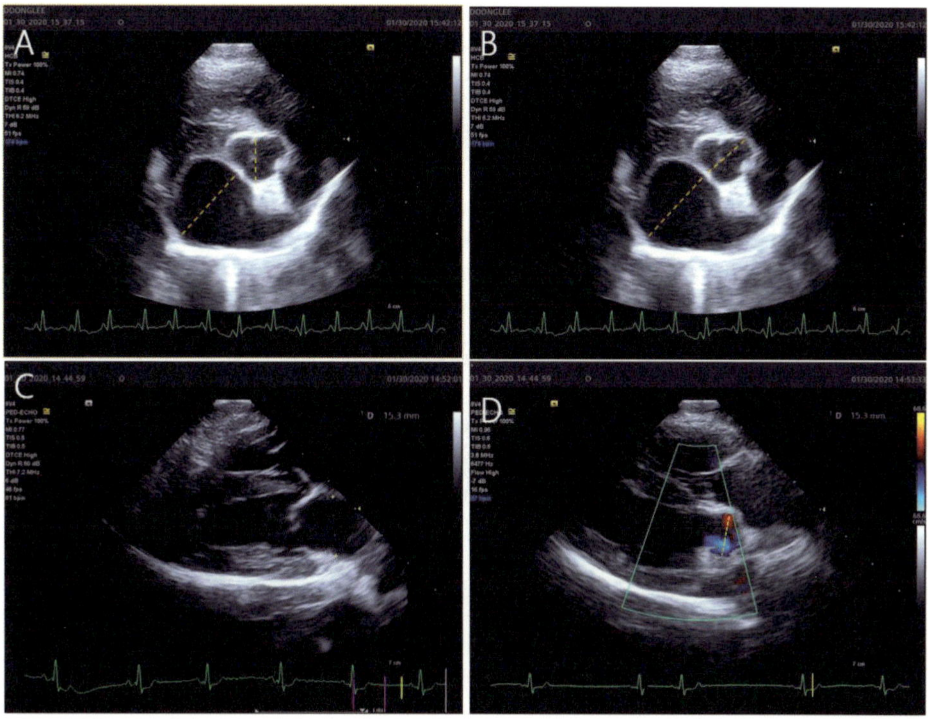

Figure 2.
The method for measurement of left atrial to aortic root ratio (LA/Ao). (A) A LA/Ao obtained from a right parasternal short axis (LA/AoSx) by method 1 (see text). (B) A LA/Ao obtained from a right parasternal short axis (LA/AoSx) by method 2 (see text). (C and D) A LA/Ao obtained from a right parasternal long axis (LA/AoLx). For LA diameter (C), the measurement was made at end-systole 1 to 2 frames before the opening of the mitral valve leaflets. The measurement bisects the atrium extending from the mid-atrial septum in the near field to the bright pericardial echo of the LA lateral wall in the far field and is roughly parallel to the mitral annulus. For Ao diameter (D), the measurement of the aortic valve was made between the opened aortic valve leaflets in an early systolic frame when the Ao diameter is the greatest.

To overcome the problem of LA/Ao at the short axis (LA/AoSx), the LA/Ao was also measured at the long axis (LA/AoLx) [34]. The method measuring LA/AoLx standardized and thus minimized the inconsistency of measurement of LA and Ao (**Figure 2C** and **D**). Several canine studies found cut-offs for LA/AoLx > 2.6 and LA/AoSx > 1.6 indicate hemodynamically relevant MMVD and timing of therapeutic intervention (e.g. enalapril and pimobendan administration) [27, 33].

Indexed LA diameter (iLA) is a good alternative for assessing LA dilation [19]. The iLA is calculated by using the following formula: LA diameter (mm)/(0.795 × body weight [kg])$^{1/3}$. In this study, the iLA diameter had higher sensitivity and specificity for detecting heart disease (healthy control vs. ACVIM B2), despite lower specificity for detecting heart failure (ACVIM B vs. ACVIM C) in dogs with MMVD. Cut-off for iLA > 12.7 indicates the risk of heart failure (ACVIM C) in dogs with MMVD [19].

Because the actual structure of LA is three-dimensional (3D), the LA dilation may occur in all direction (e.g. cranio-caudal, medio-lateral, and ventrodorsal). Therefore, the degree of LA dilation may be overestimated or underestimated, depending on the direction of LA dilation [38, 39]. For this reason, traditional estimation of LA diameter using 2D assessment of LA with linear methods (e.g. LA/AoSx, LA/AoLx, iLA) may not be enough to provide an accurate and consistent measurement. One study measured the LA volume to detect mild LA enlargement using the three-dimensional echocardiography (3D-EC) and found this method provided a more accurate measurement of LA size than the 2D echocardiography (2D-EC) [40]. Furthermore, the estimation of LA diameter and area by the 2D-EC was shown to have a poor correlation with the 3D-LA volume in humans [41]. However, it is more time-consuming, and substantial off-line analysis is required. Furthermore, the 3D-EC underestimated the LA volumes compared with magnetic resonance imaging (MRI) in human patients [42].

The area-length method (ALM; **Figure 3A**) or monoplane or biplane Simpson's modified method of discs (SMOD; **Figure 3B**) is currently recommended to measure LA area derived from the LA volume [43–46]. In human, the biplane method from four- and two-chamber views is preferred to measure the LA volume [47]. One study evaluated the difference of LA volume measurement by comparing 3D-LA volume measurement to two different 2D-LA volume measurements (using the SMOD and ALM) [48]. In this study, the SMOD and ALM systematically underestimated the LA volume by 7% and overestimated by 24%, respectively, compared with 3D-LA volume (**Figure 3C**). One human study also found the SMOD underestimated the LA volume compared to the 3D-LA volume [49]. Therefore, the 2D-SMOD may be a better method for the estimation of LA volume, if the 3D-EC is not available. One study found the LA volume indices including LA maximal volume (LAVmax) and LA minimal volume (LAVmin) using the ALM was useful to predict survival time when cardiac-related death was only considered [50]. In this study, the LAVmax > 3.53 mL/kg indicated high mortality risk in dogs with MMVD.

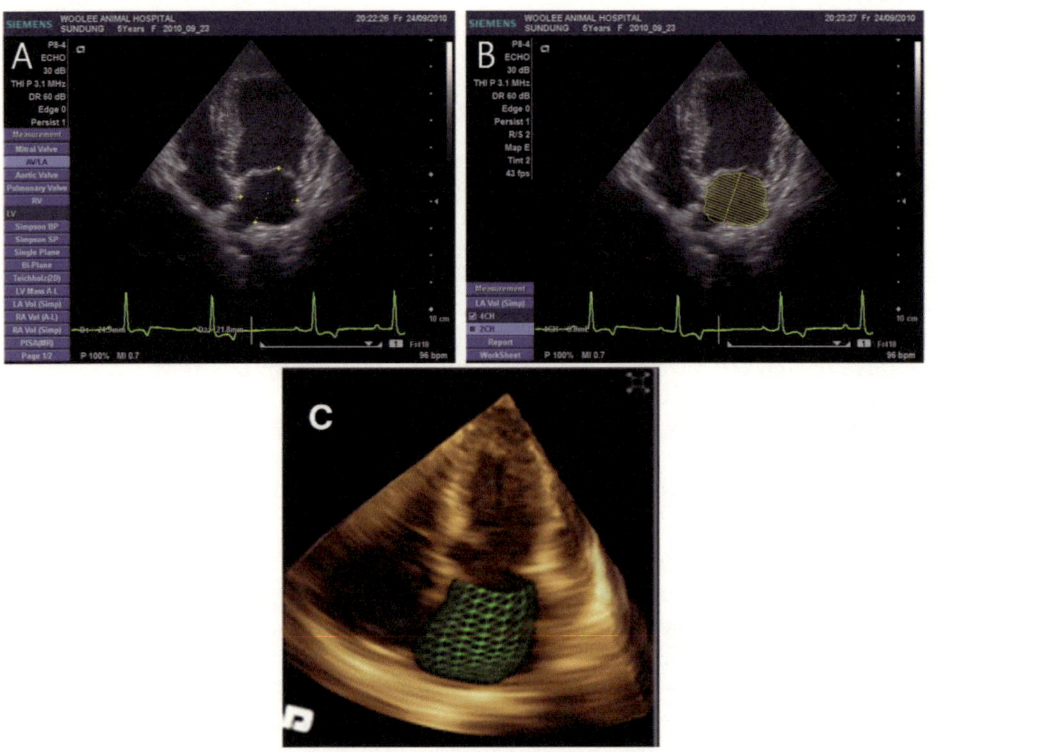

Figure 3.
Left atrial (LA) volume measured for three different methods at a left apical four-chamber view. (A) Area-length method (ALM), (B) Simpson's modified method of discs (SMOD), (C) real-time three-dimensional echocardiography (RT3DE).

Evaluation of the LA function may help to determine the severity of heart failure in dogs with MMVD [40, 44]. The LA function consists of three components: it acts as a reservoir for pulmonary venous (PV) return during ventricular systole (atrial diastole), as a conduit for the passage of stored blood from LA to LV during early ventricular diastole and diastasis, and as an active pump delivering 15–30% of LV filling during late ventricular diastole (atrial systole) [51]. One study established reference intervals for the LA function using 2D linear and area-based estimates and evaluated the diagnostic value to differentiate dogs with asymptomatic (ACVIM B) from symptomatic (ACVIM C) MMVD [52]. This study evaluated four LA functional indices (**Figure 4**): the LA expansion index for LA reservoir, the LA active emptying fraction for LA contractile, the LA passive emptying fraction for LA conduit, and the LA total emptying fraction for LA reservoir. This study demonstrated estimates of LA function except LA passive emptying fraction worsened with the severity of heart failure, although these indices were not sensitive enough to differentiate dogs with asymptomatic from symptomatic MMVD [52].

3.2 LV assessment

Chronic and hemodynamically significant MR can lead to the enlargement of the LV dimension. The degree of LV dilation was strongly correlated with the severity of heart failure in dogs with MMVD [53]. The LV internal dimension can be measured from the 2D or M-mode echocardiography by freezing the image at the

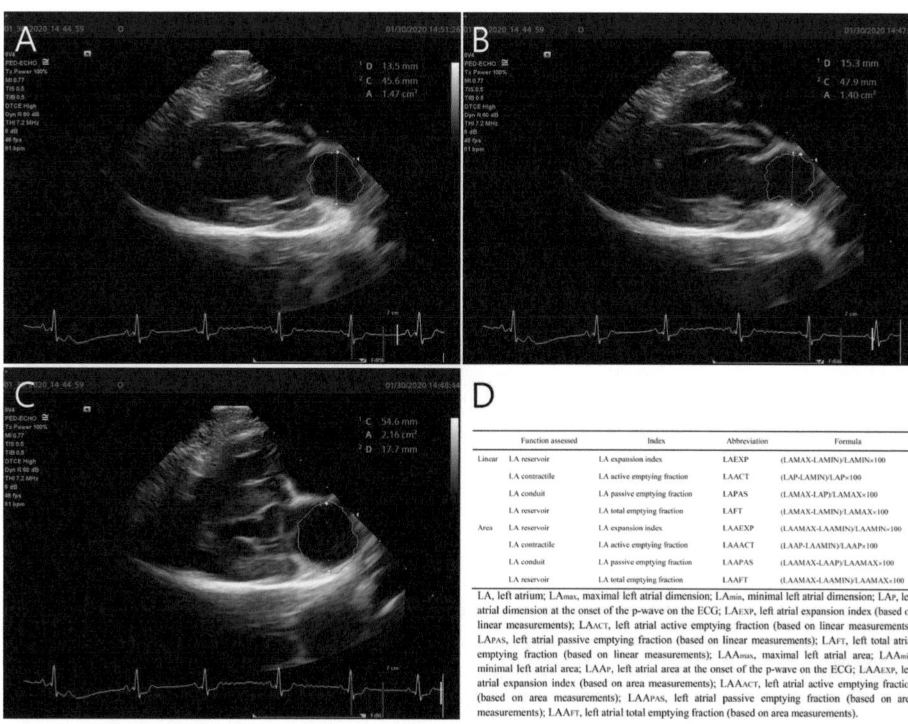

	Function assessed	Index	Abbreviation	Formula
Linear	LA reservoir	LA expansion index	LAEXP	(LAMAX-LAMIN)/LAMIN×100
	LA contractile	LA active emptying fraction	LAACT	(LAP-LAMIN)/LAP×100
	LA conduit	LA passive emptying fraction	LAPAS	(LAMAX-LAP)/LAMAX×100
	LA reservoir	LA total emptying fraction	LAFT	(LAMAX-LAMIN)/LAMAX×100
Area	LA reservoir	LA expansion index	LAAEXP	(LAAMAX-LAAMIN)/LAAMIN×100
	LA contractile	LA active emptying fraction	LAAACT	(LAAP-LAAMIN)/LAAP×100
	LA conduit	LA passive emptying fraction	LAAPAS	(LAAMAX-LAAP)/LAAMAX×100
	LA reservoir	LA total emptying fraction	LAAFT	(LAAMAX-LAAMIN)/LAAMAX×100

LA, left atrium; LA_{max}, maximal left atrial dimension; LA_{min}, minimal left atrial dimension; LA_{P}, left atrial dimension at the onset of the p-wave on the ECG; LA_{EXP}, left atrial expansion index (based on linear measurements); LA_{ACT}, left atrial active emptying fraction (based on linear measurements); LA_{PAS}, left atrial passive emptying fraction (based on linear measurements); LA_{FT}, left total atrial emptying fraction (based on linear measurements); LAA_{max}, maximal left atrial area; LAA_{min}, minimal left atrial area; LAA_{P}, left atrial area at the onset of the p-wave on the ECG; LAA_{EXP}, left atrial expansion index (based on area measurements); LAA_{ACT}, left atrial active emptying fraction (based on area measurements); LAA_{PAS}, left atrial passive emptying fraction (based on area measurements); LAA_{FT}, left atrial total emptying fraction (based on area measurements).

Figure 4.
Two-dimensional echocardiographic estimates of left atrial function. (A) the minimal left atrial diameter/area was obtained at the first frame after mitral valve closure (late ventricular diastole), (B) maximal left atrial diameter were obtained at the last frame before opening of the mitral valve (early ventricular diastole), and (C) the mid-left atrial diameter/area was obtained at the onset of the p-wave on the ECG (diastasis). (D) The formula for LA function index.

end-diastole and the end-systole (**Figure 5**). As described above, the LV internal dimension was significantly larger in dogs with MMVD [34]. However, the LV dimensions noticeably vary among breeds of dogs. Therefore, one study evaluated the allometric scaling of M-mode cardiac measurements in normal adult dogs and found a good correlation between M-mode measurements and BW after logarithmic transformation of the data [54]. Therefore, the M-mode-derived LV internal dimension at systole (LVIDs) and diastole (LVIDd) can be transformed into body weight-indexed (normalized) LV internal dimension using the following formulas to obtain a more accurate estimation of LV dilation in dogs with MMVD:

- LV end-diastolic diameter normalized for body weight (LVIDdN) = LVIDd (cm)/weight (kg)$^{0.294}$
- LV end-systolic diameter normalized for body weight (LVIDsN) = LVIDs (cm)/weight (kg)$^{0.315}$

LVIDdN $\geq$1.7 indicates dogs requiring cardiac medication (>ACVIM B2) [55].

Several studies also found that body surface area (BSA) indexed LV dimensions including end-diastolic index (EDVI) and end-systolic volume index (ESVI) could detect myocardial systolic dysfunction in dogs with MMVD [10, 11, 56]. The EDVI and ESVI can be obtained by the Teichholz formula [57]:

- EDVI = $[7 \times (\text{LVIDd})^3/(2.4 + \text{LVIDd})]/\text{BSA}$
- ESVI = $[7 \times (\text{LVIDs})^3/(2.4 + \text{LVIDs})]/\text{BSA}$

End-diastolic volume index and end-systolic volume index are obtained by dividing BSA, respectively [57]. Normal values of EDVI and ESVI are <100 and <30 mL/m^2, respectively [57]. One study evaluated the diagnostic accuracy of ESVI using two different methods (i.e. the geometric [GM, based on Teichholz formula] and two planimetric methods [PM, Simpson's derived and area-length methods]) and found that the GM overestimates ESVI in a nonlinear way [11]. However, the

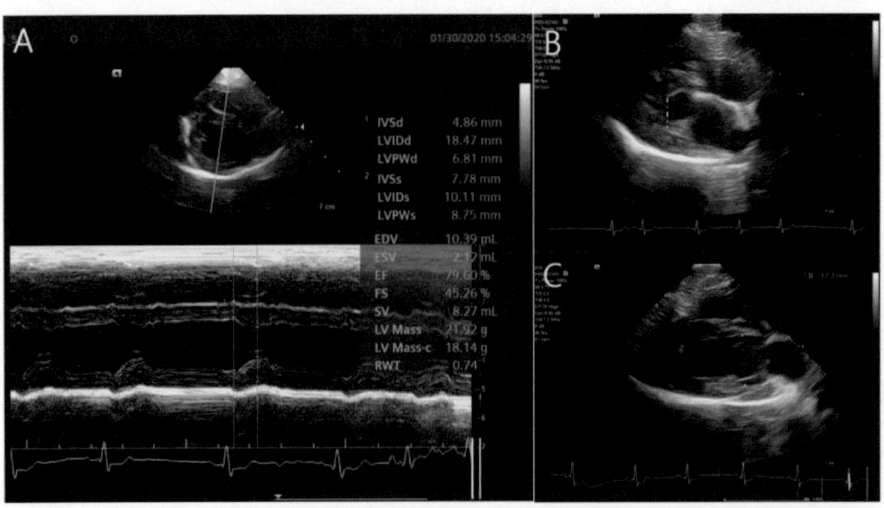

Figure 5.
Measurement of left ventricular internal dimension. (A) M-mode echocardiography obtained from a right parasternal short axis at the papillary muscle level and (B and C) 2D echocardiography obtained from a right parasternal long axis at systole (B) and diastole (C).

	Dog
Diastolic volume	LVd^3 X 7/[2.4 + 3.7 X LVd/(0.795 X W$^{1/3}$)]
Systolic volume	LVs^3 X 7/[2.4 + 5.9 X LVs/(0.795 X W$^{1/3}$)]

LVd, Left ventricle end-diastolic diameter (in cm); LVs, left ventricle end-systolic diameter (in cm); W, weight in kilograms. From "Clinical Echocardiography of the Dog and Cat - E-Book (edited by Madron E, Chetboul V and Bussadori C), St Louis: Elsevier; 2016. pp. 115.

Table 1.
Veterinary Teichholz method formulas for dogs.

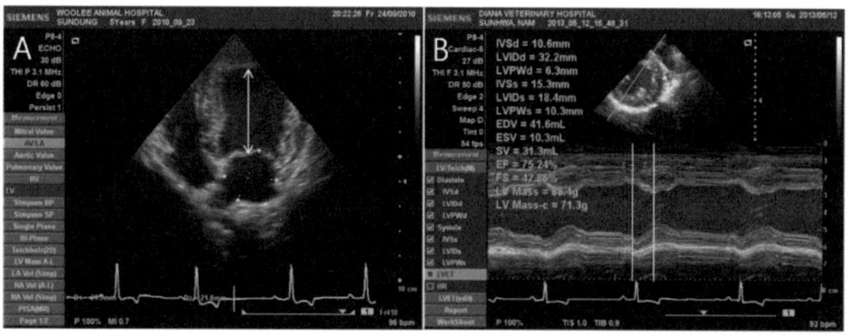

Figure 6.
The left ventricular (LV) sphericity index was calculated by the ratio of LV end-diastolic length (at left apical four-chamber plane; A) to the M-mode LV end-diastolic diameter (B).

ESVI was correlated with the severity of CHF in dogs with MMVD [11]. A recent study also found the EDVI and ESVI obtained from the GM were overestimated and had poor diagnostic values in dogs with MMVD [19]. To overcome this limitation, the veterinary Teichholz formula has been proposed (**Table 1**).

Because sole use of LV dimension often leads to the misestimation of LV dilation, the 2D and M-mode-derived LVIDd/Ao ratio is more appropriate and simpler for evaluating the degree of LV enlargement [14]. However, a recent study found the LVIDd/Ao ratio had high specificity and low sensitivity for detecting asymptomatic dogs from healthy control dogs and symptomatic dogs from asymptomatic dogs with MMVD [19].

Due to the LV dilation, the sphericity of the LV can be increased. One study revealed a significant decrease in the LV sphericity index in dogs with advanced MMVD [11]. The LV sphericity index can be calculated by the ratio of LV end-diastolic length (at left apical two- or four-chamber plane; **Figure 6A**) to the M-mode LV end-diastolic diameter (**Figure 6B**).

4. Assessment of myocardial dysfunction

LV systolic function can be reduced on serial 2D-EC in some dogs with MMVD [10], as noticed in human with advanced CHF [58]. However, LV measurement for systolic function often complicates depending on the LV loading condition, and thus fractional shortening (%FS) and LV ejection fractions (%LVEF) are often increased in dogs with advanced MMVD. In many cases of canine MMVD, when cardiac output is reduced with the progression of MMVD, the LV wall motion becomes more hyperdynamic [10]. Therefore, echocardiographic indices with Doppler for assessing LV functions and filling pressures are often ambiguous by age-related impairment of LV relaxation, LA pressure overload by MR, and impact on myocardial tissue velocities by LV loading condition. Therefore, echocardiographic indices for LV systolic and diastolic function often lead to the misinterpretation of LV function.

4.1 %FS and %LVEF

LV remodeling caused by chronic and hemodynamically significant MR is characterized by changes in LV geometry in response to chronic volume overload. The common echocardiographic indices for LV systolic myocardial function are %LVEF and %FS. The EF is the volumetric fraction of blood ejected from the LV in each heartbeat (LVEF = [end-diastolic volume – end-systolic volume]/end-diastolic volume × 100). The %FS is defined by the percent change in the dimension from end-diastole to end-systole (FS% = [LVIDd – LVIDs]/LVIDd × 100) [59]. As discussed earlier, %FS and %LVEF are reduced in human with myocardial dysfunction [58]; they are often increased in dogs with advanced MMVD due to hyperdynamic LV contraction from elevated preload and reduced afterload [19, 56]. Therefore, these two indices do not have good diagnostic value for detecting the progression of heart failure in dogs with MMVD [19].

4.2 Spectral Doppler studies

More advanced Doppler and tissue echocardiographic methods are being used for detecting LV dysfunction in dogs with MMVD to overcome problems encountered with the simple measurement of LV geometry.

Continuous-wave Doppler interrogation of MR flow profile can be affected by LA pressure, LV systolic function, and loading condition as well as systemic arterial pressure (SAP) (**Figure 7A**). Although the peak velocity of MR is closely related to MR fraction in the LA but not related to the severity of MMVD in dogs [19], dogs with LV systolic impairment and high LA pressure (as well as markedly reduced SAP) may have decreased peak MR velocity [14]. This may help to differentiate dogs with end-stage CHF from those with ACVIM C and D MMVD. Asymmetric MR flow profiles and a cut-off sign in mid to late systole are often noticed in dogs with the advanced stage of MMVD and are caused by reduction in MR flow due to high LA pressure (**Figure 7B**). The dp/dt is the rate of pressure change over time during isovolumic contraction and closely related to LV systolic function in humans (**Figure 7A**) [60]. However, the dp/dt in dogs with MMVD has limited

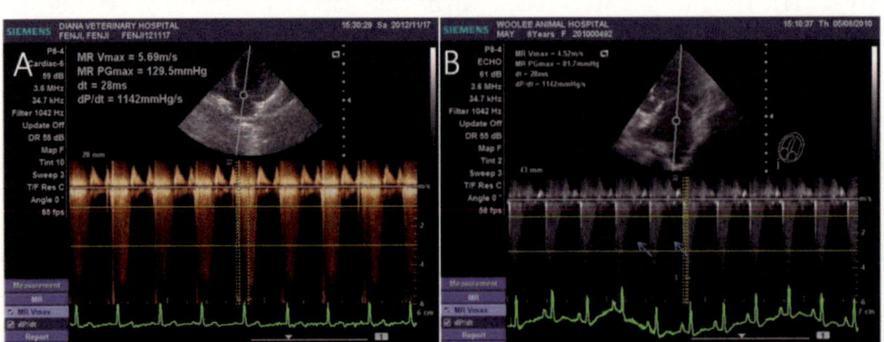

Figure 7.
Continuous-wave (CW) Doppler flow profile obtained from dogs with severe mitral regurgitation (MR). (A) The MR peak velocity and pressure gradient were 5.69 m/s and 129.5 mmHg, respectively, in this dog. (B) Asymmetric MR flow profiles and cut-off signs (arrow) in mid to late systole obtained from the advanced stage of mitral valve disease (see text).

value, because most MMVD dogs may have high peak velocity and asymmetric MR profiles, regardless of the severity of MMVD [18], although some authors proposed its use for detecting LV systolic function [2].

Pulse-wave Doppler interrogation of transmitral flow profile is closely correlated with the stage of MMVD in dogs [14, 18, 19]. The transmitral flow profile consists of an early E-peak (rapid LV filling) and a late diastolic A-peak (atrial contraction) and is closely related to diastolic LV function (LV relaxation/compliance, LV volume overload/pressure overload, and recoil) as well as LV filling pressure (**Figure 8A**) [61, 62]. Although E/A reversal (E/A < 1) is common in the aged canine population, E-peak is higher than A-peak in general canine population (i.e. E/A < 1). One study found 0.87 ± 0.13 m/s (E-peak) and 0.61 ± 0.12 m/s (A-peak) in 100 healthy dogs [63]. A high-velocity E-peak (>1.5 m/s) indicates marked elevation of LA pressure [10] and is correlated with severity of CHF and survival time in dogs with MMVD [18, 19, 23, 25]. Generally, a higher E-peak with a shorter E deceleration time (<80 ms in dogs older than 10–12 years) indicates marked LA pressure overload and non-compliant LV, while an E/A ratio <1 and/or a prolonged E deceleration time indicates impaired relaxation [10]. Because the E-peak velocity is increased with the elevation of LA pressure whereas decreased with impairment of LV relaxation, transmitral flow profile sometimes misleads the severity of LV myocardial dysfunction. However, myocardial and annular velocities are less load-dependent than transmitral flow profile, and thus the E/e (the early longitudinal mitral annular velocity measured by tissue Doppler imaging) ratio is found to better reflect LV filling pressure in dogs with MMVD [61]. A decrease in e-peak at mitral annulus

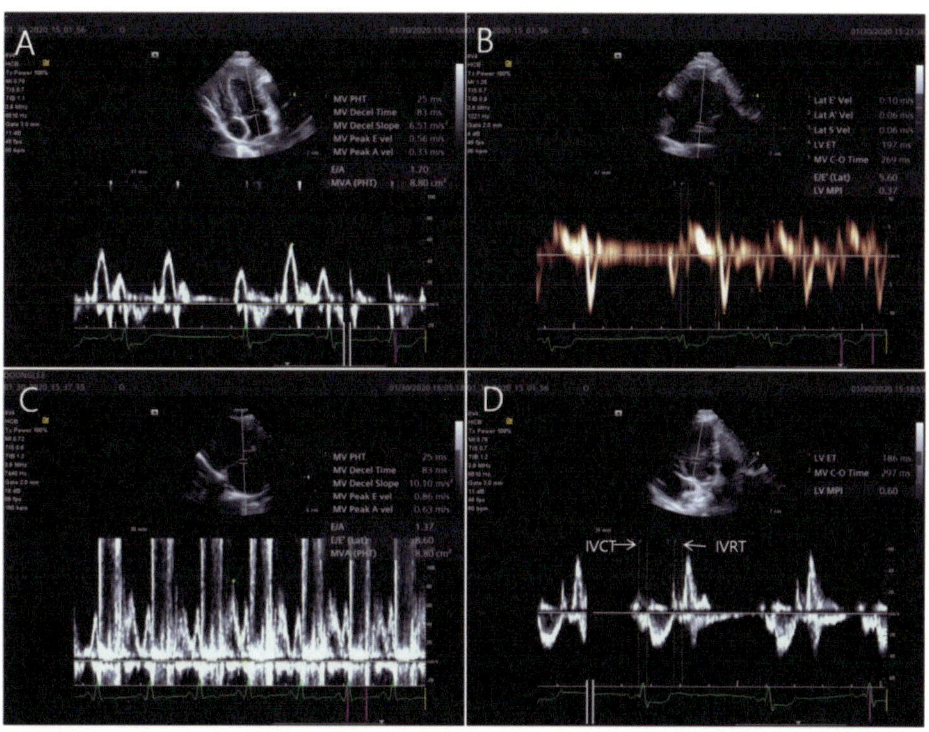

Figure 8.
Transmitral E/e ratio and E/IVRT (the isovolumic relaxation time). (A and B) Transmitral E-peak obtained from a left apical four-chamber plane and tissue Doppler imaging of lateral e-peak obtained from a left apical four-chamber plane. (C and D) Transmitral E-peak obtained from a left apical four-chamber plane. By moving sampling gate towards the midline of the aorta and mitral annulus, aortic and mitral flows were obtained simultaneously. The IVRT was measured from the end of the aortic flow to the beginning of the mitral E-peak.

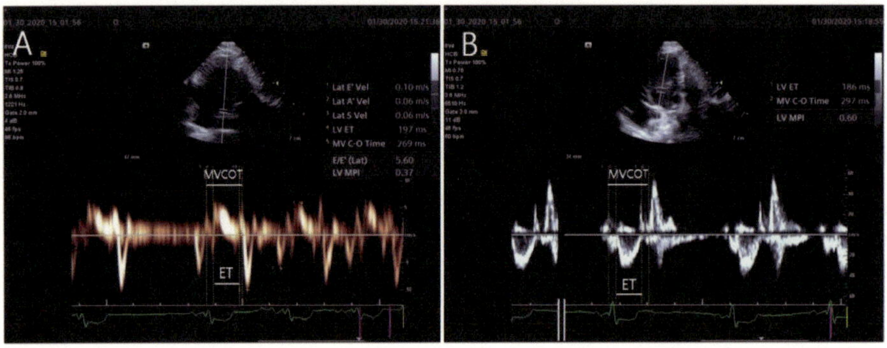

Figure 9.
Two methods for measuring left ventricular (LV) Tei index. (A) Tissue Doppler imaging at the mitral annulus and (B) Pulse-wave Doppler interrogation at the midline of the aorta and mitral annulus (see ***Figure 8D*** *for the measurement). (See text for more information).*

indicates impaired relaxation. One study revealed an E/e ratio >9 was equivalent to >20 mmHg of LA pressure (95% probability in a canine model of acute MR) (**Figure 8B**) [61]. Furthermore, >12 of E/e along with a high E-peak velocity was able to detect the presence of CHF in this study population [61]. One recent study also demonstrated an E/e cut-off value of 13 identifies CHF with high sensitivity (80%) and high specificity (83%) [64]. Although the e-peak is less affected by LV loading condition, it can be also affected by age and severe LV volume overload, and thus the E/e ratio may have limited value in this situation [14]. Several studies demonstrated E-peak/isovolumic relaxation time (E/IVRT) was correlated with LA pressure and end-diastolic LV pressure in dogs (**Figure 8C** and **D**) [62, 65, 66]. The IVRT may be decreased with the elevation of LV filling pressure. One study suggested the E/IVRT ratio >2.5 and an IVRT <45 ms might indicate the presence of CHF in dogs with advanced MMVD [62]. PW Doppler interrogation of the pulmonary venous flow profile gains popularity to determine LA volume and pressure overload by severe MR in humans [67]. However, it has limited value in dogs with MMVD, due to technical difficulty (e.g. PV usually locates at the far-end of an echocardiographic window) and poor-quality PV profiles (e.g. MR flow often enters into the PV) [14]. The LV Tei index (LV Tei = [IVRT + IVCT + LVET]/LVET, IVCT stands for the isovolumic contraction time) is a valuable index for detecting LV systolic and diastolic dysfunction simultaneously in human with CHF (**Figure 9**) [68]. A human study found shortened LVET/increased LV Tei index in patients with systolic dysfunction and increased mitral valve closure time and Tei index in humans with diastolic dysfunction [69, 70]. One canine study found the LV Tei was closely related to LV dp/dt and was increased with the severity of MMVD [71]. However, in dogs with moderate to severe MR, the IVRT and IVCT are often too short or not detectable [14]. Therefore, the Tei index is rarely used in veterinary fields.

5. Assessment of pulmonary hypertension

Pulmonary venous hypertension (PVH) is a common cause of pulmonary hypertension (PH) in dogs and is prevalent in dogs with MMVD, especially in dogs with the advanced stage of CHF [7, 62, 72]. Gold standard methods detecting PH in dogs are Doppler assessment of peak tricuspid regurgitation (TR) and pulmonic regurgitation (PR) jet velocities [7]. One study demonstrated the Doppler evidence of PH was more evidenced in dogs with more advanced MMVD [7]. Another study also found that dogs having moderate to severe PH had a poorer outcome than in MMVD dogs [72].

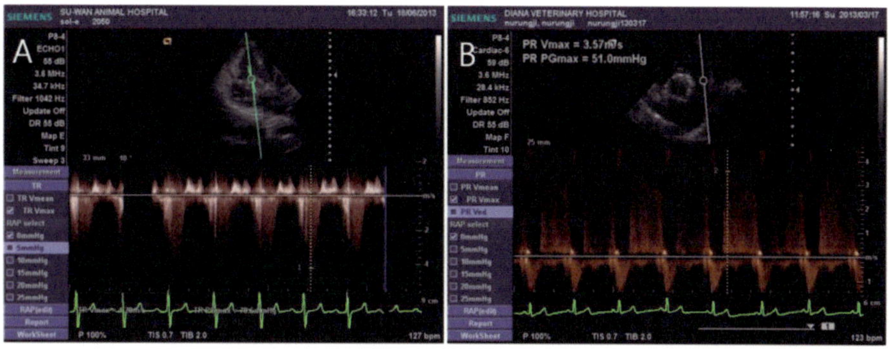

Figure 10.
Echocardiographic evidence of pulmonary hypertension. Continuous-wave Doppler study showing severe tricuspid regurgitation (A) and pulmonic regurgitation (B). (See text for more information).

5.1 Doppler interrogation of TR and PR jets

The peak velocity of TR jet (obtained from either a right parasternal short-axis view or a left parasternal four-chamber view) represents the systolic pulmonary artery pressure (sPAP) if there is no right ventricular outflow tract (RVOT) obstruction [73]. The systolic pulmonary artery pressure can be calculated by applying the modified Bernoulli equation ($\Delta P = 4 \times velocity^2$) to the peak velocity of TR (**Figure 10A**) or PR jets (**Figure 10B**) and adding the right atrial pressure (RAP): $\Delta P + \pi$ right atrium. The estimated right atrial pressure is 5 mmHg in dogs without any evidence of RA dilation; 10 mmHg in dogs with evidence of RA dilation, but no signs of right-sided heart failure (R-HF); and 15 mmHg in dogs with evidence of RA dilation and clinical signs of R-HF. Then mean pulmonary arterial pressure (mPAP) can be calculated using the following equation: $mPAP = 0.61 \times sPAP + 2$. In dogs having the only PR, the mPAP can be calculated using the following equation: PR peak pressure gradient + RAP. A mPAP <25 mmHg is considered normal, while mPAP 25–40 (equivalent to 2.8–3.4 m/s of peak TR velocity), 41–55 (3.4–4.3 m/s), and >55 mmHg (>4.3 m/s) are considered mild, moderate, and severe, respectively [73]. Because the peak velocity is closely correlated with the beam alignment of jet, it often underestimates the severity of PH, if the beam is not parallel to jet [18]. Another study also claimed that the Doppler estimation of SAP often overestimated PH in dogs with MMVD [73]. Since some dogs with PH may have no or insufficient Doppler evidence of PH (e.g. TR or PR jets), other echocardiographic evidence of PH should be pursued in dogs having R-CHF signs or persistent coughing [14]. Despite these limitations, canine studies found the SAP showed good prognostic value for detecting the progression of CHF and the survival time in dogs with MMVD [7, 62, 72].

5.2 2D-EC evidence of PA/RVOT dilation

The 2D-EC evidence of PA/RVOT dilation is the simplest way to detect the existence of PH in dogs with MMVD [35, 74–77]. Since chronic pressure overload and volume overload in RV can cause RV concentric hypertrophy (thickened RV free wall) and eccentric hypertrophy (RV dilation), respectively, simple 2D measurements of RV free wall thickness and dimension may help to identify dogs with PH [74, 78]. Furthermore, LV eccentricity (obtained from right parasternal short-axis view at papillary level; a ratio of longitudinal to the transverse length of LV chamber; **Figure 11C**) is also a simple echocardiographic index for detecting the existence of PH in dogs [78]. Two studies found the LV eccentricity becomes <1, as

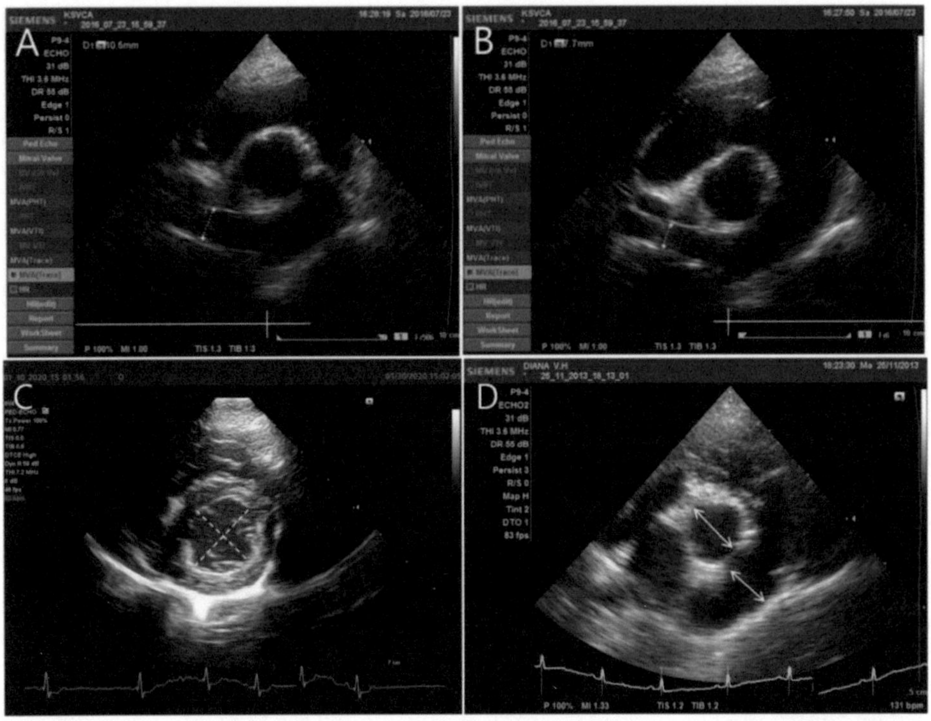

Figure 11.
2D echocardiographic interrogation of pulmonary hypertension. (A and B) right pulmonary artery distensibility index (RPADi) is the difference in diameters of the right pulmonary artery (RPA) at systole (A) and diastole (B) obtained from either 2D or M-mode echocardiography at a right parasternal short axis of PA. (C) Left ventricular (LV) eccentricity obtained from right parasternal short-axis view at papillary level (a ratio of longitudinal to the transverse length of LV chamber). (D) The ratio of main pulmonary artery diameter to aortic root diameter obtained at a right parasternal short axis of PA. (See text for more information).

the RV pressure becomes higher than the LV pressure (as commonly seen in dogs with PH) [74, 79].

In normal dogs, the diameters of the main pulmonary artery (MPA) are roughly identical, and thus MPA/Ao ratio should be close to 1 (**Figure 11D**). Therefore, MPA/Ao ratio > 1 indicates the PA dilation meaning the existence of PH, unless there is RVOT obstruction. Many studies revealed the dilation of MPA in dogs with PH [35, 74–77].

Right pulmonary artery distensibility index (RPADi) is the difference in diameters of the right pulmonary artery (RPA) at systole and diastole obtained from either M-mode right parasternal short-axis (**Figure 11A** and **B**) or long-axis four-chamber view (**Figure 12A**) of PA [77, 80]. One canine study suggested that a RPADi <35 is indicative of PH, while values of 28–35, 23–27, and <23 are indicative of mild (30–55 mmHg), moderate (56–79 mm Hg), and severe PH (>79 mm Hg), respectively [80]. Further study also found that the RPADi was closely correlated with the sPAP [77]. However, the reference range of RPADi was significantly different, depending on the echocardiographic views [77, 80].

RVOT-%FS indicates RV systolic function and can be obtained from M-mode measurement of the RVOT of the right parasternal short-axis view at the level of the aortic root using the following formula: ([RVOT dimensions at end-diastole – RVOT dimensions at end-systole]/RVOT dimensions at end-diastole) × 100 (**Figure 12B**) [81]. One recent canine study found the RVOT-%FS is significantly decreased (<45%) in dogs with PH [82]. However, the RVOT-%FS can be affected by other diseases causing RV systolic dysfunction.

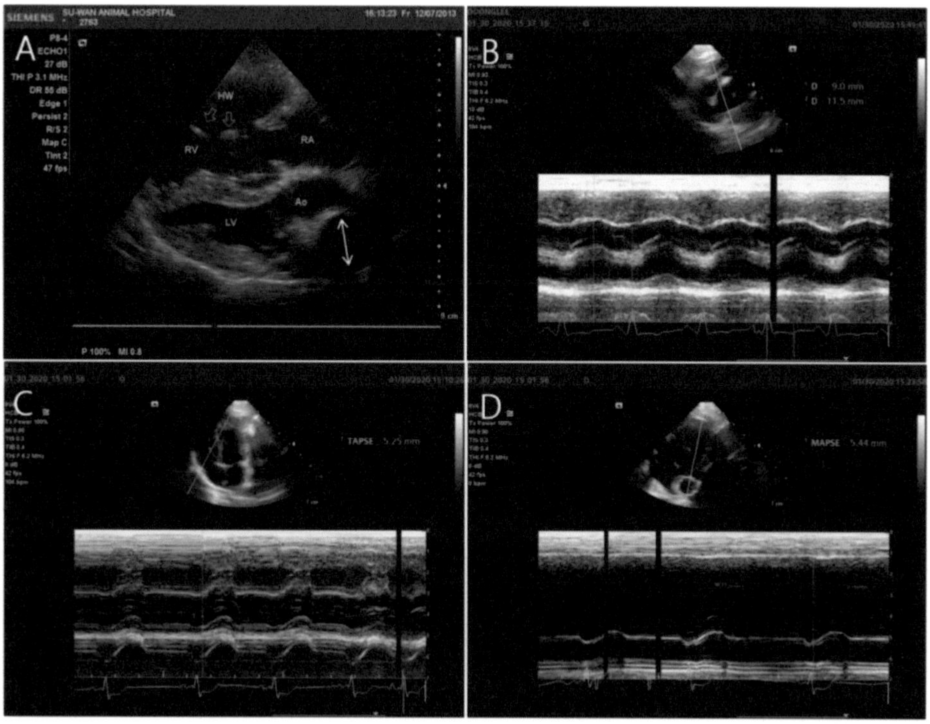

Figure 12.
2D and M-mode echocardiographic interrogation of pulmonary hypertension. (A) Right pulmonary artery distensibility index (RPADi) can be obtained from a right parasternal long axis of four-chamber plane (arrow). (B) Right ventricular outflow tract fractional shortening (RVOT-%FS) obtained from M-mode measurement of the RVOT of the right parasternal short-axis view at the level of the aortic root. Tricuspid (TAPSE; C) and mitral (MAPSE; D) annular plane systolic excursion obtained from a left apical four-chamber plane of M-mode echocardiography. (See text for more information).

Tricuspid annular plane systolic excursion (TAPSE) also reflects RV systolic function, which can be significantly affected by RV pressure overload [83]. Recent canine studies found dogs with PH had lower TAPSE, indicating pressure overload in the RV chamber [75, 84]. The TAPSE can be obtained from M-mode echocardiography that aligned the beam to the lateral tricuspid annulus in the left apical long-axis four-chamber view by calculating the maximal and the minimal excursion of lateral tricuspid annulus motion (**Figure 12C**) as similar to the measurement of mitral annular plane systolic excursion (MAPSE; **Figure 12D**). However, the TAPSE is influenced from the size of dogs; recent studies used body weight-normalized TAPSE (nTAPSE = $TAPSE/[BW(kg)]^{1/3}$) and TAPSE to Ao ratio to overcome the influence of body size [82, 85]. The median (range) of nTAPSEs were 0.60 (0.53–0.66) in ACVIM B1, 0.71 (0.64–0.84) in B2, and 0.73 (0.58–0.80) in C and D MMVD dogs [85]. Other study found the TAPSE/Ao ratio was closely correlated with the size of the LA in dogs with MMVD and PH [82]. The TAPSE/Ao ratio <0.65 was indicative of the presence of PH in dogs with MMVD, although it showed low sensitivity for detecting PH [82].

5.3 Doppler interrogation of PA flow profiles and related variables

Several studies evaluated quantitative echocardiographic variables related to PH in humans and dogs [78, 86–89]. Among those echocardiographic variables, PW Doppler-derived acceleration time to peak PA flow velocity (AT), AT to the ejection time of PA flow ratio (AT/ET) (**Figure 13A**) [86], the right ventricular Tei

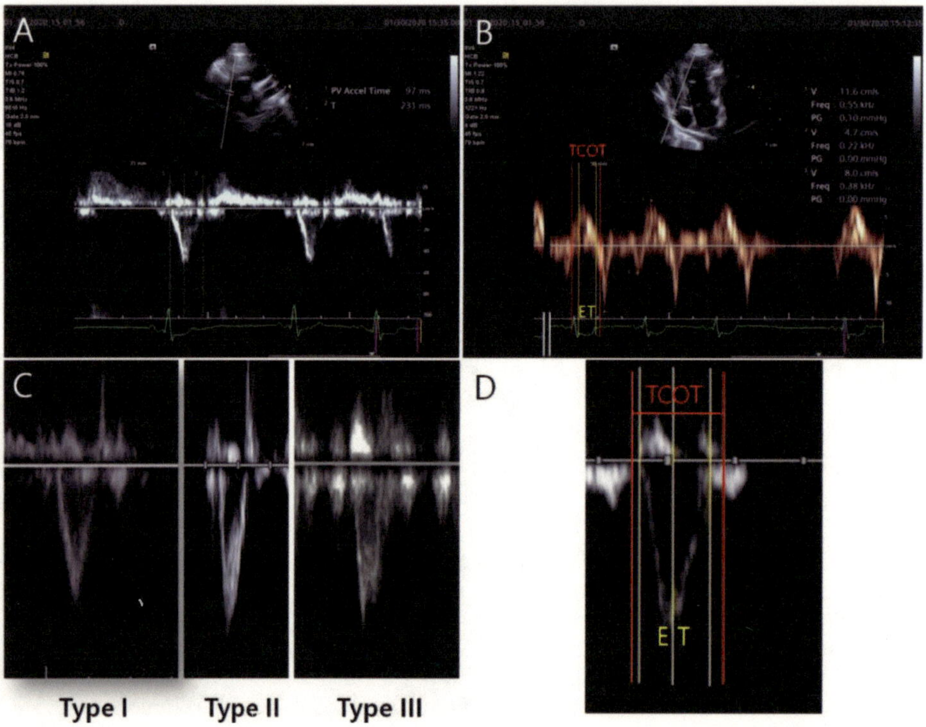

Figure 13.
Pulse-wave and tissue Doppler interrogation of pulmonary hypertension. (A) PW Doppler-derived acceleration time (AT) to peak pulmonary artery (PA) flow velocity (AT), AT to the ejection time (ET) of PA flow ratio (AT/ET). (B) Tissue Doppler-derived right ventricular Tei index (RV Tei), (C) PW Doppler-derived pulmonic outflow profiles, (D) PW Doppler-derived RV Tei index. (See text for more information).

index (RV Tei) (**Figure 13B** and **D**) [89], and Doppler pulmonic outflow profiles (**Figure 13C**) [90] are being used to interrogate PH in dogs. One study found AT, AT/ET ratio, and RV Tei index are strongly correlated with sPAP in dogs without detectable PR [35]. Especially, AT/ET ratios ≤0.25 were predictive of PH, whereas AT/ET ratios >0.42 ruled out PH [86]. However, other study found Doppler estimated mPAP was strongly associated with AT and AT/ET, but weakly associated with RV Tei index [90]. Over 50% of dogs in International Small Animal Cardiac Health Council (ISACHC) II and III had equivocal value of AT/ET indicating PH (0.25–0.42) in this study, suggesting low sensitivity for detecting PH, although most dogs having <0.25 had detectible TR or PR on echocardiography, indicating high specificity for detecting clinically significant PH [90]. This study also found Doppler pulmonic outflow profiles were closely associated with severity of PH in dogs with MMVD, since the Doppler pulmonic outflow profiles (type I/II/III) were 18/0/0 in control, 22/5/1 in ISACHC I, 21/24/2 in ISACHC II, and 17/40/4 in ISACHC III MMVD dogs [90]. The PW Doppler-derived echocardiographic variables of PA flow may have limited value in dogs with hyperdynamic RV condition because Doppler pulmonic outflow profiles can be influenced by RV loading conditions and systolic function [90]. Although RV-TDI may not be a direct indicator of PH, it can be used to evaluate RV systolic and diastolic function in PH patients. It can be obtained from the basal segment of the internal mid-portion of the RV wall in the left parasternal long-axis four-chamber view (**Figure 13D**). One study evaluated the diagnostic value of peak RV myocardial velocities at systole (Stdi), early (Etdi), and late (Atdi) diastole [35]. Also the global TDI index was calculated using the following formula in this study: global TDI index = Stdi × Etdi/Atdi [35].

This study demonstrated the decrement of the global TDI index and Etdi/Atdi in dogs with PH [35]. Furthermore, global TDI index of <11.8 showed sensitivity of 89% and specificity of 90%, while Etdi/Atdi of <1.12 showed sensitivity of 89% and specificity of 93% for detecting PH in the study population [35].

6. Assessment of cardiac chamber deformation/dyssynchrony

Strain and strain rate imaging is an advanced echocardiographic technique for estimating myocardial segmental deformation, respectively [12, 91]. Myocardial strain (i.e., deformation of a myocardial segment over time; % change from its original dimension) and strain rate (the rate of myocardial deformation; S^{-1}) can evaluate more direct intrinsic myocardial function and are less angle-dependent than TDI-based methods [92–94]. Strain and strain rate can be obtained from LV, LA, and RV wall using STE, feature-tracking echocardiography (FTE), or color TDI technology in the longitudinal, radial, and circumferential planes (**Figure 14**) [83]. Speckle tracking can detect the degree of myocardial deformation from the continuous frame-by-frame tracking of speckles (acoustic markers). By tracking these speckles in the myocardium throughout the cardiac cycle, the direction and velocity of myocardial motion can be determined. By comparing the motion of each speckle, the degree of deformation on each segment of the myocardium can be assessed.

Although precise assessment of LV systolic dysfunction is critical for therapeutic intervention and prediction of progression of CHF in dogs with MMVD, assessment of LV function using conventional echocardiography is often complicated

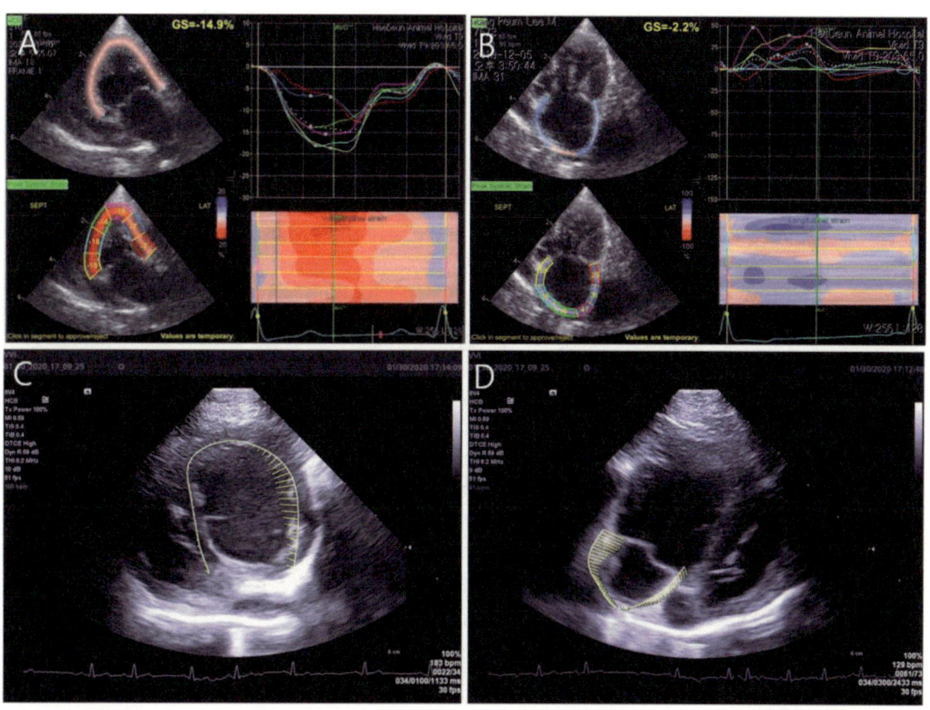

Figure 14.
Representative images of left atrial (LA) and ventricular (LV) strain and strain rate imaging for LA and LV deformation analysis in dogs with mitral regurgitation. (A and B) LV (A) and LA (B) strain profiles obtained from GE analysis software algorithm (EchoPAC). (C and D) LV (C) and LA (D) strain profiles obtained from Siemens vector velocity imaging (VVI). (See text for more information).

with loading conditions [95]. Several studies demonstrated strain and strain rate obtained from the 2D-STE were useful to grade the progression of dogs with MMVD [95–98]. One study claimed the longitudinal strain with the GE analysis software algorithm (EchoPAC) was inconsistent and less repeatable, while radial strain curves from short-axis images were more consistent and more repeatable (**Figure 14A** and **B**) [95]. Since the software algorithm for strain is automated, special attention should be focused on "(1) timing of the ECG to select the cardiac cycle and the onset and duration of analysis; (2) tracing of the endocardial border for automated detection; (3) inspecting the region of interest; (4) following the tissue tracking in real-time and slow-motion; and (5) inspecting the generated curves relative to the R-waves and aortic valve closure (AVC)" as described in Smith et al. [95]. A velocity vector imaging (VVI) is another form of strain analysis, which can display tissue velocity as a vector showing the amplitude and direction of the movement (**Figure 14C** and **D**) [99].

Atrial myocardial deformation profiles estimated by TDI and 2D-STE (e.g. strain and strain rate) have been recently emerged as a good alternative method of exploring LA mechanics in both humans and dogs [100–103]. Although many drawbacks of this approach were noticed (e.g. suboptimal reproducibility, angle dependence, and the confounding effect of noise artifacts), 2D-STE can be a more advanced angle-independent echocardiographic technique for the direct evaluation of LA function than standard grayscale echocardiographic images [100–103]. The specific STE variables subject to the LA function include peak atrial longitudinal average strain (PALS), peak atrial contraction average strain (PACS), and contraction strain index (CSI), which reflect the LA function during its reservoir, booster pump phase, and the contribution of LA active contraction to the LV filling phase (**Figure 14B**) [104]. In humans, LA strain analysis has been useful for grading patients with valvular diseases, atrial fibrillation, or acute coronary disease [105–107]. However, a recent canine study found the STE variables were not significantly different between ACVIM B1 and B2 groups, although those (especially, PALS) were significantly different between ACVIM B2 and C groups [108]. The use of cut-off for PALS <27.9% enables to perfectly differentiate dogs in ACVIM stage B2 from those in ACVIM stage C with a sensitivity of 100% and specificity of 100% [108]. Another study also demonstrated the STE variables including PALS, PACS, and CSI were significantly decreased with the progression of MMVD [103]. A further study from this study group also found the STE variables (PALS <30% and CSI per 1% increase) were predictors of cardiac death in the univariate analysis [109].

Since the RV chamber is crescent-shaped and is wrapped around the LV, precise echocardiographic assessment of RV function is often difficult. The TDI and STE can overcome this limitation as reported in human studies [110, 111]. Recent canine study found the STE on RV was applicable and repeatable in healthy dogs [93]. Furthermore, other study demonstrated the RV longitudinal strain and the dyssynchrony index were significantly different from control dogs [75]. In this study, the global, free wall, and septal RV longitudinal strain in dogs with precapillary PH were significantly lower than those in control, while free wall and septal systolic shortening time strain were significantly slower [75].

7. Conclusion

In this chapter, we described echocardiographic features of MMVD in dogs along with human echocardiographic criteria of MR. Although there are many similarities for diagnosing and grading the severity of MR in both species, veterinary cardiologists are more focused on the severity of cardiac remodeling and cardiac dysfunction caused by MR, because surgical restoration of defected mitral apparatus is rarely done in dogs. Recent canine studies also found advanced ultrasound technologies, such as strain and strain rate imaging, and two-dimensional speckle tracking echocardiography were also applicable for dogs with MMVD, although more studies are warranted for standardizing the method of assessment in dogs. The authors believe that this chapter would be a valuable reference for veterinary and human cardiologists and researchers for understanding mitral valve disease.

Acknowledgements

The authors express great gratitude to Siemens Healthineers (Ms. UnWook Park) for technical support and Drs Jae-Min Suhl and Jin-Hee Noh for sharing space and resources for preparing echocardiographic images on this chapter.

Conflict of interest

There is no conflict for this publication.

Author details

Sang-Il Suh[1], Ta-Li Lu[2], Ran Choi[3] and Changbaig Hyun[4*]

1 Cardiology Section, Haedeun Animal Medical Center, Bucheon, Korea

2 Cardiology Section, Chuan Animal Hospital, Taipei City, Taiwan

3 Cardiology Section, Dasom Animal Medical Center, Busan, Korea

4 Changbaig Hyun Special Animal Clinic, Seoul, Korea

*Address all correspondence to: changbaig@gmail.com

References

[1] Buchanan JW. Prevalence of cardiovascular disorders. In: Fox PR, Sisson D, Moise NS, editors. Textbook of Canine and Feline Cardiology. 2nd ed. Philadelphia: WB Saunders; 1999. pp. 457-470

[2] Kvart C, Häggström J. Acquired valvular heart disease. In: Ettinger SJ, Feldman EC, editors. Textbook of Veterinary Internal Medicine. 6th ed. Philadelphia: WB Saunders; 2005. pp. 1022-1039

[3] Atkins C, Bonagura J, Ettinger S, Fox P, Gordon S, Häggström J, et al. Guidelines for the diagnosis and treatment of canine chronic valvular heart disease. Journal of Veterinary Internal Medicine. 2009;**23**:1142-1150. DOI: 10.1111/j.1939-1676.2009.0392.x

[4] Fox PR. Pathology of myxomatous mitral valve disease in the dog. Journal of Veterinary Cardiology. 2012;**14**:103-126. DOI: 10.1016/j.jvc.2012.02.001

[5] Pedersen HD, Häggström J. Mitral valve prolapse in the dog: A model of mitral valve prolapse in man. Cardiovascular Research. 2000;**47**:234-243. DOI: 10.1016/s0008-6363(00) 00113-9

[6] Boon JA. Acquired heart disease: Mitral insufficiency. In: Boon JA, editor. Manual of Veterinary Echocardiography. 1st ed. Baltimore: Williams and Wilkins; 1998. pp. 261-286

[7] Serres FJ, Chetboul V, Tissier R, Carlos Sampedrano C, Gouni V, Nicolle AP, et al. Doppler echocardiography-derived evidence of pulmonary arterial hypertension in dogs with degenerative mitral valve disease: 86 cases (2001-2005). Journal of the American Veterinary Medical Association. 2006;**229**:1772-1778. DOI: 10.2460/javma.229.11.1772

[8] Stepien RL. Pulmonary arterial hypertension secondary to chronic left-sided cardiac dysfunction in dogs. The Journal of Small Animal Practice. 2009;**50**(Suppl 1):34-43. DOI: 10.1111/j.1748-5827.2009.00802.x

[9] Chiavegato D, Borgarelli M, D'Agnolo G, Santilli RA. Pulmonary hypertension in dogs with mitral regurgitation attributable to myxomatous valve disease. Veterinary Radiology & Ultrasound. 2009;**50**:253-258. DOI: 10.1111/j.1740-8261.2009.01529.x

[10] Bonagura JD, Schober KE. Can ventricular function be assessed by echocardiography in chronic canine mitral valve disease? The Journal of Small Animal Practice. 2009;**50**(Suppl 1):12-24. DOI: 10.1111/j.1748-5827.2009.00803.x

[11] Serres F, Chetboul V, Tissier R, Poujol L, Gouni V, Carlos Sampedrano C, et al. Comparison of 3 ultrasound methods for quantifying left ventricular systolic function: Correlation with disease severity and prognostic value in dogs with mitral valve disease. Journal of Veterinary Internal Medicine. 2008;**22**:566-577. DOI: 10.1111/j.1939-1676.2008.0097.x

[12] Chetboul V. Advanced techniques in echocardiography in small animals. The Veterinary Clinics of North America. Small Animal Practice. 2010;**40**:529-543. DOI: 10.1016/j.cvsm.2010.03.007

[13] Lancellotti P, Tribouilloy C, Hagendorff A, Popescu BA, Edvardsen T, Pierard LA, et al. Zamorano JL; scientific document Committee of the European Association of cardiovascular imaging: Recommendations for the echocardiographic assessment of native valvular regurgitation: An executive summary from the European Association of Cardiovascular Imaging.

European Heart Journal Cardiovascular Imaging. 2013;**14**:611-644. DOI: 10.1093/ehjci/jet105

[14] Chetboul V, Tissier R. Echocardiographic assessment of canine degenerative mitral valve disease. Journal of Veterinary Cardiology. 2012;**14**:127-148. DOI: 10.1016/j.jvc.2011.11.005

[15] Muzzi RA, de Araujo RB, Muzzi LA, Pena JL, Silva EF. Regurgitant jet area by Doppler color flow mapping: Quantitative assessment of mitral regurgitation severity in dogs. Journal of Veterinary Cardiology. 2003;**5**:33-38. DOI: 10.1016/S1760-2734(06)70050-9

[16] Gouni V, Serres FJ, Pouchelon JL, Tissier R, Lefebvre HP, Nicolle AP, et al. Quantification of mitral valve regurgitation in dogs with degenerative mitral valve disease by use of the proximal isovelocity surface area method. Journal of the American Veterinary Medical Association. 2007;**231**:399-406. DOI: 10.2460/javma.231.3.399

[17] Zoghbi WA, Enriquez-Sarano M, Foster E, Grayburn PA, Kraft CD, Levine RA, et al. Recommendations for evaluation of the severity of native valvular regurgitation with two-dimensional and Doppler echocardiography. Journal of the American Society of Echocardiography. 2003;**16**:777-802. DOI: 10.1016/S0894-7317(03)00335-3

[18] Hyun C. Acquired heart valvular diseases. In: Hyun C, editor. Case Studies in Small Animal Cardiology. 1st ed. Seoul: Panmun Education; 2013. pp. 353-398

[19] Kim H, Suh S, Hyun C. Diagnostic value of echocardiographic indices and cardiac biomarkers in dogs with chronic mitral valve insufficiency. The Thai Journal of Veterinary Medicine. 2017;**47**:373-382

[20] Di Marcello M, Terzo E, Locatelli C, Palermo V, Sala E, Dall'Aglio E, et al. Assessment of mitral regurgitation severity by Doppler colour flow mapping of the vena contracta in dogs. Journal of Veterinary Internal Medicine. 2014;**28**:1206-1213. DOI: 10.1111/jvim.12380

[21] Sargent J, Muzzi R, Mukherjee R, Somarathne S, Schranz K, Stephenson H, et al. Echocardiographic predictors of survival in dogs with myxomatous mitral valve disease. Journal of Veterinary Cardiology. 2015;**17**:1-12. DOI: 10.1016/j.jvc.2014.11.001

[22] Tidholm A, Bodegård-Westling A, Höglund K, Häggström J, Ljungvall I. Real-time 3-dimensional echocardiographic assessment of effective regurgitant orifice area in dogs with myxomatous mitral valve disease. Journal of Veterinary Internal Medicine. 2017;**31**:303-310. DOI: 10.1111/jvim.14642

[23] Chetboul V, Serres F, Tissier R, Lefebvre HP, Carlos Sampedrano C, Gouni V, et al. Association of plasma N-terminal pro-B-type natriuretic peptide concentration with mitral regurgitation severity and outcome in dogs with asymptomatic degenerative mitral valve disease. Journal of Veterinary Internal Medicine. 2009;**23**:984-994. DOI: 10.1111/j.1939-1676.2009.0347.x

[24] Serres F, Pouchelon JL, Poujol L, Lefebvre HP, Trumel C, Daste T, et al. Plasma N-terminal pro-B-type natriuretic peptide concentration helps to predict survival in dogs with symptomatic degenerative mitral valve disease regardless of and in combination with the initial clinical status at admission. Journal of Veterinary Cardiology. 2009;**11**:103-121. DOI: 10.1016/j.jvc.2009.07.001

[25] Borgarelli M, Savarino P, Crosara S, Santilli RA, Chiavegato D,

Poggi M, et al. Survival characteristics and prognostic variables of dogs with mitral regurgitation attributable to myxomatous valve disease. Journal of Veterinary Internal Medicine. 2008;**22**:120-128. DOI: 10.1111/j.1939-1676.2007.0008.x

[26] Borgarelli M, Crosara S, Lamb K, Savarino P, La Rosa G, Tarducci A, et al. Survival characteristics and prognostic variables of dogs with preclinical chronic degenerative mitral valve disease attributable to myxomatous degeneration. Journal of Veterinary Internal Medicine. 2012;**26**:69-75. DOI: 10.1111/j.1939-1676.2011.00860.x

[27] Boswood A, Häggström J, Gordon SG, Wess G, Stepien RL, Oyama MA, et al. Effect of pimobendan in dogs with preclinical myxomatous mitral valve disease and cardiomegaly: The EPIC study-a randomized clinical trial. Journal of Veterinary Internal Medicine. 2016;**30**:1765-1779. DOI: 10.1111/jvim.14586

[28] Haendchen RV, Povzhitkov M, Meerbaum S, Maurer G, Corday E. Evaluation of changes in left ventricular end-diastolic pressure by left atrial two-dimensional echocardiography. American Heart Journal. 1982;**104**:740-745. DOI: 10.1016/0002-8703(82)90005-9

[29] Bonagura JD, Herring DS. Echocardiography. Acquired heart disease. The Veterinary Clinics of North America. Small Animal Practice. 1985;**15**:1209-1224. DOI: 10.1016/S0195-5616(85)50366-6

[30] Reynolds CA, Brown DC, Rush JE, Fox PR, Nguyenba TP, Lehmkuhl LB, et al. Prediction of first onset of congestive heart failure in dogs with degenerative mitral valve disease: The PREDICT cohort study. Journal of Veterinary Cardiology. 2012;**14**:193-202. DOI: 10.1016/j.jvc.2012.01.008

[31] Lord P, Hansson K, Kvart C, Häggström J. Rate of change of heart size before congestive heart failure in dogs with mitral regurgitation. The Journal of Small Animal Practice. 2010;**51**:210-218. DOI: 10.1111/j.1748-5827.2010.00910.x

[32] Hezzell MJ, Boswood A, Moonarmart W, Elliott J. Selected echocardiographic variables change more rapidly in dogs that die from myxomatous mitral valve disease. Journal of Veterinary Cardiology. 2012;**14**:269-279. DOI: 10.1016/j.jvc.2012.01.009

[33] Atkins CE, Keene BW, Brown WA, Coats JR, Crawford MA, DeFrancesco TC, et al. Results of the veterinary enalapril trial to prove reduction in onset of heart failure in dogs chronically treated with enalapril alone for compensated, naturally occurring mitral valve insufficiency. Journal of the American Veterinary Medical Association. 2007;**231**:1061-1069. DOI: 10.2460/javma.231.7.1061

[34] Strohm LE,Visser LC, Chapel EH, Drost WT, Bonagura JD. Two-dimensional, long-axis echocardiographic ratios for assessment of left atrial and ventricular size in dogs. Journal of Veterinary Cardiology. 2018;**20**:330-342. DOI: 10.1016/j.jvc.2018.07.008

[35] Serres F, Chetboul V, Tissier R, Sampedrano CC, Gouni V, Nicolle AP, et al. Chordae tendineae rupture in dogs with degenerative mitral valve disease: Prevalence, survival, and prognostic factors (114 cases, 2001-2006). Journal of Veterinary Internal Medicine. 2007;**21**:258-264. DOI: 10.1892/0891-6640(2007)21[258:ctridw]2.0.co;2

[36] Rishniw M, Erb HN. Evaluation of four 2-dimensional echocardiographic methods of assessing left atrial size in dogs. Journal of Veterinary Internal

Medicine. 2000;**14**:429-435. DOI: 10.1892/0891-6640(2000)014<0429:eofemo>2.3.co;2

[37] Lee MH. Diagnostic features of chronic mitral valve insufficiency in dogs [Master thesis]. Chuncheon: Kangwon National University; 2011

[38] Suh IW, Song JM, Lee EY, Kang SH, Kim MJ, Kim JJ, et al. Left atrial volume measured by realtime 3-dimensional echocardiography predicts clinical outcome in patients with severe left ventricular dysfunction and in sinus rhythm. Journal of the American Society of Echocardiography. 2008;**21**:439-445. DOI: 10.1016/j.echo.2007.09.002

[39] De Castro S, Caselli S, Di Angelantonio E, Del Colle S, Mirabelli F, Marcantonio A, et al. Relation of left atrial maximal volume measured by real-time 3D echocardiography to demographic, clinical, and Doppler variables. The American Journal of Cardiology. 2008;**101**:1347-1352. DOI: 10.1016/j.amjcard.2008.01.005

[40] Tidholm A, Höglund K, Häggström J, Bodegård-Westling A, Ljungvall I. Left atrial ejection fraction assessed by real-time 3-dimensional echocardiography in normal dogs and dogs with myxomatous mitral valve disease. Journal of Veterinary Internal Medicine. 2013;**27**:884-889. DOI: 10.1111/jvim.12113

[41] Badano LP, Pezzutto N, Marinigh R, Cinello M, Nucifora G, Pavoni D, et al. How many patients would be misclassified using M-mode and two-dimensional estimates of left atrial size instead of left atrial volume? A three-dimensional echocardiographic study. Journal of Cardiovascular Medicine. 2008;**9**:476-484. DOI: 10.2459/JCM.0b013e3282f194f0

[42] Artang R, Migrino RQ, Harmann L, Bowers M, Woods TD. Left atrial volume measurement with automated border detection by 3-dimensional echocardiography: Comparison with Magnetic Resonance Imaging. Cardiovascular Ultrasound. 2009;**7**:16. DOI: 10.1186/1476-7120-7-16

[43] Höllmer M, Willesen JL, Tolver A, Koch J. Comparison of four echocardiographic methods to determine left atrial size in dogs. Journal of Veterinary Cardiology. 2016;**18**:137-145. DOI: 10.1016/j.jvc.2016.02.001

[44] Höllmer M, Willesen JL, Tolver A, Koch J. Left atrial volume and function in dogs with naturally occurring myxomatous mitral valve disease. Journal of Veterinary Cardiology. 2017;**19**:24-34. DOI: 10.1016/j.jvc.2016.08.006

[45] Wesselowski S, Borgarelli M, Bello NM, Abbott J. Discrepancies in identification of left atrial enlargement using left atrial volume versus left atrial-to-aortic root ratio in dogs. Journal of Veterinary Internal Medicine. 2014;**28**:1527-1533. DOI: 10.1111/jvim.12410

[46] Höllmer M, Willesen JL, Tolver A, Koch J. Left atrial volume and phasic function in clinically healthy dogs of 12 different breeds. Veterinary Journal. 2013;**197**:639-645. DOI: 10.1016/j.tvjl.2013.05.045

[47] Lang RM, Bierig M, Devereux RB, Flachsk-ampf FA, Foster E, Pellika PA, et al. Recommendations for chamber quantification. European Journal of Echocardiography. 2006;**7**:79-108. DOI: 10.1016/j.euje.2005.12.014

[48] Tidholm A, Bodegård-Westling A, Höglund K, Häggström J, Ljungvall I. Comparison between real-time 3-dimensional and 2-dimensional biplane echocardiographic assessment of left atrial volumes in dogs with myxomatous mitral valve disease. Journal of Veterinary Internal Medicine. 2019;**33**:455-461. DOI: 10.1111/jvim.15408

[49] Badano LP, Miglioranza MH, Mihăilă S, Peluso D, Xhaxho J, Marra MP, et al. Left atrial volumes and function by three-dimensional echocardiography: Reference values, accuracy, reproducibility, and comparison with two-dimensional echocardiographic measurements. Circulation. Cardiovascular Imaging. 2016;**9**:e004229. DOI: 10.1161/CIRCIMAGING.115.00422

[50] Baron Toaldo M, Romito G, Guglielmini C, Diana A, Pelle NG, Contiero B, et al. Prognostic value of echocardiographic indices of left atrial morphology and function in dogs with myxomatous mitral valve disease. Journal of Veterinary Internal Medicine. 2018;**32**:914-921. DOI: 10.1111/jvim.15093

[51] Spencer KT, Mor-Avi V, Gorcsan J III, DeMaria AN, Kimball TR, Monaghan MJ, et al. Effects of aging on left atrial reservoir, conduit, and booster pump function: A multi-institution acoustic quantification study. Heart. 2001;**85**:272-277. DOI: 10.1136/heart.85.3.272

[52] Dickson D, Caivano D, Matos JN, Summerfield N, Rishniw M. Two-dimensional echocardiographic estimates of left atrial function in healthy dogs and dogs with myxomatous mitral valve disease. Journal of Veterinary Cardiology. 2017;**19**:469-479. DOI: 10.1016/j.jvc.2017.09.003

[53] Kittleson MD, Brown WA. Regurgitant fraction measured by using the proximal isovelocity surface area method in dogs with chronic myxomatous mitral valve disease. Journal of Veterinary Internal Medicine. 2003;**17**:84-88. DOI: 10.1892/0891-6640(2003)017<0084:RFMBUT>2.3.CO;2

[54] Cornell CC, Kittleson MD, Della Torre P, Häggström J, Lombard CW, Pedersen HD, et al. Allometric scaling of M-mode cardiac measurements in normal adult dogs. Journal of Veterinary Internal Medicine. 2004;**18**:311-321. DOI: 10.1892/0891-6640(2004)18<311:asomcm>2.0.co;2

[55] Keene BW, Atkins CE, Bonagura JD, Fox PR, Häggström J, Fuentes VL, et al. ACVIM consensus guidelines for the diagnosis and treatment of myxomatous mitral valve disease in dogs. Journal of Veterinary Internal Medicine. 2019;**33**:1127-1140. DOI: 10.1111/jvim.15488

[56] Kittleson MD, Eyster GE, Knowlen GG, Bari Olivier N, Anderson LK. Myocardial function in small dogs with chronic mitral regurgitation and severe congestive heart failure. Journal of the American Veterinary Medical Association. 1984;**184**:455-459

[57] Lombard CW. Normal values of the canine M-mode echocardiogram. American Journal of Veterinary Research. 1984;**45**:2015-2018

[58] Enriquez-Sarano M, Tajik AJ, Schaff HV, Orszulak TA, McGoon MD, Bailey KR, et al. Echocardiographic prediction of left ventricular function after correction of mitral regurgitation: Results and clinical implications. Journal of the American College of Cardiology. 1994;**24**:1536-1543. DOI: 10.1016/0735-1097(94)90151-1

[59] Richard D, Thomas WP. Echocardiography. In: Nyland TG, Mattoon JS, editors. Small Animal Diagnostic Ultrasound. 2nd ed. Philadelphia: WB Saunders; 2002. p. 370

[60] Kolias TJ, Aaronson KD, Armstrong WF. Doppler-derived dP/dt and −dP/dt predict survival in congestive heart failure. Journal of the American College of Cardiology. 2000;**5**:1594-1599. DOI: 10.1016/S0735-1097(00)00908-6

[61] Oyama MA, Sisson DD, Bulmer BJ, Constable PD. Echocardiographic estimation of mean left atrial pressure in a canine model of acute mitral valve insufficiency. Journal of Veterinary Internal Medicine. 2004;**18**:667-672. DOI: 10.1892/0891-6640(2004)18<667:eeom la>2.0.co;2

[62] Schober KE, Hart TM, Stern JA, Li X, Samii VF, Zekas LJ, et al. Detection of congestive heart failure in dogs by Doppler echocardiography. Journal of Veterinary Internal Medicine. 2010;**24**:1358-1368. DOI: 10.1111/j.1939-1676.2010.0592.x

[63] Chetboul V, Sampedrano CC, Concordet D, Tissier R, Lamour T, Ginesta J, et al. Use of quantitative two-dimensional colour tissue Doppler imaging for assessment of left ventricular radial and longitudinal myocardial velocities in dogs. American Journal of Veterinary Research. 2005;**66**:953-961. DOI: 10.2460/ajvr.2005.66.953

[64] Teshima K, Asano K, Sasaki Y, Kato Y, Kutara K, Edamura K, et al. Assessment of left ventricular function using pulsed tissue Doppler imaging in healthy dogs and dogs with spontaneous mitral regurgitation. The Journal of Veterinary Medical Science. 2005;**67**:1207-1215. DOI: 10.1292/jvms.67.1207

[65] Schober KE, Bonagura JD, Scansen BA, Stern JA, Ponzio NM. Estimation of left ventricular filling pressure by use of Doppler echocardiography in healthy anesthetized dogs. American Journal of Veterinary Research. 2008;**69**:1034-1049. DOI: 10.2460/ajvr.69.8.1034

[66] Schober KE, Stern JA, DaCunha DN, Pedraza-Toscano AM, Shemanski D, Hamlin RL. Estimation of left ventricular filling pressure by Doppler echocardiography in dogs with pacing-induced heart failure. Journal of Veterinary Internal Medicine. 2008;**22**:578-585. DOI: 10.1111/j.1939-1676.2008.0099.x

[67] Enriquez-Sarano M, Dujardin KS, Tribouilloy CM, Seward JB, Yoganathan AP, Bailey KR, et al. Determinants of pulmonary venous flow reversal in mitral regurgitation and its usefulness in determining the severity of regurgitation. The American Journal of Cardiology. 1999;**83**:535-541. DOI: 10.1016/s0002-9149(98)00909-6

[68] Tei C. New non-invasive index for combined systolic and diastolic ventricular function. Journal of Cardiology. 1995;**26**:135-136

[69] Moskowitz RL, Wechsler BM. Left ventricular ejection time in aortic and mitral valve disease. The American Journal of Cardiology. 1965;**15**:809-814. DOI: 10.1016/0002-9149(65)90383-8

[70] Haque A, Otsuji Y, Yoshifuku S, Kumanohoso T, Zhang H, Kisanuki A, et al. Effects of valve dysfunction on Doppler Tei index. Journal of the American Society of Echocardiography. 2002;**15**:877-883. DOI: 10.1067/mje.2002.121198

[71] Teshima K, Asano K, Iwanaga K, Koie H, Uechi M, Kato Y, et al. Evaluation of left ventricular Tei index (index of myocardial performance) in healthy dogs and dogs with mitral regurgitation. The Journal of Veterinary Medical Science. 2007;**69**:117-123. DOI: 10.1292/jvms.69.117

[72] Borgarelli M, Abbott J, Braz-Ruivo L, Chiavegato D, Crosara S, Lamb K, et al. Prevalence and prognostic importance of pulmonary hypertension in dogs with myxomatous mitral valve disease. Journal of Veterinary Internal Medicine. 2015;**29**:569-574. DOI: 10.1111/jvim.12564

[73] Kellihan HB, Stepien RL. Pulmonary hypertension in canine degenerative mitral valve disease. Journal of Veterinary Cardiology. 2012;**14**:149-164. DOI: 10.1016/j.jvc.2012.01.001

[74] Kellum HB, Stepien RL. Sildenafil citrate therapy in 22 dogs with pulmonary hypertension. Journal of Veterinary Internal Medicine. 2007;**21**:1258-1264. DOI: 10.1892/07-006.1

[75] Morita T, Nakamura K, Osuga T, Morishita K, Sasaki N, Ohta H, et al. Right ventricular function and dyssynchrony measured by echocardiography in dogs with precapillary pulmonary hypertension. Journal of Veterinary Cardiology. 2019;**23**:1-14. DOI: 10.1016/j.jvc.2018.12.005

[76] Serrano-Parreño B, Carretón E, Caro-Vadillo A, Falcón-Cordón S, Falcón-Cordón Y, Montoya-Alonso JA. Pulmonary hypertension in dogs with heartworm before and after the adulticide protocol recommended by the American Heartworm Society. Veterinary Parasitology. 2017;**236**:34-37. DOI: 10.1016/j.vetpar.2017.02.001

[77] Visser LC, Im MK, Johnson LR, Stern JA. Diagnostic value of right pulmonary artery distensibility index in dogs with pulmonary hypertension: Comparison with Doppler echocardiographic estimates of pulmonary arterial pressure. Journal of Veterinary Internal Medicine. 2016;**30**:543-552. DOI: 10.1111/jvim.13911

[78] Johnson L, Boon J, Orton EC. Clinical characteristics of 53 dogs with Doppler-derived evidence of pulmonary hypertension. Journal of Veterinary Internal Medicine. 1999;**13**:440-447. DOI: 10.1892/0891-6640(1999)013<0440:ccodwd>2.3.co;2

[79] Pyle RL, Abbott J, MacLean H. Pulmonary hypertension and cardiovascular sequelae in 54 dogs. The International Journal of Applied Research in Veterinary Medicine. 2004;**2**:99-109

[80] Venco L, Mihaylova L, Boon JA. Right Pulmonary Artery Distensibility Index (RPAD Index). A field study of an echocardiographic method to detect early development of pulmonary hypertension and its severity even in the absence of regurgitant jets for Doppler evaluation in heartworm-infected dogs. Veterinary Parasitology. 2014;**206**:60-66. DOI: 10.1016/j.vetpar.2014.08.016

[81] Lindqvist P, Henein M, Kazzam E. Right ventricular outflow-tract fractional shortening: An applicable measure of right ventricular systolic function. European Journal of Echocardiography. 2003;**4**:29-35. DOI: 10.1053/euje.2002.0177

[82] Caivano D, Dickson D, Pariaut R, Stillman M, Rishniw M. Tricuspid annular plane systolic excursion-to-aortic ratio provides a bodyweight-independent measure of right ventricular systolic function in dogs. Journal of Veterinary Cardiology. 2018;**20**:79-91. DOI: 10.1016/j.jvc.2018.01.005

[83] Visser LC. Right ventricular function: Imaging techniques. The Veterinary Clinics of North America. Small Animal Practice. 2017;**47**:989-1003. DOI: 10.1016/j.cvsm.2017.04.004

[84] Pariaut R, Saelinger C, Strickland KN, Beaufrère H, Reynolds CA, Vila J. Tricuspid annular plane systolic excursion (TAPSE) in dogs: Reference values and impact of pulmonary hypertension. Journal of Veterinary Internal Medicine. 2012;**26**:1148-1154. DOI: 10.1111/j.1939-1676.2012.00981.x

[85] Poser H, Berlanda M, Monacolli M, Contiero B, Coltro A,

Guglielmini C. Tricuspid annular plane systolic excursion in dogs with myxomatous mitral valve disease with and without pulmonary hypertension. Journal of Veterinary Cardiology. 2017;**19**:228-239. DOI: 10.1016/j.jvc.2017.03.007

[86] Schober KE, Baade H. Doppler echocardiographic prediction of pulmonary hypertension in West Highland white terriers with chronic pulmonary disease. Journal of Veterinary Internal Medicine. 2006;**20**:912-920. DOI: 10.1892/0891-6640(2006)20[912:depop h]2.0.co;2

[87] Vonk MC, Sander MH, van den Hoogen FH, van Riel PL, Verheugt FW, van Dijk AP. Right ventricle Tei-index: A tool to increase the accuracy of non-invasive detection of pulmonary arterial hypertension in connective tissue diseases. European Journal of Echocardiography. 2007;**8**:317-321. DOI: 10.1016/j.euje.2006.06.002

[88] Paradies P, Spagnolo PP, Amato ME, Pulpito D, Sasanelli M. Doppler echocardiographic evidence of pulmonary hypertension in dogs: A retrospective clinical investigation. Veterinary Research Communications. 2014;**38**:63-71. DOI: 10.1007/s11259-013-9588-4

[89] Nakamura K, Morita T, Osuga T, Morishita K, Sasaki N, Ohta H, et al. Prognostic value of right ventricular tei index in dogs with myxomatous mitral valvular heart disease. Journal of Veterinary Internal Medicine. 2016;**30**:69-75. DOI: 10.1111/jvim.13820

[90] Ju S-E. Valuation of Doppler echocardiographic variables indicating pulmonary hypertension in dogs with chronic mitral valvular insufficiency [thesis]. Chuncheon: Kangwon National University; 2017

[91] Chetboul V, Sampedrano CC, Gouni V, Nicolle AP, Pouchelon JL, Tissier R. Ultrasonographic assessment of regional radial and longitudinal systolic function in healthy awake dogs. Journal of Veterinary Internal Medicine. 2006;**20**:885-893. DOI: 10.1892/0891-6640(2006)20[885:uaorr a]2.0.co;2

[92] Takano H, Fujii Y, Ishikawa R, Aoki T, Wakao Y. Comparison of left ventricular contraction profiles among small, medium, and large dogs by use of two-dimensional speckle-tracking echocardiography. American Journal of Veterinary Research. 2010;**71**:421-427. DOI: 10.2460/ajvr.71.4.421

[93] Chetboul V, Damoiseaux C, Lefebvre HP, Concordet D, Desquilbet L, Gouni V, et al. Quantitative assessment of systolic and diastolic right ventricular function by echocardiography and speckle-tracking imaging: A prospective study in 104 dogs. Journal of Veterinary Science. 2018;**19**:683-692. DOI: 10.4142/jvs.2018.19.5.683

[94] Griffiths LG, Fransioli JR, Chigerwe M. Echocardiographic assessment of interventricular and intraventricular mechanical synchrony in normal dogs. Journal of Veterinary Cardiology. 2011;**13**:115-126. DOI: 10.1016/j.jvc.2011.02.001

[95] Smith DN, Bonagura JD, Culwell NM, Schober KE. Left ventricular function quantified by myocardial strain imaging in small-breed dogs with chronic mitral regurgitation. Journal of Veterinary Cardiology. 2012;**14**:231-242. DOI: 10.1016/j.jvc.2011.11.002

[96] Zois NE, Tidholm A, Nägga KM, Moesgaard SG, Rasmussen CE, Falk T, et al. Radial and longitudinal strain and strain rate assessed by speckle-tracking echocardiography in dogs with myxomatous mitral valve disease. Journal of Veterinary Internal Medicine. 2012;**26**:1309-1319. DOI: 10.1111/j.1939-1676.2012.01017.x

[97] Zois NE, Olsen NT, Moesgaard SG, Rasmussen CE, Falk T, Häggström J, et al. Left ventricular twist and circumferential strain in dogs with myxomatous mitral valve disease. Journal of Veterinary Internal Medicine. 2013;**27**:875-883. DOI: 10.1111/jvim.12114

[98] Mantovani MM, Muzzi RA, Pereira GG, Yamato RJ, Silva AC, Reis GF, et al. Systolic cardiac function assessment by feature tracking echocardiography in dogs with myxomatous mitral valve disease. The Journal of Small Animal Practice. 2015;**56**:383-392. DOI: 10.1111/jsap.12347

[99] Petrini J, Eriksson MJ, Caidahl K, Larsson M. Circumferential strain by velocity vector imaging and speckle-tracking echocardiography: Validation against sonomicrometry in an aortic phantom. Clinical Physiology and Functional Imaging. 2018;**38**:269-277. DOI: 10.1111/cpf.12410

[100] To AC, Flamm SD, Marwick TH, Klein AL. Clinical utility of multimodality LA imaging. Assessment of size, function, and structure. JACC: Cardiovascular Imaging. 2011;**4**:788-798. DOI: 10.1016/j.jcmg.2011.02.018

[101] Vizzardi E, D'Aloia A, Rocco E, Lupi L, Rovetta R, Quinzani F, et al. How should we measure left atrial size and function? Journal of Clinical Ultrasound. 2012;**40**:155-166. DOI: 10.1002/jcu.21871

[102] Rosca M, Lancellotti P, Popescu BA, Piérard LA. Left atrial function: Pathophysiology, echocardiographic assessment, and clinical applications. Heart. 2011;**97**:1982-1989. DOI: 10.1136/heartjnl-2011-300069

[103] Baron Toaldo M, Guglielmini C, Diana A, Sarcinella F, Cipone M. Feasibility and reproducibility of echocardiographic assessment of regional left atrial deformation and synchrony by tissue Doppler ultrasonographic imaging in healthy dogs. American Journal of Veterinary Research. 2014;**75**:59-66. DOI: 10.2460/ajvr.75.1.59

[104] Cameli M, Lisi M, Righini FM, Mondillo S. Novel echocardiographic techniques to assess left atrial size, anatomy and function. Cardiovascular Ultrasound. 2012;**10**:4. DOI: 10.1186/1476-7120-10-4

[105] Vieira MJ, Teixeira R, Gonçalves L, Gersh BJ. Left atrial mechanics: Echocardiographic assessment and clinical implications. Journal of the American Society of Echocardiography. 2014;**27**:463-478. DOI: 10.1016/j.echo.2014.01.021

[106] Di Salvo G, Caso P, Lo Piccolo R, Fusco A, Martiniello AR, Russo MG, et al. Atrial myocardial deformation properties predict maintenance of sinus rhythm after external cardioversion of recent-onset lone atrial fibrillation. Circulation. 2005;**112**:387-395. DOI: 10.1161/CIRCULATIONAHA.104.463125

[107] Cameli M, Lisi M, Giacomin E, Caputo M, Navarri R, Malandrino A, et al. Chronic mitral regurgitation: Left atrial deformation analysis by two-dimensional speckle tracking echocardiography. Echocardiography. 2011;**28**:327-334. DOI: 10.1111/j.1540-8175.2010.01329.x

[108] Caivano D, Rishniw M, Birettoni F, Patata V, Giorgi ME, Porciello F. Left atrial deformation and phasic function determined by two-dimensional speckle-tracking echocardiography in dogs with myxomatous mitral valve disease. Journal of Veterinary Cardiology. 2018;**20**:102-114. DOI: 10.1016/j.jvc.2018.01.002

[109] Baron Toaldo M, Romito G, Guglielmini C, Diana A, Pelle NG, Contiero B, et al. Assessment of left atrial deformation and function by 2-dimensional speckle tracking echocardiography in healthy dogs and dogs with myxomatous mitral valve disease. Journal of Veterinary Internal Medicine. 2017;**31**:641-649. DOI: 10.1111/jvim.14722

[110] Burgess MI, Bright-Thomas RJ, Ray SG. Echocardiographic evaluation of right ventricular function. European Journal of Echocardiography. 2002;**3**:252-262

[111] Portnoy SG, Rudski LG. Echocardiographic evaluation of the right ventricle: A 2014 perspective. Current Cardiology Reports. 2015;**17**:21. DOI: 10.1007/s11886-015-0578-8

Chapter 4

Cardio-Oncology: The Role of Echocardiography in Cancer Patients

Theodoros Ntoskas

Abstract

Cardio-oncology is a rapidly emerging medical field that focusses on the improvement of the quality of life of cancer patients by preventing and treating the adverse cardiovascular complications of cancer therapy. Early recognition of cancer therapy-related cardiac dysfunction (CTRCD) provides an opportunity to mitigate cardiac injury and risk of developing late cardiac events. Cardiac imaging, and in particular, transthoracic echocardiography, plays an essential role in the baseline assessment, the detection and the surveillance of CRTCD in patients during and after the cancer therapy. Although the frequency of screening for the cardiotoxicity in patients undergoing active treatments and cancer survivors remains a topic of debate and ongoing research, echocardiography continues to be the leader for continuous monitoring by imaging due to the wide availability, lack of exposure to radiation, ability to recognise the effects on cardiac function and assess haemodynamics and other cardiac structures. The cardiac imaging applied to cardio-oncology includes standard and advanced (speckle tracking and three-dimensional (3D)) echocardiography.

Keywords: cardio-oncology, echocardiography, cancer, cardiotoxicity, heart failure, global longitudinal strain

1. Introduction

Advances in treatment have led to improved survival of patients with cancer but have also increased morbidity and mortality due to treatment side effects [1, 2]. Chemotherapy and radiation therapy can put patients at risk for a variety of cardiovascular complications including heart failure, coronary artery disease, peripheral vascular disease, thromboembolism, pericardial disease and valvular heart disease. Cardiovascular disease is now the second leading cause of morbidity and mortality in cancer survivors [3]. Cancer patients receiving therapy with known cardiac risk require close monitoring during and after treatment. In current cardio-oncology practice, echocardiography is the most widely used technique in the diagnosis, prevention and risk stratification of CTRCD in patients during and after cancer therapy. The utility of the advanced echocardiography is emerging as the three-dimensional echocardiography derived left ventricular ejection fraction (LVEF) has an excellent correlation with cardiac magnetic resonance imaging and can be used to monitor LVEF and the two-dimensional speckle tracking echocardiography

(2D-STE) derived strain and strain rate can detect changes in myocardial mechanics before changes in LVEF occur.

2. Cardiovascular complications of cancer therapy

Cancer treatment can cause various types of cardiovascular (CV) complications. Different cancer therapies have different CV complications. Cancer therapy toxicity is related to the mechanism of action of the drugs, the doses, the manner of administration and the underlying predisposing factors such as cardiac conditions, genetic pattern and age, and it can manifest itself immediately or many years after the treatment. **Table 1** summarises a variety of anti-cancer therapies and their associated complications, including myocardial dysfunction, heart failure, coronary artery disease, valvular heart disease, arrhythmias, hypertension, peripheral vascular disease, stroke and pulmonary hypertension [4].

Echocardiography is a non-invasive method that can perform a comprehensive evaluation in all stages of cancer treatment and detect myocardial, coronary, valve, pulmonary hypertension and pericardial disease complications secondary to the therapeutic regimen used (radiotherapy and/or chemotherapy).

Cardiovascular toxicity	Anti-cancer therapy
Myocardial dysfunction and heart failure	Anthracyclines (doxorubicin, idarubicin and epirubicin), anti-HER2 (trastuzumab), VEGF inhibitors, cyclophosphamide, cisplatin, ifosfamide and taxanes (paclitaxel and docetaxel)
Vasospasm or vasoocclusion resulting in angina or myocardial infarction	Fluoropyrimidines (5-FU, capecitabine and gemcitabine), platinum compounds (cisplatin), VEGF inhibitors (bevacizumab, sorafenib and sunitinib) and radiotherapy
Valvular disease	Radiotherapy
Arrhythmias	Anthracyclines, histone deacetylase inhibitors, tyrosine kinase inhibitors (TKIs) (especially vandetanib high incidence of QT prolongation)
Arterial hypertension	VEGF inhibitors
Peripheral vascular disease and stroke	Nilotinib, ponatinib or BCR-ABL tyrosine kinase inhibitors, radiotherapy. L-asparaginase, cisplatin, methotrexate, 5-FU and paclitaxel can cause Raynaud's phenomenon
Pulmonary hypertension	TKI (dasatinib), the TKI imatinib improved haemodynamics in patients with advanced pulmonary arterial hypertension

Abbreviations: HER2, human epidermal growth factor receptor 2; VEGF, vascular endothelial growth factor.

Table 1.
Cancer drug agents associated with cardiovascular toxicity.

3. Definition of CTRCD

Myocardial dysfunction and heart failure are the most concerning cardiovascular complications of cancer therapies and cause an increase in morbidity and mortality. Different definitions of CTRCD have been used historically [5]. Guidelines from cardiac societies [4, 6] define cardiotoxicity when the left ventricular (LV) ejection fraction (EF) falls to a value below the lower limit of normal (e.g. 53% in American Society of Echocardiography [ASE] guidelines) with more than a 10-percentage point reduction. As per the ESMO guidelines, the cut-off is 50% [7], at which

	Type I	**Type II**
Anti-cancer characteristic chemotherapy agents	Doxorubicin	Trastuzumab
Clinical manifestation	New onset of heart failure and LV systolic dysfunction	Asymptomatic decrease in LVEF and less often clinical heart failure
Dose effects	Cumulative, dose dependent	Not dose related
Clinical course	May stabilise with heart failure therapy (ACE inhibitors and beta-blockers), but underlying myocyte destruction appears to be permanent and irreversible	Often reversible with treatment discontinuation (to or near baseline cardiac status in 2–4 months)
Effect of rechallenge	High probability of recurrent dysfunction that is progressive	Rechallenge is often tolerated after recovery

Abbreviation: ACE, angiotensin-converting enzyme; LV, left ventricle; EF, ejection fraction.

Table 2.
Characteristics of type I and II cancer therapeutics-related cardiac dysfunction.

point cardio-protection should be considered [8]. ASE/European Association of Cardiovascular Imaging (EACVI) further classifies CRTCD into either those associated with anthracyclines or trastuzumab use. Anthracycline-related CRTCD is cumulative, dose dependent and often progressive and irreversible at cell level. On the other hand, trastuzumab-related CRTCD is dose independent, does not lead to cell death and is often reversible (**Table 2**).

4. Cancer therapy-related cardiac dysfunction (CTRCD) and echocardiography

4.1 LV systolic function

The need for a timely diagnosis of subclinical and clinical heart failure by using cardiac imaging has been addressed by the Expert Consensus of the ASE and EACVI [6] and more recently reinforced by the ESC Position Paper on cancer treatments and cardiovascular toxicity [4]. The quickest and most available imaging tool in detecting cancer therapy-related cardiac dysfunction (CTRCD) is transthoracic echocardiography.

Exposure to potentially cardiotoxic chemotherapeutic agents is a well-recognised indication for baseline and longitudinal evaluation of LV function [9, 10]. The most commonly used parameter for monitoring LV function with echocardiography is LVEF. Traditionally, an echo determination of LVEF is requested by the oncologists in all cancer patients at baseline and in any situation in which the suspicion of heart failure is plausible, during and after completion of the anti-cancer therapy. 2D-derived LVEF is also used to start cardio protection and to establish the interruption from anti-cancer therapies. The calculation of LVEF should be done with the best method available as per the skills and experience of the operators in a given echocardiography department. The same method needs to be maintained for surveillance during and after treatment. Importantly, the digital images obtained should be available for visually comparison with the previous studies and further discussion at multimodality echocardiographic and cardio-oncology team meetings. According to joint recommendations from the ASE/EACVI, the method of choice for LV volume quantification and LVEF calculation is the modified biplane

Simpson's technique by 2D echocardiography, with an LVEF of ≥55% as a normal reference range. Calculation of LVEF should be also combined with assessment of the wall motion score index, which is based on a 16-segment model of the left ventricle [11]. Resting wall motion score index based on a 16-segment model of the left ventricle has been demonstrated to be a more sensitive marker of anthracycline-induced CTRCD than relying on the LVEF alone [12]. When two contiguous LV segments are not well visualised on non-contrast apical images, the use of myocardial contrast agents is recommended [13].

Although LVEF is a commonly accepted measure of cardiac systolic function and an accepted indicator of prognosis in patients with heart failure [14], it has low sensitivity for the detection of small changes in LV function. LVEF measurement using the 2D biplane technique has a temporal coefficient of variation of 7.4% [15], which is important to highlight because the measurement variability is close to the definition of CRTCD (drop in LVEF of 10% or more). This variability is the result of a number of factors including the operator's skills and the geometric assumptions used to estimate three-dimensional (3D) volumes from 2D images. 3D echocardiography has been shown to be more accurate than the 2D echocardiography in the measurement of the LV volumes [16]. However, the feasibility of the 3D technique can be reduced in some cancer patients because of the negative influence of factors such as concomitant radiotherapy (breast cancer and lymphoma) and surgery (mastectomies of left breast cancer, breast expanders or implants), which makes the ultrasound windows under these circumstances suboptimal [17]. The ASE recommends 3D echocardiography as the preferred technique for monitoring LV function and detecting CRTCD. However, it is important to realise that this technology has several limitations as well. It is recommended that calculation of LVEF by 2D biplane Simpson's method also be included in all the oncologic patients echocardiographic report to allow comparison with previous studies if this method was used.

To minimise the risk of irreversible cardiomyopathy, the goal is to identify signs of toxicity as early as possible. Echocardiography-based deformation imaging techniques (strain) have become an essential tool to detect CRTCD. Changes in strain are more sensitive, appear prior to LVEF reduction and before the CRTCD manifests as symptomatic heart failure. Global longitudinal strain (GLS) is of particular interest because it can be incorporated into a clinical echocardiographic examination relatively efficiently with currently available technology [18]. The EACVI and ASE recommend assessing GLS as a routine component of clinical echocardiograms in patients at risk for type 1 or type 2 cardiotoxicity [6]. A relative percentage decrease in GLS > 15% is indicative of subclinical LV dysfunction and could be utilised as the starting point for timely cardio protection therapy.

4.2 LV diastolic function

A comprehensive assessment of LV diastolic function, including grading of diastolic function and providing an estimate of LV filling pressure (by using the E/e′ ratio), should be performed in addition to the assessment of LV systolic function [19]. Although abnormal diastolic function parameters may reflect subclinical LV dysfunction, it has not been found to be prognostic of cardiotoxicity, and its clinical significance remains uncertain.

4.3 Right ventricular (RV) function

The frequency of the RV dysfunction during cancer therapy-related cardiotoxicity has not been accurately examined. As early studies of CRTCD included

RV biopsies, there is a suggestion that the RV is affected by cancer therapies [20]. However, the prognostic value of RV dysfunction at the time of cardiotoxicity warrants further investigation.

5. Coronary artery disease (CAD)

The diagnostic capability of rest echocardiography in CAD is limited to the assessment of the presence and magnitude of regional wall motion abnormalities.

Stress echocardiography, an established technique for the detection and prognostication of stable CAD as recommended by guidelines, may be useful in the evaluation of patients who are undergoing regimens that may be associated with ischemia, as fluoropyrimidines, platinum compounds (cisplatin), vascular endothelial growth factor inhibitors and radiotherapy.

Stress echocardiography is also being used to unmask subclinical abnormalities of the LV function induced by chemotherapeutic agents. Although both exercise [12] and dobutamine stress echocardiography [21–23] have been applied to patients with cancer for the identification of anthracycline-induced CTRCD, the results of these studies appear to be inconclusive and contradictory. Further studies are needed to better understand the prognostic role of stress echocardiography, before can be routinely used into clinical practice.

6. Valvular disease

Patients who have received radiation therapy are at risk of long-term cardiovascular toxicity including radiation-induced heart valve disease, pericardial disease and coronary artery disease.

Transthoracic echocardiography is the main tool to identify valvular damage in these patients. There are distinct echocardiographic characteristics of radiotherapy-induced valvular disease. The main distinguishing features between radiotherapy-induced valvular heart disease and rheumatic heart disease are the presence of commissural fusion after radiotherapy, while the involvement of the mitral leaflet tips is an indication of rheumatic disease.

The EACVI and ASE expert consensus statement recommendations for long-term follow-up after radiation therapy suggest a yearly physical examination to assess for symptoms or signs of radiation-induced heart disease, which if present should prompt further evaluation. In asymptomatic patients, a transthoracic echocardiogram is recommended 5 years after exposure in high-risk individuals and 10 years after exposure in all others [24]. High risk individuals are defined the patients who received anterior or left-side chest irradiation and have at least one additional risk factor (smoking, diabetes mellitus, hypertension, hyperlipidemia and obesity).

7. Pericardial disease

Pericardial disease in cancer patients is relatively common. Pericardial effusion, cardiac tamponade and pericarditis can appear during several types of chemotherapy (anthracyclines [25], cyclophosphamide [26] and cytarabine [27]) but are especially due to radiotherapy. Constrictive pericarditis is more often associated with radiation-induced cardiotoxicity [28]. Additionally, pericardial disease may be secondary to cardiac metastasis.

Echocardiography is the first-line cardiac imaging for the diagnosis of cancer therapy-related pericarditis. It is useful for evaluating the degree of pericardial thickening, the presence of constrictive physiology and the presence and quantification of a pericardial effusion, as guidance of pericardiocentesis and for patient follow-up.

8. Conclusions

CV complications of cancer and its treatment have become increasingly recognised as an important clinical issue, with the potential to cause acute complications during therapy. The field of cardio-oncology is relatively new but developing rapidly. The goal of this emerging subspecialty is to continue anti-cancer therapy without interruption, aiming at cancer cure and remission, or alternatively support the oncologist's choice between different anti-cancer therapies, in order to maintain survival free from cardiovascular morbidity and mortality. In this context, standard and advanced echocardiography plays a pivotal role as the first-line imaging tool.

Acknowledgements

I would like to thank Dr. Charles Spencer, Dr. Paul Woodmansey, Dr. Sandeep Hothi and Dr. Elisa McAlindon, consultant cardiologists, Mrs. Farhanda Ahmad, consultant echocardiographer and Dr. Nataliya Martynyuk, consultant oncologist for their help to set up the cardio-oncology services in the New Cross Hospital, Wolverhampton, UK. I would also like to thank Jo-Anne Connolly, Gemma Priest and Veena Bhatti, senior echocardiographers and Sue Wycherley, medical secretary for their enthusiasm, hardworking and excellent cooperation in running the cardio-oncology clinic.

Conflict of interest

The author declares that he has no conflict of interest.

Author details

Theodoros Ntoskas
Department of Cardiology, Heart and Lung Centre, New Cross Hospital, Wolverhampton, United Kingdom

*Address all correspondence to: theodoros.ntoskas@nhs.net

References

[1] Siegel R, DeSantis C, Virgo K, Stein K, Mariotto A, Smith T, et al. Cancer treatment and survivorship statistics, 2012. CA: A Cancer Journal for Clinicians. 2012;**62**(4):220-241. DOI: 10.3322/caac.21149

[2] Ferlay J, Steliarova-Foucher E, Lortet-Tieulent J, Rosso S, Coebergh JWW, Comber H, et al. Cancer incidence and mortality patterns in Europe: Estimates for 40 countries in 2012. European Journal of Cancer. 2013;**49**(6):1374-1403. Available from: https://www.clinicalkey.es/playcontent/1-s2.0-S0959804913000075

[3] Reulen RC, Winter DL, Frobisher C, Lancashire ER, Stiller CA, Jenney ME, et al. Long-term cause-specific mortality among survivors of childhood. Cancer. 2010;**304**(2):172-179. DOI: 10.1001/jama.2010.923

[4] Zamorano JL, Lancellotti P, Rodriguez Muñoz D, Aboyans V, Asteggiano R, Galderisi M, et al. 2016 ESC Position Paper on cancer treatments and cardiovascular toxicity developed under the auspices of the ESC Committee for Practice Guidelines: The Task Force for cancer treatments and cardiovascular toxicity of the European Society of Cardiology (ESC). European Heart Journal. 2017;**19**(1):9-42. Available from: https://www.ncbi.nlm.nih.gov/pubmed/27565769

[5] Khouri MG, Douglas PS, Mackey JR, Martin M, Scott JM, Scherrer-Crosbie M, et al. Cancer therapy-induced cardiac toxicity in early breast cancer: Addressing the unresolved issues. Circulation. 2012;**126**(23):2749-2763 Available from: https://www.ncbi.nlm.nih.gov/pubmed/23212997

[6] Plana JC, Galderisi M, Barac A, Ewer MS, Ky B, Scherrer-Crosbie M, et al. Expert consensus for multimodality imaging evaluation of adult patients during and after cancer therapy: A report from the American Society of Echocardiography and the European Association of Cardiovascular Imaging. European Heart Journal. 2014;**27**(9):911-939. Available from: https://www.clinicalkey.es/playcontent/1-s2.0-S0894731714005343

[7] Curigliano G, Cardinale D, Suter T, Plataniotis G, De Azambuja E, Sandri MT, et al. Cardiovascular toxicity induced by chemotherapy, targeted agents and radiotherapy: ESMO Clinical Practice Guidelines. Annals of Oncology. 2012. Available from: https://boris.unibe.ch/115250/

[8] Chang H-M, Moudgil R, Scarabelli T, Okwuosa TM, Yeh ETH. Cardiovascular complications of cancer therapy: Best practices in diagnosis, prevention, and management: Part 1. Journal of the American College of Cardiology. 2017;**70**(20):2536-2551. Available from: https://www.ncbi.nlm.nih.gov/pubmed/29145954

[9] Cheitlin MD, Armstrong WF, Aurigemma GP, Beller GA, Bierman FZ, Davis JL, et al. ACC/AHA/ASE 2003 guideline update for the clinical application of echocardiography: Summary article: A report of the American college of cardiology/American heart association task force on practice guidelines (ACC/AHA/ASE committee to update the 1997 guidelines for the clinical application of Echocardiography). Circulation. 2003;**42**(5):954-970. DOI: 10.1016/S0735-1097(03)01065-9

[10] Douglas PS, Garcia MJ, Haines DE, Lai WW, Manning WJ, Patel AR, et al. ACCF/ASE/AHA/ASNC/HFSA/HRS/SCAI/SCCM/SCCT/SCMR 2011 Appropriate Use Criteria for Echocardiography: A Report of the American College of Cardiology

Foundation Appropriate Use Criteria Task Force, American Society of Echocardiography, American Heart Association, American Society of Nuclear Cardiology, Heart Failure Society of America, Heart Rhythm Society, Society for Cardiovascular Angiography and Interventions, Society of Critical Care Medicine, Society of Cardiovascular Computed Tomography, and Society for Cardiovascular Magnetic Resonance Endorsed by the American College of Chest Physicians. Journal of the American Society of Echocardiography. 2011;**57**(9):1126-1166. Available from: https://search.proquest.com/docview/1811901848

[11] Lang RM, Bierig M, Devereux RB, Flachskampf FA, Foster E, Pellikka PA, et al. Recommendations for chamber quantification: A report from the American Society of Echocardiography's guidelines and standards committee and the chamber quantification writing group, developed in conjunction with the European Association of Echocardiography, a branch of the European Society of Cardiology. Journal of the American Society of Echocardiography. 2005;**18**(12):1440. Available from: https://www.ncbi.nlm.nih.gov/pubmed/16376782

[12] Bountioukos M, Doorduijn JK, Roelandt JRTC, Vourvouri EC, Bax JJ, Schinkel AFL, et al. Repetitive dobutamine stress echocardiography for the prediction of anthracycline cardiotoxicity. European Heart Journal. 2003;**4**(4):300-305. Available from: https://www.ncbi.nlm.nih.gov/pubmed/14611826

[13] Mulvagh SL, Rakowski H, Vannan MA, Abdelmoneim SS, Becher H, Bierig S et al. American Society of Echocardiography consensus statement on the clinical applications of ultrasonic contrast agents in echocardiography. Journal of the American Society of Echocardiography. 2008;**21**(11):1179-1201. Available at: https://www.clinicalkey.es/playcontent/1-s2.0-S0894731708005695

[14] Curtis JP, Sokol SI, Wang Y, Rathore SS, Ko DT, Jadbabaie F, et al. The association of left ventricular ejection fraction, mortality, and cause of death in stable outpatients with heart failure. Journal of the American College of Cardiology. 2003;**42**(4):736-742. DOI: 10.1016/S0735-1097(03)00789-7

[15] Thavendiranathan P, Grant AD, Negishi T, Plana JC, Popović ZB, Marwick TH. Reproducibility of echocardiographic techniques for sequential assessment of left ventricular ejection fraction and volumes: Application to patients undergoing cancer chemotherapy. Journal of the American College of Cardiology. 2013;**61**(1):77-84. Available from: https://www.ncbi.nlm.nih.gov/pubmed/23199515

[16] Jacobs LD, Salgo IS, Goonewardena S, Weinert L, Coon P, Bardo D, et al. Rapid online quantification of left ventricular volume from real-time three-dimensional echocardiographic data. European Heart Journal. 2006;**27**(4):460-468. Available from: https://www.ncbi.nlm.nih.gov/pubmed/16319085

[17] Santoro C, Arpino G, Esposito R, Lembo M, Paciolla I, Cardalesi C, et al. 2D and 3D strain for detection of subclinical anthracycline cardiotoxicity in breast cancer patients: A balance with feasibility. European Heart Journal. 2017;**18**(8):930-936. Available from: https://www.ncbi.nlm.nih.gov/pubmed/28379383

[18] Farsalinos KE, Daraban AM, Ünlü S, Thomas JD, Badano LP, Voigt J-U. Head-to-head comparison of global longitudinal strain measurements among nine different vendors: The EACVI/ASE inter-vendor comparison study. Journal of the American Society of Echocardiography.

2015;**28**(10):1171-1181. Available from: https://www.ncbi.nlm.nih.gov/pubmed/26209911

[19] Nagueh SF, Smiseth OA, Appleton CP, Byrd BF, Dokainish H, Edvardsen T. et al, Recommendations for the evaluation of left ventricular diastolic function by echocardiography: An update from the American Society of Echocardiography and the European Association of Cardiovascular Imaging. Journal of the American Society of Echocardiography. 2016;**29**(4):277-314. Available from: https://www.clinicalkey.es/playcontent/1-s2.0-S0894731716000444

[20] Mason JW, Bristow MR, Billingham ME, Daniels JR. Invasive and non invasive methods of assessing adriamycin cardiotoxic effects in man: Superiority of histiopathologic assessment using endomyocardial biopsy. Cancer Treatment Reports. 1978;**62**:857-886

[21] Jarfelt M, Kujacic V, Holmgren D, Bjarnason R, Lannering B. Exercise echocardiography reveals subclinical cardiac dysfunction in young adult survivors of childhood acute lymphoblastic. Leukemia. 2007;**49**(6):835-840. DOI: 10.1002/pbc.21289

[22] Cottin Y, L'huillier I, Casasnovas O, Geoffroy C, Caillot D, Zeller M, et al. Dobutamine stress echocardiography identifies anthracycline cardiotoxicity. European Journal of Echocardiography. 2000;**1**(3):180-183. Available from: https://www.ncbi.nlm.nih

[23] Hamada H, Ohkubo T, Maeda M, Ogawa S. Evaluation of cardiac reserved function by high-dose dobutamine-stress echocardiography in asymptomatic anthracycline-treated survivors of childhood. Cancer. 2006;**48**(3):313-320. DOI: 10.1111/j.1442-200X.2006.02210.x

[24] Lancellotti P, Nkomo VT, Badano LP, Bergler-Klein J, Bogaert J, Davin L, et al. Expert consensus for multi-modality imaging evaluation of cardiovascular complications of radiotherapy in adults: A report from the European Association of Cardiovascular Imaging and the American Society of Echocardiography. Journal of the American Society of Echocardiography. 2013;**14**(12):1217

[25] Casey DJ, Kim AY, Olszewski AJ. Progressive pericardial effusion during chemotherapy for advanced Hodgkin lymphoma. American Journal of Hematology. 2012;**87**(5):521-524. DOI: 10.1002/ajh.22239

[26] Yamamoto R, Kanda Y, Matsuyama T, Oshima K, Nannya Y, Suguro M, et al. Myopericarditis caused by cyclophosphamide used to mobilize peripheral blood stem cells in a myeloma patient with renal failure. Bone Marrow Transplantation. 2000;**26**(6):685-688. Available from: https://www.ncbi.nlm.nih.gov/pubmed/11041571

[27] Gähler A, Hitz F, Hess U, Cerny T. Acute pericarditis and pleural effusion complicating cytarabine chemotherapy. Onkologie. 2003;**26**(4):348-350. Available from: https://www.karger.com/Article/Abstract/72094

[28] Kane GC, Edie RN, Mannion JD. Delayed appearance of effusive-constrictive pericarditis after radiation for Hodgkin lymphoma. Annals of Internal Medicine. 1996;**124**(5):534. Available from: https://www.ncbi.nlm.nih.gov/pubmed/8602719

Chapter 5

Tropheryma whipplei Endocarditis

Lara García-Álvarez and José Antonio Oteo

Abstract

Tropheryma whipplei mainly known as the causative agent of classical Whipple's disease, also produces acute, sub-acute and chronic localized forms of infection such as endocarditis. The development of molecular tools has allowed increasing the number of cases of endocarditis due to blood culture use to be negative in *T. whipplei* endocarditis and most of the cases are confirmed post-surgery when molecular analyses of heart valves are performed. Although, *T. whipplei* endocarditis is an uncommon condition with an atypical presentation it must be considered in the diagnosis of blood culture negative endocarditis and in patients with heart failure in which valve affectation is present. Other clinical features such as long lasting arthralgia can be present in a high percentage of the patients. It is important to know that few cases are diagnosed in the context of the classical Whipple's disease. The prognosis is very good when an appropriate surgical management and antimicrobial-specific treatment is given. This chapter describes the epidemiological, clinical characteristics, diagnosis and treatments for *T. whipplei* endocarditis.

Keywords: *Tropheryma whipplei*, *Tropheryma whipplei* endocarditis, endocarditis, blood culture negative endocarditis, infectious endocarditis

1. Introduction

Tropheryma whipplei, formerly *Tropheryma whipplei, i*s an intracellular gram-positive Actinobacteria ubiquitous in the environment that is involved in a large variety of clinical forms [1, 2]. The initial name was proposed by Relman *et al.* in 1992, and comes from the Greek *trophe,* nourishment, and *eryma*, barrier, due to the malabsorption it causes, and from the surname of George Hoyt Whipple [3]. In 2001, the name of the bacterium was slightly modified to conform to the proper spelling of Dr. George H. Whipple's name [4].

Dr. Whipple was the first who reported, in 1907, a "hitherto undescribed disease" he named "intestinal lipodystrophy" in a 36-year-old man with malabsorption, weight loss, diarrhea, migratory polyarthritis, cough and mesenteric lymphadenopathy [5]. Now, we refer to this disease as Whipple's disease. Although this disease was first described at the beginning of the last century, the hypothesis of its bacterial origin goes back to the late 40's and was supported with use of periodic acid-Schiff (PAS) staining and the success of the first antibiotic treatment [6, 7]. Subsequently, the presence of the microorganism was confirmed by electron microscopy (rod-shaped organism), polymerase chain reaction (PCR) of the 16S rRNA and finally by culture [1, 3, 8–12]. The isolation and later sequencing of its genome made possible to define its antibiotic susceptibility [13–16].

Until recently, *T. whipplei* was known to be only the causative agent of Whipple's disease, now called by some authors "classical Whipple disease", a rare chronic multisystemic infection [5]. Incidence of Whipple's disease was reported in approximately 1 per 1.000.000, although it remains unclear and epidemiological estimates varies among different studies [17–19]. Classical form of Whipple's disease usually involves the gastrointestinal tract, joints and central nervous system with malabsorption, diarrhea, abdominal pain and/or weight loss and arthralgia as prominent manifestations. Cardiac, ocular or other organs involvement has been also reported in patients with Whipple's disease [20–29]. The knowledge of the genome of *T. whipplei* has allowed developing specific and sensible tools that have let to involve this microorganism in a broad spectrum of clinical conditions [13, 14]. Therefore, *T. whipplei* can produce acute localized forms of infection such as pneumonia [30, 31], bacteremia [32], acute diarrhea [33, 34], uveitis [35, 36]; sub-acute forms such as adenitis [37] and chronic forms as uveitis [38], and, overall, endocarditis [39, 40].

T. whipplei has also been detected in asymptomatic carriers based, mainly, on stools and saliva analysis with very different prevalence among populations [41–52]. The carriage of *T. whipplei* varies considerably across studies and subjects. Many factors are involved in those differences such as the geographical region, exposure or the age of the studied subjects. The prevalence of asymptomatic carriers of *T. whipplei* in Africa and Asia is higher than in Europe and it is also higher in children than in adults [49–51, 53]. Actinobacteria are environmental microorganisms that can be found in freshwater, soil or seawater sediments, this fact could explain the high prevalence of *T. whipplei* in people expose to sewage and sewage plant workers [2, 41, 47, 54, 55]. People in contact with patients with Whipple's disease, as patients' relatives or carriers, or those with poor hygiene conditions such as homeless, also presents higher prevalences [56–59]. Differences between the targets used for the PCR and the samples used have been also observed and could explain these reported differences [52, 60]. Li *et al.* assessed that genomic variants of *T. whipplei* are associated with neither the organotropism of the bacteria nor the geographical residence of the individuals [61], however later studies show that different genotypes are more frequent in some populations [34, 56, 58, 62]. Therefore, despite Whipple's disease is rare, the high number of healthy carriers, the ubiquitous presence of the bacteria in the environment [41, 47, 57, 59] and the possibility of interhuman transmission [49, 56–59, 63, 64] make *T. whipplei* a common bacterium in humans.

2. Epidemiology

First implication of *T. whipplei* as causative agent of infective endocarditis was reported in Switzerland in 1997, in a patient with blood culture negative endocarditis (BCNE) using a broad-range PCR followed by sequencing [64]. Curiously, first stable cultivation of the bacterium of Whipple's disease was carried out in 2000, from the mitral valve of a patient with BCNE [1]. Since then, the number of cases has increased and to date *T. whipplei* endocarditis is one of the more frequent causes of BCNE in some areas [65, 66].

BCNE is a relative frequent condition among endocarditis representing 5–30% in big series [67–70]. The main reasons are the previous administration of antimicrobials and fastidiously culture microorganisms [67, 68, 71–75]. The application of molecular tools has allowed doing new approximations to the etiology of BCNE and new agents have been involved [69].

Sporadic cases of *T. whipplei* endocarditis have been reported from different countries, but there are few published series of *T. whipplei* endocarditis. France, Spain, Germany and Switzerland have the largest number of diagnosed cases

[39, 64, 65, 70]. This fact could be due to their larger experience in the knowledge and use of the molecular tools to heart valves [40]. The incidence of *T. whipplei* endocarditis among BCNE varies depending on the series. The incidence rate estimated varies between 2.6% and 7.1% depending on the country (France: 2.6% [76], Spain and Denmark: 3.5% [70, 77], Switzerland: 4.3% [78], Germany: 6.3% [65], Czech Republic: 7.1% [79]). However, it is difficult to know the true incidence of *T. whipplei* endocarditis since its study by molecular tools is not the rule in all hospitals. Thus, several parameters seem to affect the incidence of *T. whipplei* endocarditis such as the diagnostic tools available, the working group experience and the true incidence itself [39].

A total of 174 cases of *T. whipplei* endocarditis have been reported between 1999 and 2020 [21, 39, 65, 70, 78–117]. The vast majority of cases were men (>85% of the cases) and the average age was around 57 years (range: 33–81 years).

3. Clinical features

Comorbidities or other predisposing risk factors have been not uniformly reported in the literature [118]. Previous valvular affectation has been documented in 21% of the diagnosed cases, while prosthetic valve replacement previously to the event seems not an important condition (<5% of the available series). Alcohol abuse has been reported in very few cases, however alcohol intake (>60 g/d) was referred by the 23.5% of the patients in the Spanish series [70]. Previous cardiac condition or a cardiac event (i.e., coronary heart disease) has been observed in 50% of cases [66]. Data of historical immunosuppression forms (autoimmune disease or immunosuppressive therapies such as steroids or tumor necrosis factor inhibitors) have been reported in 21 cases (12%).

Classical Whipple's disease has been reported as concomitant with the diagnose of endocarditis in few cases (6%) [66, 70]. However, in lot of cases this data is not available and in some of them although, classical Whipple's Disease has not been diagnosed, it cannot be excluded.

The signs and symptoms *T. whipplei* endocarditis are not the typical ones. Fever has been only reported in 21% of the cases. Cardiac failure and arthralgia have been shown as the main presenting symptoms and have been described in 43% and 52% of patients, respectively. Cardiac failure is of special interest because it is the first manifestation in a high percentage of patients. Long lasting arthralgias presence as a prominent symptom varies depending on the series. While in the French series arthralgias were present in 75% of patients [39], in the Spanish one this condition was present in 53% [70]. These variations could be due to this symptom is sometimes weak and only detected after an exhaustive clinical research. Some authors suggest that, in those patients with sub-acute endocarditis and low-grade fever or not fever, if arthralgias are present, *T. whipplei* as causative agent should be suspected [39, 103]. Asthenia and malaise lasting more than six months were notified by the 41.2% of the patients in one series [70]. Other signs such as weight loss or gastrointestinal symptoms have been observed in 25% and 21% of the reported patients [118]. In addition, central nervous system manifestations (i.e., emboli) have been detected in 16% of patients.

The valve involved in patients with *T. whipplei* endocarditis has been predominantly the aortic (63%). Involvement of multiple valves (mainly aortic valve in combination with the mitral or tricuspid valve, and mitral-tricuspid affection) has been noticed in 23% of patients. Only mitral valve affectation has been observed in 20% of patients and tricuspid valve just in six of 174 patients (3%). Native valve was affected in the vast majority of cases.

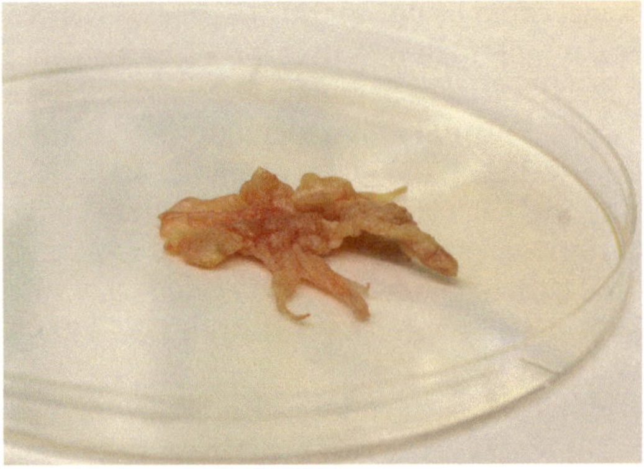

Figure 1.
Valve vegetation specimen obtained after surgery from a patient with T whipplei endocarditis.

		% (No.)
Patients (No.)	174	
Epidemiological data		
Medium Age (years)	57	
Male gender		85% (148)
Medical history		
Immunosuppression		12% (21)
Valvular abnormality		21.8% (38)
Affected valve		
Aortic		63% (110)
Mitral		20.7% (36)
Tricuspid		3.4% (6)
Multiple valves		22.9% (40)
Presenting symptoms		
Arthralgia		51.7% (90)
Heart failure		43% (75)
Weight loss		25.2% (44)
Fever		21.3% (37)
Central nervous system		16.1% (28)
Gastrointestinal symptoms		20,7% (36)
Laboratory abnormalities		
Anemia		39,1% (68)
Outcome		
Valve surgery		73.5% (128)
Death		17.8% (31)

Table 1.
Main clinical epidemiological, clinical and outcome characteristics of patients with T. whipplei *endocarditis reported in the literature. Updated from McGee et al. [118].*

Echocardiography features are one of the most valuable tools for suspecting infectious endocarditis. According to the literature, when these data were recorded, presence of vegetations was observed in more than the half of patients [66]. In our series, echocardiography was performed in all patients (both transthoracic and transesophageal in more than 80%) and allowed the diagnosis of infectious endocarditis in 70% of patients through the visualization of vegetations in the vast majority, or by indirect signs in a few [70]. Valve vegetation from a patient after cardiac valve surgery is shown in **Figure 1**. In the French series, echocardiography showed vegetations in 78% of the patients, but these data are not recorded in the German one [39, 65]. Data of vegetation appearance or size is rarely reported. Data of size vegetations when available, shown a minimum size of 5 mm and a maximum of 33 mm [118].

The main laboratory recording abnormalities at the time of the diagnosis have been anemia, which was detected in 40% of patients but this date can reach 88.2% in some series, and increasing of C-reactive protein in range from 2.3 to 137 mg/L [70]. In patients who had heart failure, B-type natriuretic peptide (BNPs) of up to 2536 ng/L has been also reported [118].

Main characteristics of patients are shown in **Table 1**.

4. Diagnosis

The suspicion and diagnosis of *T. whipplei* endocarditis is complicated. To date, 174 cases have been reported but, due to the difficulties for the identification of *T. whipplei*, the prevalence of the endocarditis it causes could be underestimated [119].

Diagnosis of *T. whipplei* endocarditis remains a challenge for several reasons. One of them is because this endocarditis does not exhibit the typical sings (no fever nor peripheral stigmata and low inflammatory response) and blood cultures used to be negative; therefore, modified Duke's criteria are ineffective for diagnosis before heart valve analysis [39]. In this sense, some series have shown that only 3.6% patients met criteria for endocarditis according to the modified Duke criteria and 60.7% met for possible endocarditis [39]. It is very difficult to perform a microbiological or histological diagnose without analyzing the surgical remove valve. Routine blood and tissue culture are not often useful for the diagnosis. Thus, the diagnosis is often made post-surgery and valve analysis requires specialized laboratories, moreover if culture of the bacteria is intended to carry out.

Different targets have been used for molecular analyses. PCR based on the 16S rRNA amplification and subsequent sequencing has been widely used and has been the first-line screening in our series. However, some authors alert that this broad-spectrum PCR could have a limited sensitivity (value sensitivity 60%, specificity 100%) [120], while specific qPCR for *T. whipplei* have showed higher sensitivities [48, 60]. So, if 16S rRNA PCR has been negative, specific targets should be used in highly suspected cases of *T. whipplei*. At least 2 of the PCRs must be positive and their sequences have to show higher identity with the bacterium studied. PCR yield in other specimen different from valves varies depending on the specimen type and should be interpreted with caution according to the clinical context [66, 118]. A positive PCR result from a non-sterile site such as stool or saliva samples has been used to diagnose classical Whipple's disease and to detect asymptomatic carriers, but is nor sensible nor specific for the diagnosis of *T. whipplei* endocarditis without clinical evidence of disease [42, 121, 122].

The role of serological tests in the diagnosis of Whipple's disease is unclear because healthy carrier patients may paradoxically have a higher immune response

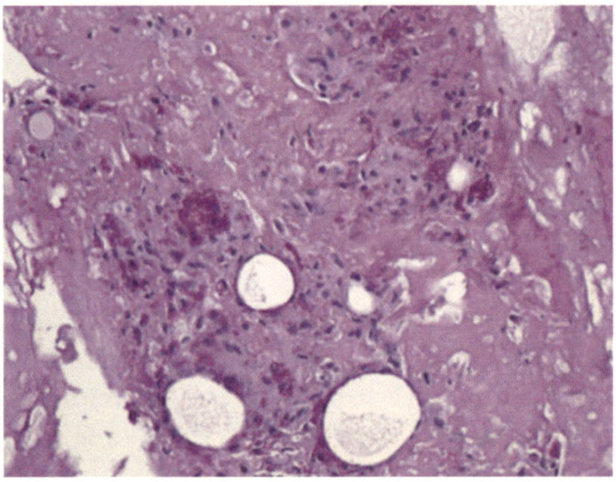

Figure 2.
PAS staining positive in valvular tissue and vegetation.

to *T. whipplei* compared with patients with active Whipple's disease [123]. Specific tools for an indirect diagnose for *T. whipplei* endocarditis are not available. This fact does not occur in other BCNE such as Q fever endocarditis or *Bartonella* spp. endocarditis. Curiously, a patient with Q fever and *T. whipplei* concomitant endocarditis has been described [124]. Valvular inflammatory infiltrates of *T. whipplei*–infected heart valves mainly consisted of foamy macrophages and lymphocytes. These macrophages have been observed in valvular tissue and in the vegetations on the surface of the heart valves. The dense and granular material that foamy histiocytes are filled with is strongly positive on PAS staining or immunopositive with a specific antibody against *T. whipplei* [39]. Thus, PAS staining and specific immunohistochemistry test (IHC) using specific antibodies against *T. whipplei* of cardiac valves could be useful for the diagnosis of *T. whipplei* endocarditis (**Figure 2**).

According to the literature, 156 patients have been diagnosed of definite *T. whipplei* endocarditis by direct examination of the valve, of which more than 70% had positive PCR, almost 40% reported PAS staining positive on valve tissue and around 50% showed positive IHC. Seven patients were diagnosed of possible endocarditis regarding to vegetations on valve imaging and classical Whipple's disease concomitant diagnosis. In these last cases, 85% had positive PCR on different specimen such as duodenal sample, stool, saliva or central nervous system samples and more than 50% had positive PAS staining in other tissue specimen [118].

In summary, definitive *T. whipplei* endocarditis could considered if positive results of PAS staining and/or specific IHC test using specific antibodies against *T. whipplei* and/or 2 positive results of PCR assays targeting 2 different sequences in a cardiac valve specimen are met [60]. It is important to notice that in patients with subacute endocarditis with negative blood cultures and low-grade fever (or not fever), if arthralgias are present, *T. whipplei* as causative agent should be suspected [39, 103].

5. Treatment

The optimal treatment of IE caused by *T. whipplei* remains uncertain. Treatment options and duration are based on previous experience and expert opinion owing to the microorganism's nature, the lack of large series (because of the low incidence) in which follow-up is documented and because clinical trials have not been developed [74]. Recommendations are mainly based on the experience obtained from the treatment of classical Whipple's disease and other types of BCNE such as Q fever endocarditis [125, 126]. Two weeks treatment with ceftriaxone, followed by 1 year of trimethoprim/sulfamethoxazole, has been the most recommended treatment for years [126]. However, *in vitro* studies have shown best results with the combination of doxycycline and hydroxychloroquine [127, 128].

According to the literature, treatments used in *T. whipplei* endocarditis include, in most cases, two weeks of parenteral high dose of ceftriaxone (others such as meropenem, penicillin G have been also used) followed by an oral treatment strategy of 12 months with sulfamethoxazole (160/800 mg BID) or, at least, 18 months of doxycycline (100 mg BID) plus hydroxychloroquine (600 mg/d), in a smaller proportion [125, 129, 130]. Available data indicate that the average treatment length (range) has been 17 months (12 months to indefinite) [118].

Last European guidelines published in 2015, recommend doxycycline (200 mg/24 h) plus hydroxychloroquine (200–600 mg/24 h) orally for at least 18 months (in the case of central nervous system involvement, sulfadiazine 1.5 g/6 h orally must be added to doxycycline). As alternative therapy, 2–4 weeks of ceftriaxone (2 g/24 h intravenously) or 2–4 weeks of penicillin G (2 million U/4 h) and streptomycin (1 g/24 h) intravenously can be used, followed by, at least, 1 year of oral trimethoprim/sulfamethoxazole (800 mg/12 h) [74]. It is likely that this recommendation was included after taking into consideration an *in vitro T. whipplei* resistant to trimethoprim, a case report of a patient with clinically acquired resistance to trimethoprim/sulfamethoxazole and the cases of *T. whipplei* endocarditis relapses after treatment with trimethoprim/sulfamethoxazole which were apparently cured after two years of doxycycline and hidroxychloroquine [109, 114, 131, 132]. Furthermore, some authors do not recommend the use of trimethoprim/sulfamethoxazole because the clinical, microbiological and genetic data analyses show that it is an antibiotic not efficient for the management of *T. whipplei* endocarditis [109]. In fact, three *T. whipplei* endocarditis relapses after treatment with trimethoprim/sulfamethoxazole have been published.

After the end of treatment, some authors recommend checking for the presence of *T. whipplei* in blood, saliva, and fecal samples every six months for two years and every year for the entire life of the patient [39]. If colonization is detected, they recommend treating again, but there is not still evidence for this procedure.

Follow-up data and long-term outcome of the treatments used in this condition have not been widely reported. These data are well documented in the Spanish series. Although in this series only the 35% of the patients received treatment according to guidelines, all the treatment lines used in this cohort in the management of *T. whipplei* endocarditis were effective and well tolerated and therapeutic failures or relapses were not detected either during the treatment or after it was finished [133]. Furthermore, no major complications were detected once the treatment was established or during the follow-up. Even though, follow-up of all patients continues in order to identify possible late relapses. It has been demonstrated that doxycycline plus hydroxychloroquine treatment of duration shorter than 18 months was not associated with either relapses or fatal outcomes. Moreover, data suggest that, with a very careful post-treatment monitoring, in patients who require the replacement of the infected valve and without classical manifestation of Whipple's disease, replacement of the affected valve and a shorter duration antimicrobial treatment might be sufficient [133].

Since *T. whipplei* is not present in the stool or saliva of patients with endocarditis caused by this microorganism and in the absence of other biological markers indicating the discontinuation of the antimicrobials, other tools are needed. In this regard, the role of PCR of urine should be explored both as a tool for monitoring patients post-treatment and the non-invasive diagnosis of *T. whipplei* endocarditis [134].

6. Conclusions

In the last years and with the development of molecular tools, new cases of *T. whipplei* endocarditis have been diagnosed. For this reason, although *T. whipplei* infective endocarditis is an infrequent condition has emerged as an important differential diagnosis for BCNE. Endocarditis due to *T. whipplei* is often slowly progressive, similar to that caused by *Coxiella burnetii* and *Bartonella* spp. and it could be diagnosed with specific procedures when BCNE undergo cardiac surgery. An early and appropriate diagnosis is required since this condition has a very good course and prognosis when the appropriate treatment is started (including surgery). In our opinion, patients with unexplained valve destruction which requires cardiac surgery, an exhaustive clinical investigation must be performed and removed valves should be studied by molecular tools for to rule out an underlying infectious endocarditis.

Conflict of interest

The authors declare no conflict of interest.

Author details

Lara García-Álvarez and José Antonio Oteo*
San Pedro University Hospital - Center for Biomedical Research of La Rioja (CIBIR), Logroño, Spain

*Address all correspondence to: jaoteo@riojasalud.es

References

[1] Raoult D, Birg ML, La Scola B, Fournier PE, Enea M, Lepidi H,, et al. Cultivation of the bacillus of Whipple's disease. N Engl J Med. 2000;342:620-625.DOI: 10.1056/NEJM200003023420903.

[2] Dutly F, Altwegg M. Whipple's disease and "Tropheryma whippelii". Clinical Microbiology Reviews. 2001;**14**:561-583. DOI: 10.1128/CMR.14.3.561-583.2001

[3] Relman DA, Schmidt TM, MacDermott RP, Falkow S. Identification of the uncultured bacillus of Whipple's disease. The New England Journal of Medicine. 1992;**327**:293-301. DOI: 10.1056/NEJM199207303270501

[4] La Scola B, Fenollar F, Fournier PE, Altwegg M, Mallet MN, Raoult D. Description of Tropheryma whipplei gen. Nov., sp. nov., the Whipple's disease bacillus. International Journal of Systematic and Evolutionary Microbiology. 2001;**51**:1471-1479. DOI: 10.1099/00207713-51-4-1471

[5] Whipple GH. A hitherto undescribed disease characterized anatomically by deposits of fat and fatty acids in the intestinal and mesenteric lymphatic tissues. Bulletin of the Johns Hopkins Hospital. 1907;**18**:382-393

[6] Black-Schaffer B. The tinctoral demonstration of a glycoprotein in Whipple's disease. Proc Soc Exp Biol. 1949;**72**:225-227. DOI: 10.3181/00379727-72-17388

[7] Paulley JW. A case of Whipple's disease (intestinal lipodystrophy). Gastroenterology. 1952;**22**:128-133

[8] WJr C, Ashworth CT. Electron microscopy study of the intestinal mucosa in Whipple's disease-demonstration of encapsulated bacilliform bodies in the lesion. Gastroenterology. 1961;**41**:129-138

[9] Yardley JH, Hendrix TR. Combined electron and light microscopy in Whipple's disease. Bulletin of the Johns Hopkins Hospital. 1961;**109**:80-98

[10] Wilson KH, Blitchington R, Frothingham R, Wilson JA. Phylogeny of the Whipple's-disease-associated bacterium. Lancet. 1991;**338**:474-475. DOI: 10.1016/0140-6736(91)90545-z

[11] Cohen AS, Schimmel EM, Holt PR, Isselbacher KJ. Ultrastructural abnormalities in Whipple's disease. Proceedings of the Society for Experimental Biology and Medicine. 1960;**105**:411-414. DOI: 10.3181/00379727-105-26126

[12] Schoedon G, Goldenberger D, Forrer R, Gunz A, Dutly F, Höchli M, et al. Deactivation of macrophages with interleukin-4 is the key to the isolation of Tropheryma whippelii. The Journal of Infectious Diseases. 1997;**176**:672-677. DOI: 10.1086/514089

[13] Raoult D, Ogata H, Audic S, Robert C, Suhre K, Drancourt M. Tropheryma whipplei twist: A human pathogenic actinobacteria with a reduced genome. Genome Research. 2003;**13**:1800-1809. DOI: 10.1101/gr.1474603

[14] Bentley SD, Maiwald M, Murphy LD, Pallen MJ, Yeats CA, Dover LG, et al. Sequencing and analysis of the genome of the Whipple's disease bacterium Tropheryma whipplei. Lancet. 2003;**361**:637-644. DOI: 10.1016/S0140-6736(03)12597-4

[15] Boulos A, Rolain JM, Raoult D. Antibiotic susceptibility of Tropheryma whipplei in MRC5 cells. Antimicrobial Agents and Chemotherapy. 2004;**48**:747-752. DOI: 10.1128/aac.48.3.747-752.2004

[16] Boulos A, Rolain JM, Mallet MN, Raoult D. Molecular evaluation of

antibiotic susceptibility of Tropheryma whipplei in axenic medium. The Journal of Antimicrobial Chemotherapy. 2005;**55**:178-181. DOI: 10.1093/jac/dkh524

[17] Sieracki JC. Whipple's disease: Observations on systemic involvement. Cytologic observations. Amer Med Asso Arch Pathol. 1958;**66**:464-467

[18] von Herbay A, Otto HF, Stolte M, Borchard F, Kirchner T, Ditton HJ, et al. Epidemiology of Whipple's disease in Germany. Analysis of 110 patients diagnosed in 1965-95. Scandinavian Journal of Gastroenterology. 1997;**32**:52-57. DOI: 10.3109/00365529709025063

[19] Biagi F, Balduzzi D, Delvino P, Schiepatti A, Klersy C, Corazza GR. Prevalence of Whipple's disease in North-Western Italy. European Journal of Clinical Microbiology & Infectious Diseases. 2015;**34**:1347-1348. DOI: 10.1007/s10096-015-2357-2

[20] Durand DV, Lecomte C, Cathebras P, Rousset H, Godeau P. Whipple disease: Clinical review of 52 cases. The SNFMI research group on Whipple disease. Société Nationale Française de Médecine interne. Medicine (Baltimore). 1997;**76**:170-184. DOI: 10.1097/00005792-199705000-00003.

[21] Fenollar F, Lepidi H, Raoult D. Whipple's endocarditis: Review of the literature and comparisons with Q fever, Bartonella infection, and blood culture-positive endocarditis. Clinical Infectious Diseases. 2001;**33**:1309-1316. DOI: 10.1086/322666

[22] Enzinger FM, Helwig EB. Whipple's disease: A review of the literature and report fifteen patients. Virchows Archiv für Pathologische Anatomie und Physiologie und für Klinische Medizin. 1963;**336**:238-269

[23] Maizel H, Ruffin JM, Dobbins WO 3rd. Whipple's disease: A review of 19 patients from one hospital and a review of the literature since 1950. Medicine (Baltimore). 1993;**72**:343-355

[24] McAllister HAJ, Fenoglio JJJ. Cardiac involvement in Whipple's disease. Circulation. 1975;**52**:152-156. DOI: 10.1161/01.cir.52.1.152

[25] Hausser-Hauw C, Roullet E, Robert R, Marteau R. Oculo-facioskeletalmyorhythmia as a cerebral complication of systemic Whipple's disease. Movement Disorders. 1988;**3**:179-184. DOI: 10.1002/mds.870030211

[26] Adler CH, Galetta SL. Oculo-facial-skeletal myorhythmia in Whipple disease: Treatment with ceftriaxone. Annals of Internal Medicine. 1990;**112**:467-469. DOI: 10.7326/0003-4819-76-3-112-6-467

[27] Simpson DA, Wishnow R, Gargulinski RB, Pawlak AM. Oculofacial-skeletal myorhythmia in central nervous system Whipple's disease: Additional case and review of the literature. Movement Disorders. 1995;**10**:195-200. DOI: 10.1002/mds.870100210

[28] Rickman LS, Freeman WR, Green WR, Feldman ST, Sullivan J, Russack V, et al. Brief report: uveitis caused by Tropheryma whippeli (Whipple's bacillus). N Engl J Med. 1995;332:363-366. DOI: 10.1056/NEJM199502093320604.

[29] Helliwella TR, Appleton RE, Mapstone NC, Davidson J, Walsh KP. Dermatomyositis and Whipple's disease. Neuromuscular Disorders. 2000;**10**:46-51. DOI: 10.1016/s0960-8966(99)00054-1

[30] Stein A, Doutchi M, Fenollar F, Raoult D. Tropheryma whipplei pneumonia in a patient with HIV-2 infection. American Journal of Respiratory and Critical Care Medicine.

2013;**188**:1036-1037. DOI: 10.1164/rccm.201304-0692LE

[31] Bousbia S, Papazian L, Auffray JP, Fenollar F, Martin C, Li W, et al. Tropheryma whipplei in patients with pneumonia. Emerging Infectious Diseases. 2010;**16**:258-263. DOI: 10.3201/eid1602.090610

[32] Fenollar F, Mediannikov O, Socolovschi C, Bassene H, Diatta G, Richet H, et al. Tropheryma whipplei bacteremia during fever in rural West Africa. Clinical Infectious Diseases. 2010;**51**:515-521. DOI: 10.1086/655677

[33] Gautret P, Benkouiten S, Parola P, Brouqui P, Memish Z, Raoult D. Occurrence of Tropheryma whipplei during diarrhea in hajj pilgrims: A PCR analysis of paired rectal swabs. Travel Medicine and Infectious Disease. 2014;**12**:481-484. DOI: 10.1016/j.tmaid.2014.04.003

[34] Raoult D, Fenollar F, Rolain JM, Minodier P, Bosdure E, Li W, et al. Tropheryma whipplei in children with gastroenteritis. Emerging Infectious Diseases. 2010;**16**:776-782. DOI: 10.3201/eid1605.091801

[35] Nishimura JK. Cook BE Jr, Pach JM (1998). Whipple disease presenting as posterior uveítis without prominent gastrointestinal symptoms. American Journal of Ophthalmology. 1998;**126**:130-132. DOI: 10.1016/s0002-9394(98)00084-1

[36] Drancourt M, Fenollar F, Denis D, Raoult D. Postoperative panophthalmitis caused by Whipple disease. Emerging Infectious Diseases. 2009;**15**:825-827. DOI: 10.3201/eid1505.081209

[37] Al-Hamoudi W, Habbab F, Nudo C, Nahal A, Flegel K. Eosinophilic vasculitis: A rare presentation of Whipple's disease. Canadian Journal of Gastroenterology. 2007;**21**:189-191. DOI: 10.1155/2007/326174

[38] Thaler S, Grisanti S, Klingel K, Raible A, Kempf VA, Schulte B. Intermediate uveitis and arthralgia as early symptoms in Whipple's disease. International Journal of Infectious Diseases. 2010;**14**:388-389. DOI: 10.1016/j.ijid.2009.11.038

[39] Fenollar F, Célard M, Lagier JC, Lepidi H, Fournier PE, Raoult D. Tropheryma whipplei endocarditis. Emerging Infectious Diseases. 2013;**19**:1721-1730. DOI: 10.3201/eid1911.121356

[40] Moos V, Schneider T. Changing paradigms in Whipple's disease and infection with Tropheryma whipplei. Eur J Clin Microbiol Infect. 2011;**30**:1151-1158. DOI: 10.1007/s10096-011-1209-y

[41] Maiwald M, Schuhmacher F, Ditton HJ, von Herbay A. Environmental occurrence of the Whipple's disease bacterium (Tropheryma whipplei). Applied and Environmental Microbiology. 1998;**64**:760-762. DOI: 10.1128/AEM.64.2.760-762.1998.

[42] Street S, Donoghue HD, Neild GH. Tropheryma whippelii DNA in saliva of healthy people. Lancet. 1999;**354**:1178-1179. DOI: 10.1016/s0140-6736(99)03065-2

[43] Ehrbar HU, Bauerfeind P, Dutly F, Koelz HR, Altwegg M. PCR-positive tests for Tropheryma whippelii in patients without Whipple's disease. Lancet. 1999;**353**:2214. DOI: 10.1016/S0140-6736(99)01776-6

[44] Dutly F, Hinrikson HP, Seidel T, Morgenegg S, Altwegg M, Bauerfeind P. Tropheryma whippelii DNA in saliva of patients without Whipple's disease. Infection. 2000;**28**:219-222. DOI: 10.1007/s150100070039

[45] Maibach RC, Dutly F, Altwegg M. Detection of Tropheryma whipplei DNA in feces by PCR using a target capture method. Journal of Clinical Microbiology. 2002;**40**:2466-2471. DOI: 10.1128/jcm.40.7.2466-2471.2002

[46] Amsler L, Bauernfeind P, Nigg C, Maibach RC, Steffen R, Altwegg M. Prevalence of Tropheryma whipplei DNA in patients with various gastrointestinal disease and in healthy controls. Infection. 2003;**31**:81-85. DOI: 10.1007/s15010-002-3083-0

[47] Schoniger-Hekele M, Petermann D, Weber B, Muller C. Tropheryma whipplei in the environment—Survey of sewage plant influxes and sewage plant workers. Applied and Environmental Microbiology. 2007;**73**:2033-2035. DOI: 10.1128/AEM.02335-06

[48] Fenollar F, Trani M, Davoust B, Salle B, Birg ML, Rolain JM, et al. Prevalence of asymptomatic Tropheryma whipplei carriage among humans and nonhuman primates. The Journal of Infectious Diseases. 2008;**197**:880-887. DOI: 10.1086/528693

[49] Fenollar F, Trape JF, Bassene H, Sokhna C, Raoult D. Tropheryma whipplei in fecal samples from children, Senegal. Emerging Infectious Diseases. 2009;**15**:922-924. DOI: 10.3201/eid1506.090182

[50] Keita AK, Bassene H, Tall A, Sokhna C, Ratmanov P, Trape JF, et al. Tropheryma whipplei: A common bacterium in rural Senegal. PLoS Neglected Tropical Diseases. 2011;**5**:e1403. DOI: 10.1371/journal.pntd.0001403

[51] Ramharter M, Harrison N, Bühler T, Herold B, Lagler H, Lötsch F, et al. Prevalence and risk factor assessment of Tropheryma whipplei in a rural Community in Gabon: A community based cross-sectional study. Clinical Microbiology and Infection. 2014;**20**:1189-1194. DOI: 10.1111/1469-0691.12724

[52] García-Álvarez L, Pérez-Matute P, Blanco JR, Ibarra V, Oteo JA. High prevalence of asymptomatic carriers of Tropheryma whipplei in different populations from the north of Spain. Enfermedades Infecciosas y Microbiología Clínica. 2016;**34**:340-345. DOI: 10.1016/j.eimc.2015.09.006

[53] Keita AK, Dubot-Peres A, Phommasone K, Sibounheuang B, Vongsouvath M, Mayxay M, et al. High prevalence of Tropheryma whipplei in Lao kindergarten children. PLoS Neglected Tropical Diseases. 2015;**9**:e0003538. DOI: 10.1371/journal.pntd.0003538

[54] Marth T, Raoult D. Whipple's disease. Lancet. 2003;**361**:239-246. DOI: 10.1016/S0140-6736(03)12274-X

[55] Marth T, Moos V, Müller C, Biagi F, Schneider T. Tropheryma whipplei infection and Whipple's disease. The Lancet Infectious Diseases. 2016;**16**:e13-e22. DOI: 10.1016/S1473-3099(15)00537-X

[56] Fenollar F, Keita AK, Buffet S, Raoult D. Intrafamilial circulation of Tropheryma whipplei, France. Emerging Infectious Diseases. 2012;**18**:949-955. DOI: 10.3201/eid1806.111038

[57] Keita AK, Raoult D, Fenollar F. Tropheryma whipplei as a commensal bacterium. Future Microbiology. 2013;**8**:57-71. DOI: 10.2217/fmb.12.124

[58] Keita AK, Brouqui P, Badiaga S, Benkouiten S, Ratmanov P, Raoult D, et al. Tropheryma whipplei prevalence strongly suggests human transmission in homeless shelters. International Journal of Infectious Diseases. 2013;**17**:e67-e68. DOI: 10.1016/j.ijid.2012.05.1033

[59] Keita AK, Mediannikov O, Ratmanov P, Diatta G, Bassene H,

Roucher C, et al. Looking for Tropheryma whipplei source and reservoir in rural Senegal. Am J Trop Med Hyg. 2013;88:339-343. DOI: 10.4269/ajtmh.2012.12-0614.

[60] Fenollar F, Laouira S, Lepidi H, Rolain JM, Raoult D. Value of Tropheryma whipplei quantitative polymerase chain reaction assay for the diagnosis of Whipple disease: Usefulness of saliva and stool specimens for first-line screening. Clinical Infectious Diseases. 2008;**47**:659-667. DOI: 10.1086/590559

[61] Li W, Fenollar F, Rolain JM, Fournier PE, Feurle GE, Müller C, et al. Genotyping reveals a wide heterogeneity of Tropheryma whipplei. Microbiology. 2008;**154**:521-527. DOI: 10.1099/mic.0.2007/011668-0

[62] Wetzstein N, Fenollar F, Buffet S, Moos V, Schneider T, Raoult D. Tropheryma whipplei genotypes 1 and 3, in Central Europe. Emerging Infectious Diseases. 2013;**19**:341-342. DOI: 10.3201/eid1902.120709

[63] Fenollar F, Lagier JC, Raoult D. Tropheryma whipplei and Whipple's disease. The Journal of Infection. 2014;**69**:103-112. DOI: 10.1016/j.jinf.2014.05.008

[64] Goldenberger D, Künzli A, Vogt P, Zbinden R, Altwegg M. Molecular diagnosis of bacterial endocarditis by broad-range PCR amplification and direct sequencing. Journal of Clinical Microbiology. 1997;**35**:2733-2739. DOI: 10.1128/JCM.35.11.2733-2739.1997

[65] Geissdörfer W, Moos V, Moter A, Loddenkemper C, Jansen A, Tandler R, et al. High frequency of Tropheryma whipplei in culture-negative endocarditis. Journal of Clinical Microbiology. 2012;**50**:216-222. DOI: 10.1128/JCM.05531-11

[66] García-Álvarez L, Sanz M, Oteo JA. Tropheryma Whipplei endocarditis. An epidemiological, clinical and treatment review. Aperito J infect dis. Vaccine. 2015;**1**:103

[67] Murdoch DR, Corey GR, Hoen B, Miró JM, Fowler VG Jr, Bayer AS, et al. Clinical presentation, etiology, and outcome of infective endocarditis in the 21st century: The international collaboration on endocarditis-prospective cohort study. Archives of Internal Medicine. 2009;**169**:463-473. DOI: 10.1001/archinternmed.2008.603.

[68] Tattevin P, Watt G, Revest M, Arvieux C, Fournier PE. Update on blood culture-negative endocarditis. Médecine et Maladies Infectieuses. 2014;**45**:1-8. DOI: 10.1016/j.medmal.2014.11.003

[69] Muñoz P, Kestler M, De Alarcon A, Miro JM, Bermejo J, Rodríguez-Abella H, et al. Current epidemiology and outcome of infective endocarditis: A multicenter, prospective. Cohort study. Med (Baltimore). 2015;**94**:e1816. DOI: 10.1097/MD.0000000000001816

[70] García-Álvarez L, Sanz MM, Marín M, Fariñas M, Montejo M, Goikoetxea J, et al. Tropheryma whipplei endocarditis in Spain: Case reports of 17 prospective cases. Medicine (Baltimore). 2016;**95**(26):e4058. DOI: 10.1097/MD.0000000000004058

[71] Cecchi E, Forno D, Imazio M, Migliardi A, Gnavi R, Dal Conte I, et al. New trends in the epidemiological and clinical features of infective endocarditis: Results of a multicenter prospective study. Italian Heart Journal. 2004;**5**:249-256

[72] López-Dupla M, Hernández S, Olona M, Mercé J, Lorenzo A, Tapiol J, et al. Clinical characteristics and outcome of infective endocarditis in individuals of the general population managed at a teaching hospital without cardiac surgery facilities.

Study of 120 cases. Rev Esp Cardiol. 2006;**59**:1131-1139

[73] Baddour LM, Wilson WR, Bayer AS, Fowler VG Jr, Tleyjeh IM, Rybak MJ, et al. Infective endocarditis in adults: Diagnosis, antimicrobial therapy, and management of complications: A scientific statement for healthcare professionals from the American Heart Association. Circulation. 2015;**132**:1435-1486. DOI: 10.1161/CIR.0000000000000296

[74] Habib G, Lancellotti P, Antunes MJ, Bongiorni MG, Casalta JP, Del Zotti F, et al. 2015 ESC guidelines for the management of infective endocarditis: The task force for the Management of Infective Endocarditis of the European Society of Cardiology (ESC). Endorsed by: European Association for Cardio-Thoracic Surgery (EACTS), the European association of NuclearMedicine (EANM). European Heart Journal. 2015;**36**:3075-3128. DOI: 10.1093/eurheartj/ehv319

[75] Díez-Villanueva P, Muñoz P, Marín M, Bermejo J, de Alarcón González A, Fariñas MC, et al. Infective endocarditis: Absence of microbiological diagnosis is an independent predictor of inhospitalmortality. International Journal of Cardiology. 2016;**220**:162-165. DOI: 10.1016/j.ijcard.2016.06.129

[76] Fournier PE, Thuny F, Richet H, Lepidi H, Casalta JP, Arzouni JP, et al. Comprehensive diagnostic strategy for blood culture–negative endocarditis: A prospective study of 819 new cases. Clinical Infectious Diseases. 2010;**51**:131-140. DOI: 10.1086/653675

[77] Voldstedlund M, Norum PL, Baandrup U, Klaaborg KE, Fuursted K. Broad-range PCR and sequencing in routine diagnosis of infective endocarditis. APMIS. 2008;**116**:190-198. DOI: 10.1111/j.1600-0463.2008.00942.x

[78] Bosshard PP, Kronenberg A, Zbinden R, Ruef C, Bottger EC, Altwegg M. Etiologic diagnosis of infective endocarditis by broadrange polymerase chain reaction: A 3-year experience. Clinical Infectious Diseases. 2003;**37**:167-172. DOI: 10.1086/375592

[79] Grijalva M, Horvath R, Dendis M, Erny J, Benedik J. Molecular diagnosis of culture negative infective endocarditis: Clinical validation in a group of surgically treated patients. Heart. 2003;**89**:263-268. DOI: 10.1136/heart.89.3.263.

[80] Pron B, Poyart C, Abachin E, Fest T, Belanger C, Bonnet C, et al. Diagnosis and follow-up of Whipple's disease by amplification of the 16S rRNA gene of Tropheryma whippelii. European Journal of Clinical Microbiology & Infectious Diseases. 1999;**18**:62-65. DOI: 10.1007/s100960050228

[81] Wolfert AL, Wright JE. Whipple's disease presenting as sarcoidosis and valvular heart disease. Southern Medical Journal. 1999;**92**:820-825. DOI: 10.1097/00007611-199908000-00017

[82] Smith MA. Whipple endocarditis without gastrointestinal disease. Annals of Internal Medicine. 2000;**132**:595. DOI: 10.7326/0003-4819-132-7-200004040-00025

[83] Ferrari Mde L, Vilela EG, Faria LC, Couto CA, Salgado CJ, Leite VR, et al. Whipple's disease. Report of five cases with different clinical features. Revista do Instituto de Medicina Tropical de São Paulo. 2001;**43**:45-50. DOI: 10.1590/s0036-46652001000100009

[84] Charniot JC, Mouthon L, Martin A, Barthelemy B, Podeva JD, Artigou JY, et al. Valvular locations in Whipple's disease: Report of two cases and review of the literature. Archives des Maladies du Coeur et des Vaisseaux. 2001;**94**:1117-1121

[85] Geissdörfer W, Wittmann I, Seitz G, Cesnjevar R, Röllinghoff M, Schoerner C, et al. A case of aortic valve disease associated with Tropheryma whippelii infection in the absence of other signs of Whipple's disease. Infection. 2001;29:44-47. DOI: 10.1007/s15010-001-0135-9.

[86] Geissdörfer W, Wittmann I, Röllinghoff M, Schoerner C, Bogdan C. Detection of a new 16S-23S rRNA spacer sequence variant (type 7) of Tropheryma whippelii in a patient with prosthetic aortic valve endocarditis. European Journal of Clinical Microbiology & Infectious Diseases. 2001;**20**:762-763. DOI: 10.1007/s100960100588

[87] Richardson DC, Burrows LL, Korithoski B, Salit IE, Butany J, David TE, et al. Tropheryma whippelii as a cause of afebrile culture-negative endocarditis: The evolving spectrum of Whipple's disease. The Journal of Infection. 2003;**47**:170-173. DOI: 10.1016/s0163-4453(03)00015-x

[88] Dreier J, Szabados F, von Herbay A, Kröger T, Kleesiek K. Tropheryma whipplei infection of an acellular porcine heart valve bioprosthesis in a patient who did not have intestinal Whipple's disease. Journal of Clinical Microbiology. 2004;**42**:4487-4493. DOI: 10.1128/JCM.42.10.4487-4493.2004

[89] Marrakchi C, Abdennadher M, Blin D. Endocarditis caused by Tropheryma whippelii. La Tunisie Médicale. 2004;**82**:781-784

[90] Lepidi H, Fenollar F, Dumler JS, Gauduchon V, Chalabreysse L, Bammert A, et al. Cardiac valves in patients with Whipple endocarditis: Microbiological, molecular, quantitative histologic, and immunohistochemical studies of 5 patients. The Journal of Infectious Diseases. 2004;**190**:935-945. DOI: 10.1086/422845

[91] Aïouaz H, Célard M, Puget M, Vandenesch F, Mercusot A, Fenollar F, et al. Whipple's disease endocarditis: Report of 5 cases and review of the literature. La Revue de Médecine Interne. 2005;**26**:784-790. DOI: 10.1016/j.revmed.2005.07.012

[92] Saba M, Rollot F, Park S, et al. Whipple disease. initially diagnosed as sarcoidosis. Presse Med. 2005;**34**:1521-1524

[93] Marín M, Muñoz P, Sánchez M, et al. Grupo de Apoyo al Manejo de la endocarditis Infecciosa del Hospital Gregorio Marañón, Madrid, Spain. Tropheryma whipplei infective endocarditis as the only manifestation of Whipple's disease. Journal of Clinical Microbiology. 2007;**45**:2078-2081

[94] West D, Hutcheon S, Kain R, Reid T, Walton S, Buchan K. Whipple's endocarditis. Journal of the Royal Society of Medicine. 2005;**98**:362-364. DOI: 10.1258/jrsm.98.8.362

[95] Williams OM, Nightingale AK, Hartley J. Whipple's disease. N Engl J Med 2007;356:1479-1480;author reply 1480-1. DOI: 10.1056/NEJMc070234.

[96] Kolek M, Zaloudíková B, Freiberger T, Brát R. Aortic and mitral valve infective endocarditis caused by Tropheryma whipplei and with no gastrointestinal manifestations of Whipple's disease. Klinická Mikrobiologie a Infekční Lékařství. 2007;**13**:213-216

[97] Le Scanff J, Gaultier JB, Durand DV, Durieu I, Celard M, Benito Y, et al. Tropheryma whipplei and Whipple disease: False positive PCR detections of Tropheryma whipplei in diagnostic samples are rare. La Revue de Médecine Interne. 2008;**29**:861-867. DOI: 10.1016/j.revmed.2008.02.020

[98] Voldstedlund M, Pedersen LN, Baandrup U, Fuursted K. Whipple's

disease–a cause of culture-negative endocarditis. Ugeskrift for Laeger. 2004;**166**:3731-3732

[99] Besnard S, Cady A, Flecher E, Fily F, Revest M, Arvieux C, et al. Should we systematically perform central nervous system imaging in patients with Whipple's endocarditis? The American Journal of Medicine. 2010;**123**:962.e1-962.e4. DOI: 10.1016/j.amjmed.2010.04.030

[100] Lagier JC, Lepidi H, Raoult D, Fenollar F. Systemic Tropheryma whipplei: Clinical presentation of 142 patients with infections diagnosed or confirmed in a reference center. Medicine (Baltimore). 2010;**89**:337-345. DOI: 10.1097/MD.0b013e3181f204a8

[101] Ansemant T, Celard M, Tavernier C, Maillefert JF, Delahaye F, Ornetti P. Whipple's disease endocarditis following anti-TNF therapy for atypical rheumatoid arthritis. Joint, Bone, Spine. 2010;**77**:622-623. DOI: 10.1016/j.jbspin.2010.07.003

[102] Escher R, Roth S, Droz S, Egli K, Altwegg M, Täuber MG. Endocarditis due to Tropheryma whipplei: Rapid detection, limited genetic diversity, and long-term clinical outcome in a local experience. Clinical Microbiology and Infection. 2010;**16**:1213-1222. DOI: 10.1111/j.1469-0691.2009.03038.x

[103] Whistance RN, Elfarouki GW, Vohra HA. Livesey SA. A case of Tropheryma whipplei infective endocarditis of the aortic and mitral valves in association with psoriatic arthritis and lumbar discitis. The Journal of Heart Valve Disease. 2011;**20**:353-356

[104] Chan V, Wang B, Veinot JP, Suh KN, Rose G, Desjardins M, et al. Tropheryma whipplei aortic valve endocarditis without systemic Whipple's disease. International Journal of Infectious Diseases. 2011;**15**:e804-e806. DOI: 10.1016/j.ijid.2011.05.020

[105] Agard C, Brisseau JM, Grossi O, Pattier S, Espitia-Thibault A, Le Goff B, et al. Two cases of atypical Whipple's disease associated with cytoplasmic ANCA of undefined specificity. Scandinavian Journal of Rheumatology. 2012;**41**:246-248. DOI: 10.3109/03009742.2011.648656

[106] Algin A, Wegdam-Blans M, Verduin K, Janssen H, van Dantzig JM. Tropheryma whipplei aortic valve endocarditis, cured without surgical treatment. BMC Research Notes. 2012;**5**:600. DOI: 10.1186/1756-0500-5-600

[107] Love SM, Morrison L, Appleby C, Modi P. Tropheryma whipplei endocarditis without gastrointestinal involvement. Interactive Cardiovascular and Thoracic Surgery. 2012;**15**:161-163. DOI: 10.1093/icvts/ivs116

[108] Weisman A, Rebick G, Morris A, Butany J, Liles WC. Whipple's endocarditis: An enigmatic cause of culture-negative bacterial endocarditis. Can J Infect Dis Med Microbiol. 2013;**24**:e29-e30. DOI: 10.1155/2013/138746

[109] Fenollar F, Lagier JC, Rolain JM, Célard M, Bouchot O, Eicher JC, et al. Tropheryma whipplei endocarditis relapses after treatment with trimethoprim/sulfamethoxazole. International Journal of Antimicrobial Agents. 2013;**41**:592-594. DOI: 10.1016/j.ijantimicag.2013.02.003

[110] Herrmann MD, Neumayr A, Essig A, Spiess J, Merk J, Möller P, et al. Isolated Whipple's endocarditis: An underestimated diagnosis that requires molecular analysis of surgical material. The Annals of Thoracic Surgery. 2014;**98**:e1-e3. DOI: 10.1016/j.athoracsur.2014.04.059

[111] Loughran D, Beale L, Lodge F, et al. Whipple's in the valleys: A case of Whipple's with thrombocytopenia and endocarditis. Journal of Clinical Pathology. 2014;**67**:445-448

[112] Borne RT, Babu A, Levi M, et al. Tropheryma whipplei endocarditis: A two-patient case series. The American Journal of Medicine. 2015;**128**:1364-1366

[113] Alozie A, Zimpfer A, Köller K, Westphal B, Obliers A, Erbersdobler A, et al. Arthralgia and blood culture-negative endocarditis in middle age men suggest Tropheryma whipplei infection: Report of two cases and review of the literature. BMC Infectious Diseases. 2015;**15**:339. DOI: 10.1186/s12879-015-1078-6

[114] Emonet S, Wuillemin T, Harbarth S, Wassilew N, Cikirikcioglu M, Schrenzel J, et al. Relapse of Tropheryma whipplei endocarditis treated by trimethoprim/sulfamethoxazole, cured by hydroxychloroquine plus doxycycline. International Journal of Infectious Diseases. 2015;**30**:17-19. DOI: 10.1016/j.ijid.2014.11.003

[115] Jos SL, Angelakis E, Caus T, Raoult D. Positron emission tomography in the diagnosis of Whipple's endocarditis: A case report. BMC Research Notes. 2015;**8**:56. DOI: 10.1186/s13104-015-1022-2

[116] Damaraju D, Steiner T, Wade J, Gin K, FitzGerald JM. Clinical problem-solving. A surprising cause of chronic cough. The New England Journal of Medicine. 2015;**373**:561-566. DOI: 10.1056/NEJMcps1303787

[117] Gruber JR, Sarro R, Delaloye J, Surmely JF, Siniscalchi G, Tozzi P, et al. Tropheryma whipplei bivalvular endocarditis and polyarthralgia: A case report. Journal of Medical Case Reports. 2015;**9**:259. DOI: 10.1186/s13256-015-0746-x

[118] McGee M, Brienesse S, Chong B, Levendel A, Lai K. Tropheryma whipplei Endocarditis: Case Presentation and Review of the Literature. Open Forum Infect Dis 2018;6:ofy330. DOI: 10.1093/ofid/ofy330

[119] Houpikian P, Raoult D. Blood culture-negative endocarditis in a reference center: Etiologic diagnosis of 348 cases. Medicine (Baltimore). 2005;**84**:162-173. DOI: 10.1097/01.md.0000165658.82869.17

[120] Greub G, Lepidi H, Rovery C, Casalta JP, Habib G, Collard F, et al. Diagnosis of infectious endocarditis in patients undergoing valve surgery. Am J Med. 2005;118:230-238. DOIi: 10.1016/j.amjmed.2004.12.014.

[121] Grasman ME, Pettersson AM, Catsburg A, Koek AG, van Bodegraven AA, Savelkoul PHM. Tropheryma whipplei, a potential commensal detected in individuals undergoing routine colonoscopy. Journal of Clinical Microbiology. 2015;**53**:3919-3921. DOI: 10.1128/JCM.02630-15

[122] Rolain JM, Fenollar F, Raoult D. False positive PCR detection of Tropheryma whipplei in the saliva of healthy people. BMC Microbiology. 2007;**7**:48. DOI: 10.1186/1471-2180-7-48

[123] Fenollar F, Amphoux B, Raoult D. A paradoxical Tropheryma whipplei Western blot differentiates patients with whipple disease from asymptomatic carriers. Clinical Infectious Diseases. 2009;**49**:717-723. DOI: 10.1086/604717

[124] Santibáñez P, Portillo A, Santibáñez S, García-Álvarez L, de Toro M, Oteo JA. Qué aporta la secuenciación masiva del gen ARNr 16S

al estudio de endocarditis infecciosa en tejido valvular? In: Programme of the VIII Congreso de la Sociedad Española de Infecciones cardiovasculares (SEICAV); 16-17 November 2018; Seville, Spain. 2018. p. 30

[125] Schneider T, Moos V, Loddenkemper C, Marth T, Fenollar F, Raoult D. Whipple's disease: New aspects of pathogenesis and treatment. The Lancet Infectious Diseases. 2008;**8**:179-190. DOI: 10.1016/S1473-3099(08)70042-2

[126] Feurle GE, Moos V, Bläker H, Loddenkemper C, Moter A, Stroux A, et al. Intravenous ceftriaxone, followed by 12 or three months of oral treatment with trimethoprim-sulfamethoxazole in Whipple's disease. The Journal of Infection. 2013;**66**:263-270. DOI: 10.1016/j.jinf.2012.12.004

[127] Fenollar F, Puéchal X, Raoult D. Whipple's disease. The New England Journal of Medicine. 2007;**356**:55-66. DOI: 10.1056/NEJMra062477

[128] Lagier JC, Fenollar F, Lepidi H, Raoult D. Failure and relapse after treatment with trimethoprim/sulfamethoxazole in classic Whipple's disease. The Journal of Antimicrobial Chemotherapy. 2010;**65**:2005-2012. DOI: 10.1093/jac/dkq263

[129] Raoult D, Ogata H, Audic S, Robert C, Suhre K, Drancourt M, et al. Tropheryma whipplei twist: A human pathogenic actinobacteria with a reduced genome. Genome Research. 2003;**13**:1800-1809. DOI: 10.1101/gr.1474603

[130] Feurle GE, Junga NS, Marth T. Efficacy of ceftriaxone or meropenem as initial therapies in Whipple's disease. Gastroenterology. 2010;**138**:478-486. DOI: 10.1053/j.gastro.2009.10.041

[131] Fenollar F, Perreal C, Raoult D. Tropheryma whipplei natural resistance to trimethoprim and sulphonamides in vitro. International Journal of Antimicrobial Agents. 2014;**43**:388-390

[132] Fenollar F, Rolain JM, Alric L, Papo T, Chauveheid MP, van de Beek D, et al. Resistance to trimethoprim/sulfamethoxazole and Tropheryma whipplei. International Journal of Antimicrobial Agents. 2009;**34**:255-259. DOI: 10.1016/j.ijantimicag.2009.02.014

[133] García-Álvarez L, Sanz MM, Marín M, Fariñas MC, Montejo M, Goikoetxea J, et al. Antimicrobial management of Tropheryma whipplei endocarditis: the Spanish Collaboration on Endocarditis (GAMES) experience. The Journal of Antimicrobial Chemotherapy. 2019;**74**:1713-1717. DOI: 10.1093/jac/dkz059

[134] Lagier JC, Raoult D. Whipple's disease and Tropheryma whipplei infections: When to suspect them and how to diagnose and treat them. Current Opinion in Infectious Diseases. 2018;**31**:463-470. DOI: 10.1097/QCO.0000000000000489

Chapter 6

Fetal Echocardiogram Normal and Abnormal

Madhavi Latha Routhu and Gudikandula Krishna

Abstract

In this chapter, the normal anatomy of the heart as well as pathologic cases is consistent with cardiac malposition and isomerism, septal defects, pulmonary stenosis/atresia/absent pulmonary valve syndrome, aortic malformation, hypoplastic left heart, conotruncal anomalies/common arterial trunk, tricuspid dysplasia, Ebstein anomaly, univentricular heart, and systemic venous abnormalities among other congenital cardio vascular defects by ultrasound images. Anatomical details of most CHD in fetus were provided by two-dimensional (2D) ultrasound with higher quality imaging, which enhances the diagnostic accuracy in a variety of CHD.

Keywords: congenital heart disease, fetal echocardiogram, ultrasound

1. Introduction

The incidence of congenital heart disease (CHD) is 8–9 per 1000 live births [1]. Including all subtle cardiac anomalies, the overall CHD incidence may be of 50 per 1000 live births (like bicuspid aortic valve, atrial septal aneurysm and Persistent left SVC) [2]. There are several risk factors for CHD which includes fetal and maternal factors. The fetal risk factors are extra cardiac abnormalities which are frequently associated with CHD even in the presence of normal karyotype [3]. About 10–20% of nonimmune hydrops is associated with CHD [4, 5]. One percent of arrhythmias are associated with CHD. Maternal factors like Diabetes mellitus, Phenylketonuria, Maternal exposure to Anticonvulsants, ethanol, nonsteroidal anti-inflammatory drugs, ACE inhibitors, indomethacin, and use of lithium increase the risk of CHD. IVF pregnancies increase CHD rates by four folds. CHD or syndromes associated with CHD in first-degree relatives increase risk of CHD. Half of the CHD cases are minor abnormalities and are easily corrected by surgery; prenatal diagnosis allows for better counseling and improved the outcome.

Guidelines for fetal echocardiogram by International society of ultrasound in obstetrics and gynecology (ISUOG), American institute of ultrasound in medicine (AIUM) and association for European pediatric cardiology (AEPC) (**Figure 1**): presence of clear guidelines for defining cardiac screening and fetal echocardiography helps to standardize the approach for the sonographic evaluation of fetal echocardiography.

Fetal echocardiogram is most optimally performed between 18 and 22 weeks gestation. The screening examination includes the upper abdomen; the four-chamber (4ch) view and outflow tracts for obtaining these planes need a sweep from four chamber view and into the upper mediastinum. Initial sweep shows five chamber (5ch) view followed by right ventricular outflow tract (RVOT),

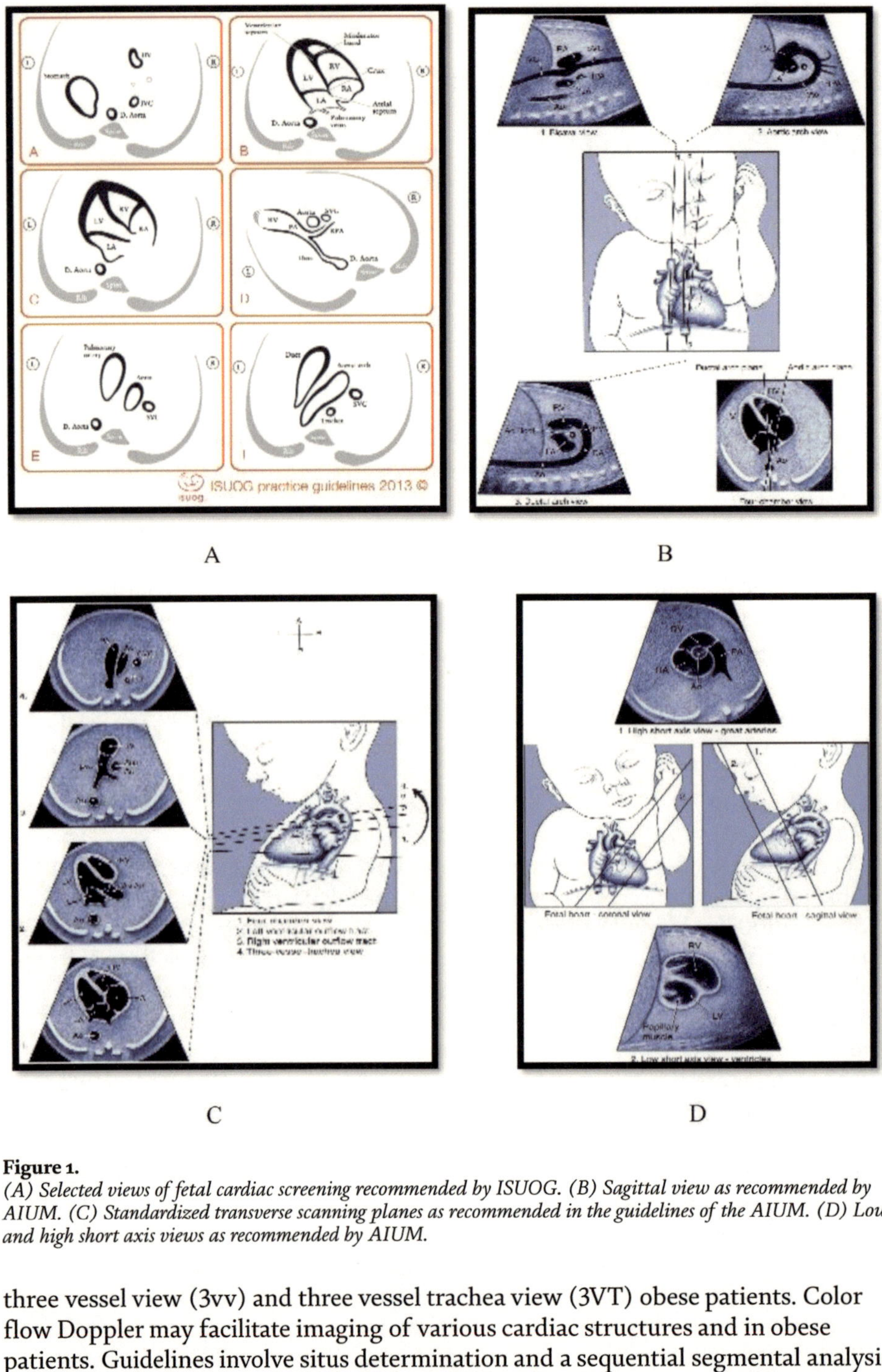

Figure 1.
(A) Selected views of fetal cardiac screening recommended by ISUOG. (B) Sagittal view as recommended by AIUM. (C) Standardized transverse scanning planes as recommended in the guidelines of the AIUM. (D) Low and high short axis views as recommended by AIUM.

three vessel view (3vv) and three vessel trachea view (3VT) obese patients. Color flow Doppler may facilitate imaging of various cardiac structures and in obese patients. Guidelines involve situs determination and a sequential segmental analysis of Atria, Ventricles and great arteries and their connections. Documentation fetal heart rhythm should be performed. Fetal echo should be performed by real time imaging with acquisition of recording or digital video clips and still images. It is important to note that screening for cardiac malformations in the low risk population includes minimum views of four chambers and outflow tracts. It is not specified to screen three vessel trachea view, but it is relatively easy plane to obtain and provides significant information on outflow tracts and arches.

2. Embryology of heart

In third week of post conception, the embryo consists of three basic germ layers–the Ectoderm, Mesoderm and Endoderm. The lateral splanchnic mesoderm involves in the formation of single heart tube. The major steps in development of embryonic heart are (1) primitive heart tube, (2) looping, (3) atria, ventricles and outflow tracts septations, (4) septation of the atria, (5) septation of ventricles, (6) septation of the outflow tracts.

During cardiac looping, the primitive ventricles move downward to the right while the primitive atrium moves upward and to the left behind the ventricle. In the folded cardiac tube various regions are recognized and are separated by transitional zones. These regions will develop into cardiac cavities and the zones will become the septa and valves. Systemic veins begin with the formation of three paired veins the vitelline, umbilical and common cardinal veins, but the pulmonary veins develop separately.

3. Genetic diseases related to cardiac anomalies

CHD and chromosomal deletion syndrome: (1) DiGeorge syndrome or 22q11microdeletion; (2) Williams-Beuren syndrome, 1p36 deletion syndrome.

CHD associated with single gene disorders: Noonan syndrome and RASopathies, Holt-Oram syndrome, Alagille syndrome, Tuberous sclerosis complex and CHARGE syndrome.

Familial recurrence of congenital heart defects: recurrence risk of 3% for two healthy nonconsanguineous parents with one affected child, risk of recurrence increases to 10% with two affected siblings.

3.1 Fetal situs

Assessment of fetal visceral situs is essential first step in fetal echocardiogram. Evaluating cardiac position and orientation in thoracic cavity and anatomical relationship of abdominal organs is the part of the fetal echocardiogram examination.

Steps for sequential segmental analysis in the fetus are identifying visceral situs, Atrial arrangement, Atrioventricular valves, ventricular arrangement, ventriculoarterial connection, Ventricular outflow tracts and systemic and pulmonary venous connections. First step is Fetal visceral situs (**Figure 2**) for this identify fetal presenting part (cephalic/breech) next step is to determine fetal lie by obtaining sagittal view of fetal spine and compare with the maternal spine after this determine the location of the fetal left side with the regard to maternal abdomen. Bronshtein et al. [6] described a method to determine situs is referred as the right-hand rule for abdominal scan and left-hand rule for transvaginal approach. Palm of the hand corresponds to the face of fetus and sonographer holds the hand according to the side of fetal face; left side of the fetus will be shown by the examiners thumb.

Types of visceral situs are situs solitus, situs inversus and situs ambiguous.

Situs solitus is normal viscerocardiac arrangement where the cardiac apex, stomach and descending Aorta should be located on the fetal left side. Inferior vena cava is located on the right side. Situs inversus is the mirror image arrangement of organs and vessels to situs solitus. Incidence is about 0.01%. There is slight increased risk of CHD and 20% association with Kartagener's syndrome which is autosomal recessive transmission.

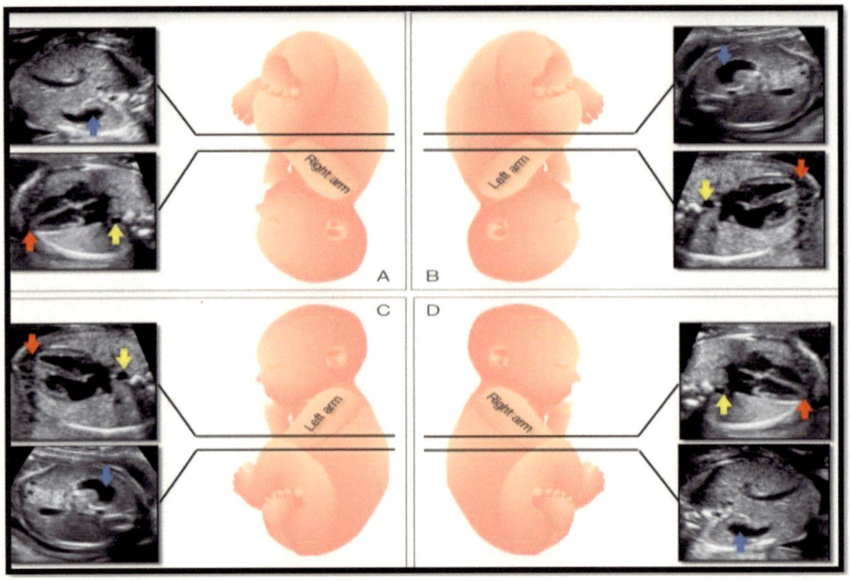

Figure 2.
Determining the fetal situs in longitudinal lie. (A) Fetus in cephalic presentation with spine close left uterine wall, results right side being anterior and left side posterior. (B) Cephalic with spine close to left uterine wall results left side being anterior and right side posterior. (C) Fetus in breech presentation with spine close to left uterine wall results left side being anterior and right side posterior. (D) Fetus in breech with spine close to right uterine wall results right side being anterior and left side posterior. The corresponding transverse ultrasound planes of the chest and abdomen. Blue arrow indicates fetal stomach, red arrow apex of heart and yellow arrow descending aorta.

Situs ambiguous, which refers to Viscerocardiac malposition, is commonly associated with complex CHD. Incidence of situs ambiguous is around 1per 10,000 infants [7]. This may be of right or left isomerism or situs ambiguous also known as visceral Heterotaxy syndrome which is very less commonly noted.

Detection of CHD on ultrasound depends on the position and axis of the cardia. Fetal cardiac axis: to determine the axis, obtain the transverse view of the chest at the level of four chamber view plane. A line is drawn from the spine to the anterior chest wall, the cardiac axis is the angle that the interventricular septum makes with this line (**Figure 3A**). Normal angle lies 45° to the left of the midline [8]. It is independent of gestational age. The axis is abnormal when it is >65° and < 25°. Study of Smith et al. [9] showed that >75° of leftward deviation are associated with CHD in 76% of fetuses which include Tetralogy of Fallot, Common arterial trunk, coarctation of aorta and Ebstein anomaly. Double outlet right ventricle, Atrioventricular septal defect and common atrium are more commonly associated with right axis deviation.

Cardiac position: depending upon the position of the heart it can be described as Levocardia Dextrocardia and mesocardia. Ectopia cordis refers when the cardia is outside the chest. As per Abuhamad et al [10] Heart positioned in right chest regardless of its axis it is termed as Dextrocardia, when the heart is placed in right chest with axis pointing to left then it is termed as Dextroposition and when the heart is positioned in right chest with axis pointing toward right side is known as dextroversion. Dextrocardia with axis to right: more commonly associated with Situs inversus, Congenital corrected transposition. Whereas Dextrocardia with left axis deviation is more commonly associated with extrinsic factors (**Figure 3B** and **C**) resulting in shift of heart to right side like Left diaphragmatic hernia, left lung mass, left pleural effusion, agenesis or hypoplasia of the right lung (scimitar syndrome). Mesocardia-Heart located in central chest

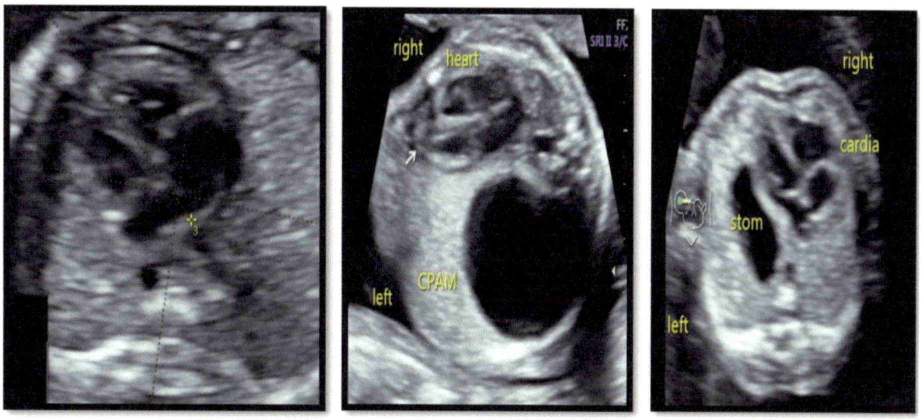

A B C

Figure 3.
(A) Measuring the cardiac axis. (B) Dextrocardia due to congenital adenomatoid malformation of left lung. (C) Dextrocardia with apex pointing to left due to congenital diaphragmatic hernia.

with cardiac apex pointing toward the midline of the chest usually associated with abnormal ventriculoarterial connections such as transposition of great arteries, Double outlet right ventricle. Bilateral increased lung volume such as laryngeal atresia is also associated with mesocardiac. Levocardia–it is more commonly used term for normal position of heart. Levoposition is noted in Right sided space occupying lesions or agenesis/hypoplasia of left lung. Levocardia with left axis deviation is commonly associated with CHD. Normal heart size should be 1/3rd to 1/2 that of thoracic cavity. The width of heart at AV valves corresponds to gestational age in weeks. Cardiothoracic (C/T) circumference is constant throughout gestation is about 0.45–0.5. Contractility of vetricles should be equal. Rhythm normal is 120–160 beats per minute.

4. Optimization of two-dimensional grayscale image in fetal echocardiography

The quality of 2D image is dependent on several factors such as choice of the transducer and presets, the angle of insonation and access to the region of interest and magnification of target region. Routinely two types of transducers are used in fetal echocardiography low frequency range (2–5 MHz) which allows good penetration and acceptable resolution. High frequency range (5–8 MHz) allows for improved resolution but limited penetration. Recently linear transducers are used for first trimester echocardiography as it gives high resolution. Image presets: (1) Harmonic imaging: in harmonic imaging, the reflected harmonic wave has a low amplitude high frequency which results in improved image and contrast with reduced artifacts. (2) Compound imaging allows the transducer to send signals at multiple angles to eliminate artifacts and improves the image resolution. (3) Speckle reduction imaging: weak signals are eliminated and strong signals are enhanced this allows the image to become smoother and reduces artifacts. (4) Focal zones: when imaging the heart chooses one focal zone at the region of interest to obtain better lateral resolution. (5) Dynamic range: narrow dynamic range provide better image as artifacts are eliminated. (6) High frame rate: high frame rate more than 25 frames per second. This can be achieved by narrowing the sector width and reducing the depth. (7) Tint or color maps. Magnify the heart in order to fill 1/3rd to 1/4th of the ultrasound image. Insonate from the apical or right lateral aspect of the fetal chest when possible. Try to use cine loop to analyze cardiac and valves motion. Optimizing color Doppler for the fetal Echo: when examining fetal heart with color Doppler a rapid frame rate with an acceptable image quality is essential. The image quality can be improved by optimizing the use of the velocity, the wall filter, persistence, gain and color line density. Velocity scale or Pulse repetition frequency is used to determine the range of velocities in the region of interest. For AV valves, semilunar valves and the great vessels use high velocity range > 30 cm/sec. Pulmonary and systemic veins need low to mid velocity scale 10–20 cm/sec. Color filter: high filter is selected for AV valves, great vessels and low filters for pulmonary and systemic veins. Color gain-color gain should be initially set on low and gradually increases until the color information is optimized. Color Doppler image resolution and color line density: high color resolution is needed at periphery pulmonary vessels and fetal echo in early pregnancy. In this condition, the smallest color box is chosen to increase frame rate. In power, Doppler or HD mode reducing balance in combination with increasing gain can demonstrate clear delineation of flow events within the chambers and vessels. Near parallel insonation to the direction of blood flow helps to optimize image when color Doppler is used. Pulse Doppler allows Doppler wave forms quantifications for the assessment of cardiac abnormalities and functions.

Scanning technique: determine the fetal situs. The anatomic markers for visualization of four chamber view are: one complete rib on each side of fetal chest wall, the two inferior pulmonary veins noted along the posterior wall of the left atrium, the apex of the heart pointing to the left upper chest about 45° and descending Aorta in front and to the left of fetal spine. Slight tilt of the medial aspect of transducer from four chamber view plane, five chamber view (LVOT view) can be imaged. Sliding the transducer cranially (while maintaining the transverse orientation in the chest) from four chamber plane three vessel view can be obtained. The larger and left most vessel is main pulmonary artery, slightly smaller aorta in the middle and smaller SVC on right side. From three vessel plane cranial tilt of transducer the transverse view of arterial duct can be obtained. Still slight cranial tilt of transducer the transverse view of the aortic arch can be obtained. Anterior to the 3VT, there is hypoechoic structure which is slightly echogenic to the lungs is identified as thymus. Further cranial movement of the transducer with slightly oblique to the left from 3VT view, SVC connecting with brachiocephalic vein is noted. In this plane great vessels are not seen as they are inferior.

Four chamber view is basic plane for detail evaluation of the fetal heart. In this plane, look for situs, size, axis of the heart. In normal heart both atria equal in size, foramen ovale in midsection of atrial septum with leaflet of foramen ovale in left atrium. Tricuspid valve septal leaflet is more apically inserted on the septum than mitral valve. Both ventricles equal in size with intact ventricular septum and moderator band in right ventricle. Based on the position and fetal lie four types of four chamber views of fetal heart can be obtained: (1) When the fetal anterior chest wall is closest to the transducer the Apical four chamber view obtained (**Figure 4A**), in which the ultrasound beam is nearly parallel to ventricular septum. (2) When fetal right posterior chest wall is closest to the transducer, a basal four chamber view is obtained ultrasound beam is nearly parallel to ventricular septum. (3) When the fetal spine is neither anterior or posterior but closer to right or left lateral uterine walls a Lateral four chamber view is obtained (**Figure 4B**), where the ultrasound beam is perpendicular to inter ventricular septum. Apex of the heart, ventricles the atrioventricular valves, atrial, Ventricular longitudinal dimensions are optimally evaluated by apical four chamber view. Basal view allows optimum visualization

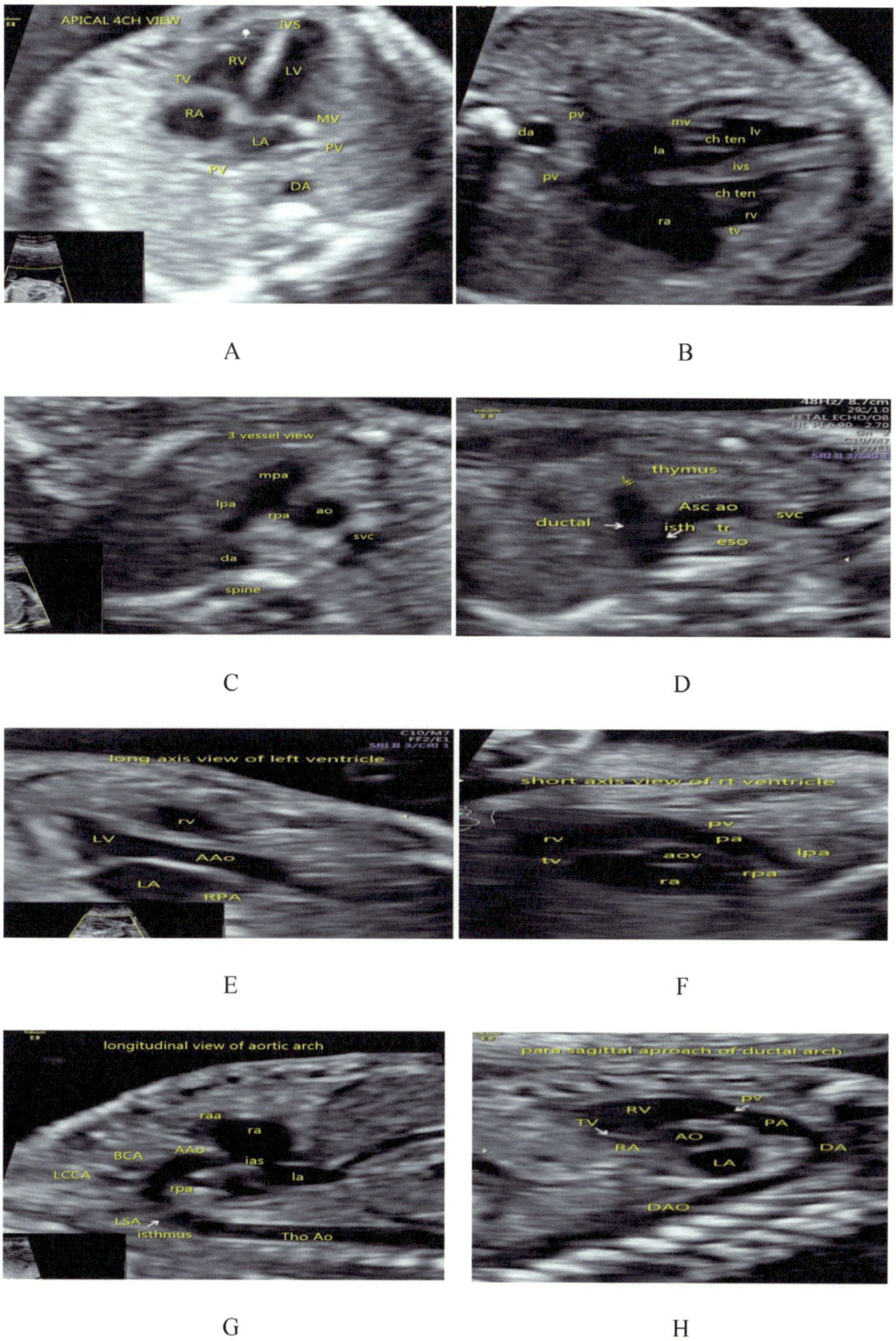

Figure 4.
(A) Apical 4ch view. (B) Lateral 4 ch view. (C) 3vv. (D) 3VT. (E) Long axis view of left ventricle. (F) Short axis view of right ventricle. (G) Longitudinal view of aortic arch. (H) Parasagittal approach of ductal arch.

of atria and atrioventricular valves. The lateral view allows adequate visualization of interventricular and interatrial septum, atrial and ventricular walls, ventricular contractility and septal thickness. From four chamber plane rotate the transducer 90° to get short axis views of the heart which provides a detail anatomic evaluation of spatial relationship of cardiac chambers and helps to evaluate ventricular size, ventricular wall and septal thickness. Origin and relationship of the great vessels can also be evaluated. In most Apical short axis plane Posteromedial and anterolateral papillary muscle of left ventricle are imaged in same plane at 8- and 5-o clock positions. Basal or more posterior short axis plane demonstrates the muscular part of ventricular septum, Mitral and tricuspid valves.in this plane mitral valve is crescent shaped and has the appearance of fish mouth. Three vessel view/transverse pulmonary trunk view (**Figure 4C**) shows the large main pulmonary artery anteriorly, ascending aorta in middle and posteriorly placed small SVC. In this plane we can assess conotruncal abnormalities and abnormalities associated with vessel size, alignment, arrangement, number and location of descending aorta. Three VT view (**Figure 4D**) demonstrates transverse main pulmonary artery and ductal arch, Transverse Aortic arch and its isthmic region, and the cross section of SVC and trachea. Trachea in this plane appears as circular structure with echogenic wall and a black lumen. In normal 3VT plane aortic and ductal arches are located left of the spine and trachea and no vessel should be seen to the right of trachea. Color Doppler reveals anteroposterior flow in both arches. By reducing velocity scale svc and azygos arch blood flow entering into SVC can be recognized. Slightly more cranial to this plane the mammary arteries running on the lateral border of thymus can be visualized which is known as thymic box. More cranial plane will show blood flow in Left Brachiocephalic vein in left to right direction, always opposite to the direction of the Aortic flow. Abnormal findings in 3VT view are (1) Narrow or absent Aortic arch—which is suggestive for Tubular hypoplasia of aortic arch or aortic coarctation. (2) Narrow or absent pulmonary artery—can typically be seen in pulmonary stenosis or atresia showing decreased antegrade or revers flow in pulmonary artery. Common anomalies associated are Tetralogy of Fallot, Ebstein anomaly, some cases of Double outlet right ventricle, Tricuspid atresia with VSD. (3) Dilated transverse Aortic arch-Aortic valve stenosis with post stenotic dilatation of Aorta can be found as isolated finding. (4) Dilated pulmonary artery—a hugely dilated pulmonary artery typically found in Tetralogy of Fallot with absent pulmonary valve. Absent pulmonary valve syndrome is commonly in association with the absence of the arterial duct. (5) Only one normal sized great vessel suggests transposition, DORV, the visualized single vessel that is seen is Aorta with a posterior non visualized pulmonary artery. Aorta shows a typical right ward convex course. (6) Only one great vessel of larger size-single enlarged great vessel may be aortic arch in case of pulmonary atresia where pulmonary artery is small tortuous or even absent. On the other hand, it could be a dilated pulmonary artery in the presence of left outflow tract obstruction such as hypoplastic left heart syndrome where on color Doppler demonstrates reverse flow in aortic arch. In an interrupted aortic arch, the pulmonary artery is less dilated than in left outflow tract obstruction. In case of common arterial trunk, a single dilated great vessel is noted. (7) Course of Aortic arch to the right of the trachea–then it is known as Right sided aortic arch. It may be isolated or associated with left ductus arteriosus which forms a U configuration (U sign) with the trachea in the middle. Rarely both the arches may be right of the trachea forming right sided V sign. (8) Tortuous course of great vessel—most commonly found at the level of the ductal arch towards the end of gestation where it appears as S configuration. Sometimes it may also present in mid gestation. Tortuous ductal arch may be a normal variant with no clinical implications. An abnormal tortuous course of aortic arch may be seen in a cervical aortic arch where the aorta runs into the upper mediastinum which is distant from the course of pulmonary artery. (9) Connection between both great vessels—this may be found in Aortopulmonary window. It is a rare condition and may be found in tetralogy of Fallot or other conotruncal anomalies or an isolated finding. (10) Demonstration of four vessels—commonly present in association with persistent left SVC. A double Aortic arch may also show four vessels, but it is generally detected by the presence of a right aortic arch. (11) Three vessels but no Right SVC – this condition may be seen with persistent left SVC. Dilated Superior vena cava: this may occur in case of Dilated Azygos vein in cases of interrupted IVC. This condition can also be depicted in the presence of supra cardiac type of total anomalous pulmonary venous drainage and also present in arteriovenous malformation of brain or vein of Galen aneurysm where increased venous drainage to SVC noted. In three VT view we can also asses the Thymus and left Brachiocephalic vein and also the other mediastinal structures like esophagus behind trachea, Bifurcation of trachea into both bronchi, the azygos vein connects to the SVC over the right bronchus referred as Azygos arch. In cases of conotruncal anomalies associated with hypoplastic or aplasia of thymus increases the suspicion for the presence of a 22q11 deletion.

Axial, oblique and sagittal views of great vessels (**Figure 3E–H**). The five chamber view displays ascending Aorta and demonstrates the left ventriculoarterial connection, the peri-membranous and muscular ventricular septa. Ascending aorta arises in between two AV valves in left to right orientation (directed toward right shoulder). There is a wide angle noted between the direction of ventricular septum and anterior wall of ascending Aorta which is absent in conotruncal anomalies where it is more parallel orientation with the septum. Fibrous–fibrous continuity of the posterior wall of the Aorta with the mitral valve and fibrous-muscular continuity of the anterior wall of Aorta and septum. This connection will be disrupted in Overriding of Aorta. At the level of five chamber view the two superior pulmonary veins enter the posterior walls of the left atrium. To obtain right ventricular outflow view (**Figure 4F**) from the mid sagittal plane of the chest by keeping the transducer in an oblique plane that is pointing from the right iliac bone to the left shoulder of the fetus. In this plane, right inflow and out flow tracts can be seen in same plane and are in perpendicular orientation. Left ventricle long axis view (**Figure 4E**)–to get this plane obtain sagittal view of fetal thoracic spine and slide the transducer from right to left parasagittal chest where we can image three planes one is superior and inferior venae cava second one is the aortic arch and lastly the ductal arch.

Longitudinal Aortic arch: by sliding the transducer to left parasagittal plane, we can obtain longitudinal aortic arch plane. In this view, aorta appears as a candy or a walking cane (**Figure 4G**) and arises centrally and superiorly in chest. Three arterial branches arise from superior aspect. Ductal arch view: it can be obtained by sliding the transducer still more left from the aortic arch view. Ductal arch (**Figure 4H**) arises from anterior aspect of chest with a wide angular curvature and is almost perpendicular to descending aorta and looks like hockey stick appearance. Ductal arch does not give any branches.

Normal variants in four Chamber view are (1) Echogenic intra cardiac focus (EIF) it may be single or multiple. In a patient at low risk of aneuploidy the presence of EIF after a normal detailed ultrasound should be considered as a normal variant; (2) pericardial fluid: if the pericardial fluid is less than 2 mm in thickness should be considered as normal variant; (3) mild ventricular disproportion in third trimester (left is smaller than right) can only be considered as normal variant after detailed ultrasound evaluation which ruled out coarctation of Aorta, TAPVC or other cardiac abnormalities associated with small left ventricle; (4) linear insertion of Atrioventricular valve could be found in normal fetuses and in fetuses with AVSD, depending on the plane in which the four chamber view is visualized (10). The area behind the 4ch view: during swallowing, esophagus may dilate and appears as a second vessel in front of Aorta but it will be decreased when swallowing ends.

Abnormal fetal echo: septal defects-Atrial septal defects-classified as Septum primum (ASD1), septum secundum (ASDII), Sinus venosus and coronary sinus defect. Septum secundum is the most common ASD which is around 80% of all ASDs and is mainly due to defect at foramen ovale. Next most common ASD is septum primum defect adjacent to both AV valves also known as partial AVSD. Sinus venosus ASD is noted posterior and superior to foramen ovale and inferior to the where IVC and **SVC** entering Right atrium. Coronary sinus ASD is rare and located at the site of the coronary sinus ostium in right atrium. Most ASDs cannot be diagnosed prenatally. ASD 1 can be identified as absent crux with linear insertion of both AV valves and Right to Left shunt noted. False positive diagnosis can be due to coronary sinus which mimics ASD1 where the flow is from left to right. Associated Cardiac and extra cardiac findings are AVSD, Anomalous pulmonary venous connections, single ventricle, Ebstein anomaly, tricuspid atresia and pulmonary atresia with intact ventricular septum. Venous abnormalities are common with sinus venosus defect (80–90%) and 10–15% with ASDII. ASD1 is associated with trisomy 21 and is also associated with Aortic coarctation. ASD secundum is associated with Holt-Oram syndrome.

Ventricular septal defect (VSD): these are the common congenital heart defects. VSDs are reported based on anatomic location on the septum. Most common VSD in neonates are perimembranous VSD (approximately 80%). Muscular, inlet and outlet VSDs are approximately reported in 5–20%, 5–8% and 5% respectively [11–13]. Whereas muscular VSDs (**Figure 5B**) are more common in prenatal period (aproxmately 80–90%) [14]. Small muscular VSDs are rarely diagnosed on gray scale color Doppler can be helpful in identifying the septal defect. Identification of VSDs is better in lateral chamber view. In Apical view drop out may mimic like VSD in such cases the borders of VSD appear echogenic. Most of the small muscular VSDs are bidirectional. On grayscale more commonly detected VSDs are perimembranous VSDs which are visualized in five chamber view where there is discontinuity between ventricular septum and medial wall of ascending Aorta. This type of VSDs is commonly associated with conotruncal abnormalities.

Atrioventricular septal defects (AVSD): common synonyms to AVSD are Endocardial cushion defect or AV canal defect. In the complete form of AVSD there is a combination of ASDI defect and VSD with common AV valve which usually have five leaflets (**Figure 5A**). Partial AVSD includes ASD1 and a cleft in mitral valve with separate AV valves but attaches at the same level. Transitional AVSD is a type of partial AVSD in this consists of two distinct AV annuli with large defect in atrial septum and small VSD.AVSDs can be classified as balanced or unbalanced.

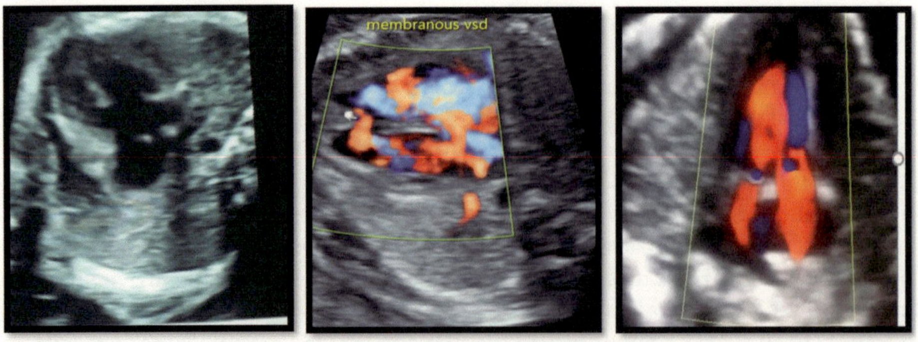

A B C

Figure 5.
(A) Atrioventricular septal defect. (B) Small membranous VSD. (C) Double inlet ventricle.

In unbalanced AVSDs the AV connections predominantly drains to one of the two ventricles results in ventricular disproportion and is typically found in Heterotaxy syndrome.

Incidence of AVSDs in infants with congenital heart diseases is 4–7.4% [15, 16]. Eighteen percent of prenatally detected CHDs are AVSDs [17]. It is best detected in Apical 4 chamber view. Ultrasound findings in AVSD in diastole are Absent Crux with a defect in the center of the heart noted. In systole the common AV valve is closed with loss of offset noted and appears like linear line across. Atrioventricular length ratio (AVL ratio) is increased in AVSD [10]. A cut off value for AVL ratio over 0.6 detects AVSD in 83% with false positive rate of 5.7% [18]. Presence of conotruncal Anomalies are more commonly associated with AVSD. Color and pulsed Doppler will demonstrate common regurgitation in complete AVSD. A regurgitant jet, which appears to arise from left ventricle should alert for the presence of a complete or partial AVSD as mitral regurgitation is rare in fetus (10). Associated cardiac findings are TOF, DORV, Right Aortic arch, aortic coarctation and other conotruncal anomalies. AVSD is also associated with Heterotaxy syndrome. Extra cardiac anomalies associated with AVSD are mainly trisomy 21 and also noted in trisomy 18 and 13. Antenatal diagnosis of AVSD, when isolated is associated with trisomy 21 in 58% of cases [19]. AVSD in combination of with hypoplastic left heart syndrome can be found in turners' syndrome (10). In a recent study 13% of CHARGE syndrome patients were associated with AVSDs [20]. AVSD may be recognized in early gestation at 11–13 weeks. Prenatal diagnosis of complete AVSD has low survival rate due to associated cardiac and extra cardiac findings whereas in isolated cases the outcome is excellent [21, 22].

Univentricular atrioventricular connection: this is due to failure of the development of bulboventricular loop stage. It describes a heart with one functioning ventricle with inflow from one or both atria. Synonymous terms for this condition are primitive ventricle, single ventricle, cor triloculare biatriatum, cor biloculare and double inlet ventricle (DIV). Three subgroups are identified in this condition, they are (1) double inlet (**Figure 5C**), where two atria connect to a single ventricle through two atrioventricular valves; (2) single inlet where one atrium connects to single ventricle through a single AV valve; (3) common inlet where both atria connected to single ventricle. Most common morphology of single ventricle is left ventricular morphology with right rudimentary chamber. Rarely right ventricular morphology with rudimentary left chamber or a ventricle of indeterminant morphology without rudimentary chamber can be seen. Cardiac anomalies which may show a single ventricle morphology are Hypoplastic left heart syndrome, Pulmonary atresia with intact septum, AVSD (large or unbalanced), single ventricle in Heterotaxy syndrome, corrected TGA with tricuspid atresia, mitral atresia with ventricular septal defect and more commonly found DIV is tricuspid atresia with ventricular septal defect. Double inlet left ventricle (DILV) presents as rudimentary right ventricle communicating with single ventricle with a VSD. Rudimentary right ventricle is a small outlet chamber. Great arteries usually arise in D or L malposition. The rudimentary outlet chamber in DILV is more commonly located on left side of the main ventricle (L looping) rarely on right side (D looping). Diagnosis is usually made on gray scale ultrasound. DIV with patent AV valves is well tolerated in fetus. Follow up ultrasound is important to look for outflow obstruction. Associated malformations are Atresia, hypoplasia or straddling of the atrioventricular valves, pulmonary outflow obstruction, subaortic outflow obstruction and conduction abnormalities.

Tricuspid Atresia with ventricular septal defect (TA): in this condition, the atrioventricular connection on right side is absent hence right ventricle is diminutive in size. Most of the cases tricuspid valve appears echogenic and thickened on ultrasound. Aliasing noted across the mitral valve due to increased blood flow. Prenatal mitral regurgitation will have poor outcome. Inlet type of VSD typically perimembranous is present in almost all cases. The size of right ventricle depends on the size of VSD. Right ventricular contractility is normal with no myocardial thickening. A large interatrial connection in the form of large patent foramen ovale or atrial septal defect. There may be redundant flap of septum secundum that is bulging into Left atrium: malaligned interatrial and interventricular septa. The right ventricular outflow stenosis is a common finding in these cases. Pulmonary stenosis in this condition shows only decreased in arterial size and it is nonturbulent. Right aortic arch may be present. TA is classified into three types depends on spatial orientation of the great vessels. TA type 1 is a normally oriented great artery, which is most common (70–80%) (**Figure 6A**). Type 2 in 12–25% associated with D transposition of great vessels. Type3 is uncommon where there may be common arterial trunk or L Transposition. Four chamber view in TA is diagnostic. Ductal dependent pulmonary circulation in TA is seen in severe pulmonary stenosis or pulmonary atresia in association of small right ventricle. Doppler study of ductus venosus shows reverse A wave in end diastole most commonly noted at second or third trimester. Associated cardiac findings are great vessel stenosis/atresia, coarctation of aorta, interrupted aortic arch, persistent LSVC, Right aortic arch, pulmonary venous abnormality and juxtaposition of atrial appendage. Sometimes it may be associated with corrected transposition of great arteries where atretic tricuspid valve is on left side. Fetal karyotyping should be offered to rule out 22q11 microdeletion.

Ebstein anomaly, Tricuspid valve dysplasia and tricuspid regurgitation: in Ebstein anomaly (**Figure 6B**) septal and posterior leaflet of TV are displaced inferiorly from TV annulus towards the apex and originates from the right ventricular myocardium. Anterior leaflet maintains its normal attachment to annulus. Proximal portion of right ventricle is then in continuous with the right atrium and forms the atrialized portion of right ventricle. Gray scale ultrasound findings in four chamber view are cardiomegaly with increased cardiothoracic ratio. Progressive dilatation of right atrium with advancing gestation is noted. Attachment of septal leaflet of TV to the ventricular wall rather than valve annulus is noted by observing TV anatomy in systole and diastole by using cine loop which is essential to differentiating Ebstein anomaly from tricuspid valve dysplasia. In severe form of Ebstein anomaly with

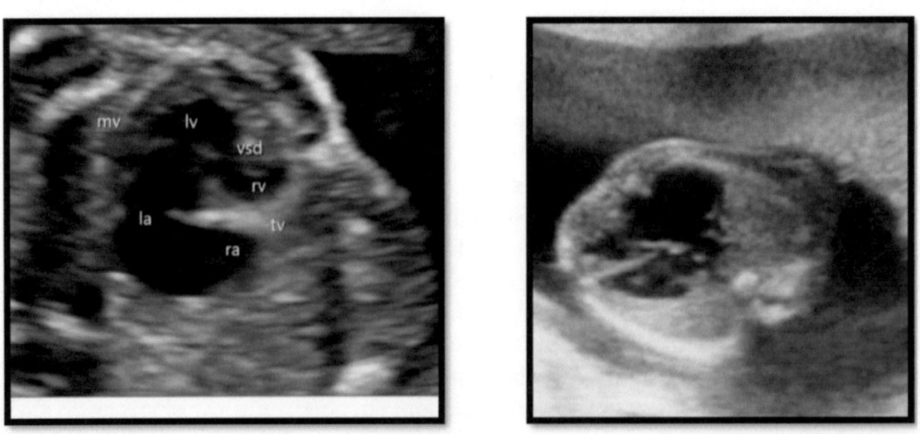

A B

Figure 6.
(A) Tricuspid atresia with VSD. (B) Ebstein anomaly demonstrating apical displacement of tricuspid valve.

large atrialized ventricle there will be paradoxical movement of ventricular septum noted and pronounced cardiomegaly with compression of both lungs results in lung hypoplasia and may results in cardiac failure and hydrops. This anomaly may be associated with pulmonary stenosis or atresia. Color Doppler confirms the tricuspid regurgitation (TR). TR occurs during entire systole (holosystolic) with peak velocities of greater than 200 cm/sec. Systolic regurgitant jet typically arises from the middle of the right ventricle in contrast to other functional tricuspid regurgitations which arises at the level of annulus. Mild Ebstein cases may be missed in utero.

Tricuspid dysplasia: it involves the abnormalities of TV with normal insertion of leaflets. It also classified as a part of the pulmonary atresia with intact septum. Ultrasound findings are thickened leaflets which do not close properly in systole. Enlarged right atrium noted. It also associated with Right ventricular outflow obstruction and atrial septal defect. Color Doppler shows regurgitant jet arising from annulus. In the presence of significant right ventricular outflow obstruction the pulmonary artery may be of normal in size with minimal valvular excursion. Color Doppler will demonstrate reverse flow in the ductus arteriosus and may be of pulmonary valve regurgitation. Outcome of fetuses with this condition is good except in severe form it may be associated with heart failure, RVOT obstruction, severe tricuspid regurgitation and high rate of neonatal mortality.

Tricuspid regurgitation (TR): the regurgitant jet is limited to early or mid or whole systole is then referred as early systolic or mid systolic or holosystolic, respectively. Mild regurgitation peak systolic velocity varies from 30 to 70 cm/sec and in severe it may vary from 180 to 350 cm/sec. Mild TR is defined as the jet that extends less than 1/3rd of the distance to opposite atrial wall and covers an area less than 25% of right atrium. Trivial TR is common finding which is mild and nonholosystolic with maximum velocity less than 200 cm/sec. As Abuhamed et al, it is reported as 83% of fetuses in low risk in 14–16 weeks. In most of the cases it resolves in second trimester. TR is main component in Ebstein anomaly and TV dysplasia. RVOT obstructions such as pulmonary atresia with intact septum, pulmonary stenosis and constriction of ductus arteriosus are commonly associated with TR. It can also present in coarctation of aorta, hypoplastic left heart syndrome, Double outlet right ventricle and absent pulmonary valve syndrome. Volume overload like fetal anemia, Vein of Galen aneurysm, sacrococcygeal teratoma, chorioangioma, in the recipient twin in twin-twin transfusion syndrome and in fetal arrhythmias. Impairment of myocardial function like cardiomyopathies, sever IUGR, fetal hypoxia and infections or autoimmune myocarditis may associate with TR. In first trimester risk assessment TR is diagnosed when peak velocity of regurgitant jet is more than 60 cm/sec and duration involves at least half of the systole.

Hypoplastic left syndrome (HLHS): there are two main classic forms of HLHS noted. One involving both mitral and aortic atresia with severely hypoplastic left ventricle. The other form involves a small left ventricle with hyperechoic wall globular shape and poor contractility (**Figure 7A**). It is often difficult to differentiate HLHS from critical aortic stenosis on fetal echo. Ultrasound findings in four chamber view shows small hypokinetic left ventricle with apex is mostly formed by right ventricle. The size of left ventricle may be hypoplastic or normal in size or sometimes it may even dilate but always associated with poor contractility with decreased function this can be demonstrated by M mode. Aortic valve is atretic the mitral valve is patent but dysplastic and left ventricle is globular, hypokinetic with bright echogenic inner wall. Small left atrium with paradoxical movement of leaflet of foramen ovale. In five chamber view, aorta size will be less than 3 mm and at three vessel view dilated pulmonary trunk with small or nonvisible aorta noted. Color Doppler conforms retrograde flow from ductus arteriosus into aortic isthmus (**Figure 7B**). Pulse Doppler shows end diastolic pronounced reverse flow of A

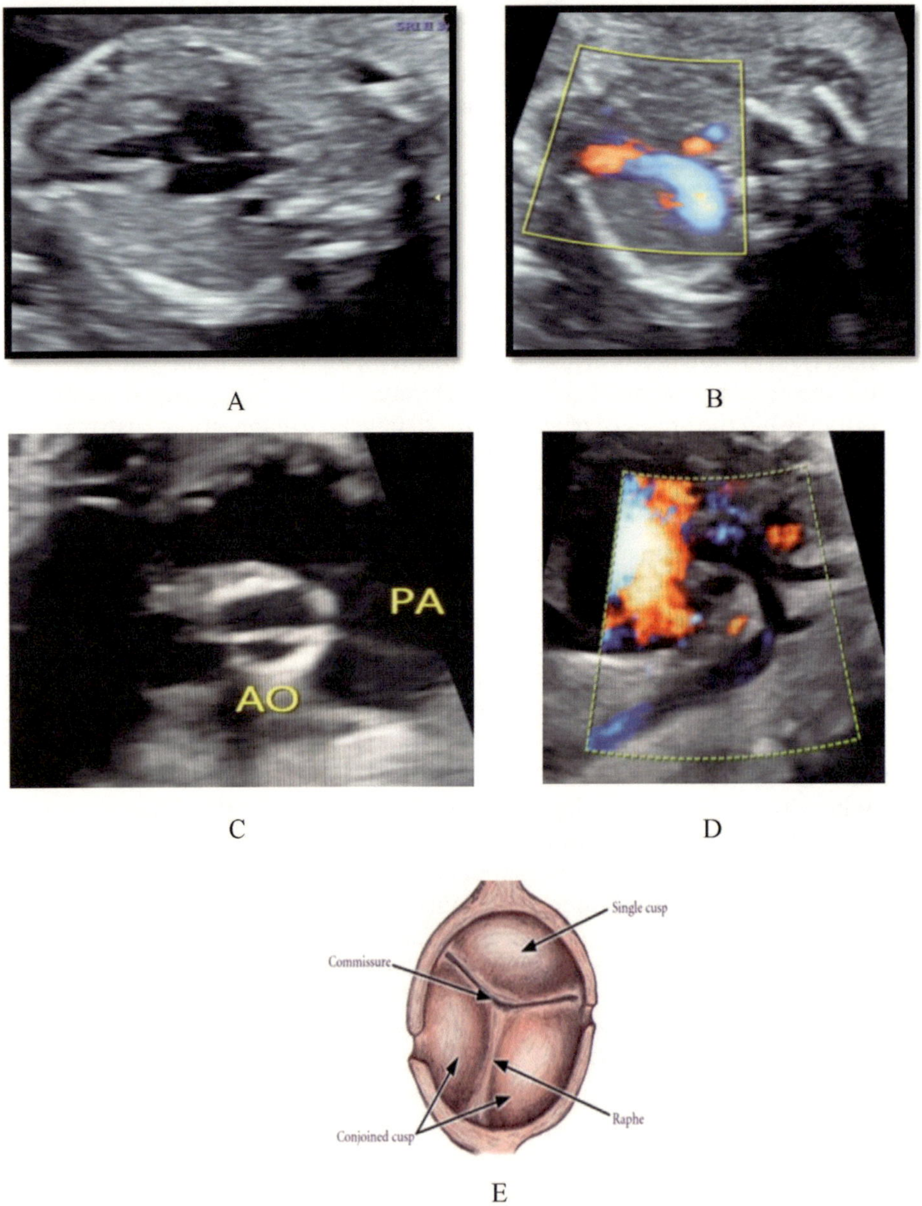

Figure 7.
(A) Hypoplastic left heart. (B) 3vessele view showing small aorta with reverse flow. (C, E) at the level of aortic root showing bicuspid aortic valve with single straight line across valve annulus. (D) Coarctation of aorta.

wave in pulmonary veins which is dependent on opening of foramen ovale size. In severe aortic stenosis left atrium may be dilated due to mitral valve regurgitation. Ascending aorta may show post stenotic dilatation. Peak velocities are generally >200 cm/sec. HLHS is associated with turner's syndrome, trisomies 13 and 18, Noonan syndrome, Smith-Lemli-Opitz syndrome and Holt-Oram syndrome. Follow up scans for every 4–6 weeks is recommended.

Aortic stenosis (AS) and Bicuspid aortic valve (BAV): it is classified as valvular, sub valvular and supra valvular depending on anatomical location of the obstruction in relation to aortic valve. Valvular AS is most diagnosed in prenatal ultrasound where the valve leaflets are dysplastic. It may be tricuspid with fused commissures, bicuspid, unicuspid or noncommissural. Mild AS is difficult to diagnose prenatally. On gray scale aortic valve is thickened valve leaflets, doming of the cusps and lack of complete valve opening during systole noted. Doppler study shows turbulent antegrade flow through a normal-size or slightly dilated aortic arch. In shone complex the combination of left ventricular inflow and outflow obstruction with a normally contractile left ventricle. In shone complex there is narrowing of mitral valve orifices with a regular filling of small normally contractile left ventricle.

Bicuspid aortic valve: —this is an autosomal dominant inheritance pattern. It can also occur in other cardiac anomalies such as coarctation of Aorta, aortic stenosis and ventricular septal defects [23]. In 80–90% cases BAV (**Figure 7C** and **E**) is made of two unequal leaflets in this larger one results from the fusion of the right and left cusps with central raphe and smaller leaflet which by itself is larger than one of the three leaflets of a normal aortic valve.

Valve leaflets are best visualized in third trimester and short axis view of aortic valve. Ultrasound findings in BAV are mildly dilated ascending aorta with increased flow velocities, echogenic aortic valve, visualization of valve leaflets in late systole.

Coarctation of Aorta (CoA) and interrupted aortic arch (IAA): —CoA involves narrowing of aorta at isthmic region typically located between left subclavian artery and ductus arteriosus (**Figure 7D**). If long segment of aorta involved, it is known as tubular hypoplasia. Recurrent rate for CoA is 2–6% for previously affected child 4% an affected mother [24, 25]. CoA is simple without associated with intra cardiac lesions and complex when it is associated with significant intra cardiac lesions like HLHS, Aortic atresia, unbalanced AV defect with a narrow-left ventricle, DORV, Tricuspid atresia with VSD and malposition of great vessels (type2), double inlet ventricle/single ventricle and corrected TGA. Ultrasound findings of CoA are ventricular disproportion left is <right. Ratio of right to left ventricular width should be more than 1.69 [26]. In this case, normal ventricular contractility and patent Mitral valve noted. Occasionally it may be associated with persistent left superior vena cava (PLSVC). In five chamber view normal ascending aorta normal or small aortic root especially if it is associated with perimembranous VSD or Aortic stenosis. On 3VT view narrowing of transverse aortic arch diameter more at isthmic region. PLSVC noted left of ductal arch. Narrowing and shelf is better assessed in longitudinal aortic arch section. Color Doppler confirms normal ventricular filling during diastole which differentiates CoA to HLHS. Narrowing of isthmus with normal flow without any aliasing noted. Look for shelf sign which is noted at the junction between the ductus arteriosus and descending aorta. An accurate diagnosis of CoA in early gestation is difficult as the ventricular disproportion found in early gestation may resolve with advancing gestation. Associated non cardiac findings are vascular anomalies like variations in brachiocephalic anatomy, berry aneurysm of circle of Willis. And nonvascular lesions involving multiple organs like Genitourinary, Musculoskeletal, Gastrointestinal and others may be present in 30% of children [27]. Associated aneuploidy rate is up to 35% (10), commonly associated with turner syndrome and occasionally with trisomy 13 and 18. CoA is difficult to detect prenatally with high false positive and false negative rates [28, 29].

Interrupted Aortic arch: it is classified into Type A, B and c in relation to brachiocephalic vessels. Type B is most common and is associated with large malaligned VSD and posterior displacement of infundibular septum. Type A is similar to Coarctation of aorta. Four chamber view usually appears on normal five chamber view shows large VSD with small aortic root showing nonturbulent flow. 3 VT view demonstrates absent continuity of aortic arch. Trachea appears to touch pulmonary artery due to absence of medially located aortic arch. It is associated with 22q11 deletion where the thymus is hypoplastic or absent in 3VT view.

Instead of candy cane appearance longitudinal aortic arch shows straight course with brachiocephalic and left common carotid vessels. Left subclavian artery arises from ductus arteriosus. Slightly dilated pulmonary trunk in 3 VT view. Occasionally associated with aberrant right subclavian artery (ARSA) or aberrant left subclavian artery (ALSA). 50% of IAA type B is associated with 22q11 microdeletion [30–32]. About 43% is associated with DiGeorge syndrome [33]. It may also associated with turner syndrome, pulmonary stenosis (PS), pulmonary atresia with intact ventricular septum (PA-IVS) and ductus arteriosus constriction.

Pulmonary stenosis: There may be infravalvular (infundibulum) narrowing or rarely supra valvular narrowing involving the main pulmonary artery or its branch. This is typically associated with tetralogy of fallot, Twin-twin transfusion syndrome. Valvular stenosis is due to fusion of valve commissures. Sometimes it may be due to unfused thickened dysplastic valve leaflets with associated pulmonary regurgitation usually associated with Noonan syndrome. Recurrence of PS is 2%in one affected sibling 6% when two siblings are affected. Ultrasound findings in PS in 4 chamber view are right ventricular hypertrophy with bulging of septum into left side TV shows normal leaflet excursion may associated with tricuspid regurgitation leads to right atrial dilatation. Right ventricular outflow view shows abnormal excursion, thickening and doming of valvular leaflets during systole. Valvular leaflets are visible within pulmonary artery throughout cardiac cycle. 3vv and 3vt view shows post stenotic dilatation. Color Doppler of PulmonaryValve shows turbulent antegrade flow with color aliasing. Pulse Doppler shows high flow velocities >200 cm/sec. Most of the cases shows antegrade flow in ductus arteriosus. Retrograde flow across the ductus arteriosus is a poor sign. In sever PS tricuspid valve shows holosystolic regurgitation. Ductus venosus shows reverse a wave. Associated cardiac lesions are tricuspid regurgitation, ASD, Aortic stenosis, Tricuspid Stenosis and Total anomalous pulmonary venous connection. Associated syndrome are Noonan, Beckwith-Wiedemann, Alagille and Williams-Beuren. Every 2–4 weeks of follow-up, scans are recommended.

Pulmonary atresia with intact ventricular septum (PA-IVS): —here, the PA is membranous type with complete fusion of commissures and normally developed infundibulum. In PA-IVS and hypoplastic right ventricle may show anomaly of coronary circulation known as ventriculocoronary arterial communication (VCAS). Systemic collateral arteries to lung are typical to PA-with VSD and not with PA-IVS. Ultrasound findings in PA-IVS (**Figure 8A** and **B**) are hypoplastic and hypokinetic right ventricle with thickened walls. The size of right ventricle May vary from nearly absent or hypoplastic or normal with poor contractility. Dysplastic tricuspid valve with narrow annulus and abnormal leaflet excursion noted. Hypoplastic main pulmonary artery noted. Color Doppler shows the lack of adequate filling of right ventricle during diastole. No antegrade flow across PV and reverse flow in ductus arteriosus. Dilated aorta with normal antegrade flow.in color Doppler VCACs which siphon right ventricular blood during systole, in the presence of Right ventricular cavity with diastolic filling and without significant regurgitation the apex or right ventricular wall as turbulent flow followed along the wall of right ventricle until the origin of the right or left coronary artery at the aortic root. Pulse Doppler demonstrates bidirectional turbulent flow with high velocities. Poor prognostic findings are severe tricuspid regurgitation, small tricuspid valve annulus (Z-score < 3or 4), small Rv/Lv length or width (<0.5), presence of VCAC, associated extracardiac abnormalities and chromosomal abnormalities.

Premature constriction of the ductus arteriosus: —DA is a muscular tube which connects the MPA at the origin of left PA to the descending aorta just distal to the left subclavian artery. It is the largest vessel in the fetus equal to that of descending aorta. In advanced gestation, increased deposition of collagen, elastin and

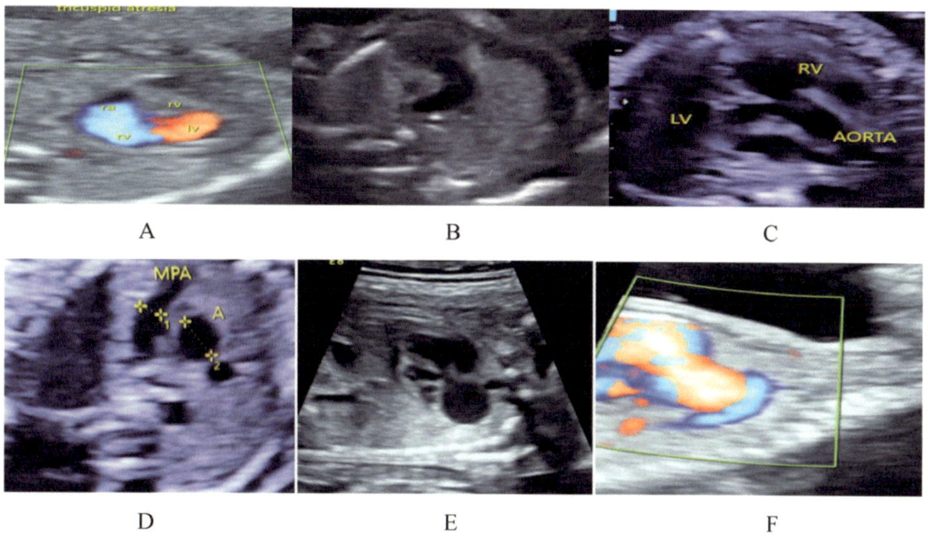

Figure 8.
(A) Pulmonary atresia with intact septum showing hypoplasia of right ventricle absence of blood flow across dysplastic tricuspid valve. (B) PA-IVS 3VT view showing small pulmonary artery. (C) Case of TOF in five chamber view showing large ventricular septal defect and dilated overriding aorta, with a parallel to the ventricular septum. (D) In TOF 3VV showing small pulmonary artery with dilated aorta and descending aorta on the right side of the spine as an associated with right aortic arch. (E, F) Absent pulmonary valve syndrome showing grossly dilated pulmonary artery showing high velocities with color aliasing.

glycoprotein with proliferation of smooth muscle to prepare for postnatal closure this narrowing can be monitored by prenatal ultrasound. Most cases of DA constriction are due to maternal drug therapy with prostaglandin synthetase inhibitors in late gestation. On gray scale it is difficult to diagnose this condition. Sometimes it may show dilated and hypokinetic right ventricle noted. Color Doppler reveals holosystolic tricuspid regurgitation. Dilated Right ventricular out flow tract, pulmonary artery and narrow ductus arteriosus by showing turbulent high diastolic and systolic velocities of around 200-300 cm/sec diastolic >35 cm/sec with PI less than 1.9. Interruption of drug therapy reverses the constriction within 24-48 hours but TR may persists longer time.

TOF (**Figure 8C** and **D**) is characterized by malaligned VSD (sub aortic), overriding aorta (aortic root overrides the VSD) assumes a parallel course to the septum, infundibular pulmonary stenosis and right ventricular hypertrophy. In 4chamber view normal or may show the VSD. Deviation of axis may be the first clue. On five chamber view shows perimembranous sub aortic VSD with overriding of aorta by demonstrating discontinuity between IVS and medial aortic wall which is known as malaligned VSD. There by the aorta is slightly shifted towards right side (Aortic dextroposition) so aorta receives blood from both right and left vetricles becomes dilated. Short axis or three vessel view shows narrow pulmonary artery. Mild TOF can be missed in second trimester scans due to subtle changes. Sometimes perimembranous VSD is evident without vessel diameter discrepancy in second trimester. Inflow of aorta shows aliased due to high perfusion where as in pulmonary artery may generally shows normal or only slightly increased flow. In TOF instead of PS, it may also associated with pulmonary atresia or absent pulmonary valve. Associated cardiac abnormalities are right sided aortic arches, sometimes TOF may associate with AVSD which increase the risk of chromosomal abnormalities [34]. A patent foramen ovale or atrial septal defect has been reported in 83% and PLSVC in 11%of new born with TOF [35]. Chromosomal abnormalities are around 30% with trisomies 21, 13 and 18 [20]. TOF may be associated with 22q11 microdeletion.

It may also found in Alagille syndrome, CHARGE syndrome [10]. Follow up scans to evaluate pulmonary artery growth and flow across the ductus arteriosus. A pulmonary valve and aortic valve ratio of<0.6 or a pulmonary valve Z-score of-3 at fetal fine echocardiogram (10) was highly sensitive but poor specific whereas classifying direction of flow in the ductus arteriosus as either normal or abnormal was both highly sensitive and specific for predicting the need for a neonatal intervention.

Pulmonary atresia with VSD: —includes atresia of PV hypoplasia of pulmonary artery and membranous or infundibular VSD, and an overriding of aorta. Distinct features that differentiate PA-VSD to TOF are no right ventricular outflow severe abnormalities of pulmonary circulation. The source of blood supply to lungs mainly depends on ductus arteriosus and systemic pulmonary collateral circulation or combination of both. Collaterals arising from descending aorta to lungs is known as major aortopulmonary collateral arteries (MAPCAs). This is commonly seen with diabetic mother.it is also commonly associated with 22q11 microdeletion. Ultrasound findings are similar to TOF except the diameter of aortic root has a larger diameter than TOF. In 3VV hypoplastic PA can occasionally visualized. In some cases, closed pulmonary valve with absent proximal pulmonary trunk noted. Ductus arteriosus tortuous and hypoplastic or may be dilated. Color Doppler demonstrates absent flow from right ventricle to pulmonary trunk and retrograde filling in branching pulmonary arteries. A longitudinal view of aorta from anterior or lateral approach may show the MAPCAs arising from descending aorta which need low velocity Doppler settings. Associated cardiac malformations are right sided aortic arch in 20–50% of cases [36]. ASD secundum type is commonly seen postnatally [37]. The absence of ductus arteriosus is in half the cases. MAPCAs are associated in about 44% of cases [38]. Extra cardiac association are with 22q11microdeletion which is found in 18–25%of fetuses [38, 39] previous type IV CAT where both the branching PA arising directly from descending aorta is currently classified as PA-VSD.

Absent pulmonary valve syndrome: absent or dysplastic or rudimentary pulmonary valve leaflets with an outlet VSD and an overriding Aorta noted in TOF-APVS. Most of the times it may be associated with absent patent ductus arteriosus. Branching arteries are grossly dilated and main pulmonary valve annulus shows signs of stenosis and severe insufficiency. It may also be associated with air way abnormalities. The rarer form of APVS with an intact septum and less dilated pulmonary trunk and a patent ductus arteriosus are reported. Four chamber may be normal or may show dilated right ventricle. Five chamber view may show VSD with overriding aorta with normal aortic root (not dilated as in TOF). Short axis and 3VT view shows aneurysmal dilatation of pulmonary artery and massively dilated branch pulmonary arteries.in most cases absent ductus arteriosus noted [40]. On color Doppler high velocities across PV annulus with typical to-and-fro flow with peak systolic velocities approx. Meas 200–250 cm/sec (**Figure 8E** and **F**). Sometimes there may be tricuspid regurgitation. A normal sized pulmonary artery may present in early gestation and full spectrum of APVS may not be evident till late gestation.so, diagnosis of APVS is difficult in early gestation. High mortality in APVS is due to cardiac failure or bronchomalacia.

Common arterial trunk (CAT): also known as persistent truncus arteriosus, aorticopulmonary trunk and truncus arteriosus communis. It is characterized by a single arterial trunk which arises from the base of the heart and gives origin to the systemic, pulmonary and coronary circulations. A large VSD is nearly absent in infundibular septum [41]. It is classified into four types. Type 1 is a short pulmonary trunk arises from the CAT and divides into right and left pulmonary arteries (**Figure 9A** and **B**). In type 2 and 3, both pulmonary arteries arise separately they may be close anatomically (from posteriorly) as in type2 or some distance from one another as in type3 (laterally) and in type 4 which is reclassified as PA-VSD.

The root is of CAT is large and has biventricular origin. In most of the cases root arise entirely from right ventricle rarely from left ventricle. On ultrasound levorotation of heart noted. Large malaligned VSD with overriding large vessel with color aliasing noted on 5 chamber view with pulmonary trunk arising from overriding vessel. Root is large with thickened dysplastic leaflets 3VT view show a single large vessel represents artic arch as the ductus arteriosus is not developed in more than 50% of cases [9]. In an interrupted aortic arch there is an absent continuity of aortic isthmus noted. Seventy percent of the cases aortic arch is left of trachea (right aortic arch). In about 1/3rd of cases hypoplastic or absent thymus noted [30, 38, 42]. Aortic arch abnormalities are commonly associated with CAT. 21–36% right sided aortic arch 15% with interrupted arch rarely hypoplasia of arch or double aortic arch noted. It may be associated with trisomies 21,18, 13 and 22q11 deletion is reported in 30–40%of the cases [43–45]. It is more commonly seen in diabetic mother.

Double outlet right ventricle (DORV): it is a type of ventriculoarterial connection, where both the great vessels arise from right ventricle. Several types of DORV (**Figure 9E** and **F**) noted, differing with regard to spatial relationship of the great arteries, location of the VSD, presence or absence of outflow obstruction. There are four types of anatomic relationships of the aorta to pulmonary artery at the level of semilunar valves [46]. They are right posterior aorta, a right anterior aorta, left anterior aorta and right lateral aorta. Location of VSD which is associated with DORV are sub aortic type, sub pulmonic type, doubly committed and remote. Ultrasound findings are abnormal ventriculoarterial connections. It may associate with atrioventricular valves like Mitral atresia, AVSD and double inlet ventricle. Five chamber view demonstrates VSD, the lack of continuity of the medial wall of the aorta with septum, origin of both vessels is from the anterior chamber. The location and relation of VSD to great arteries should be evaluated. Angle the transducer in between 5 chamber and 3VT view to demonstrate parallel course

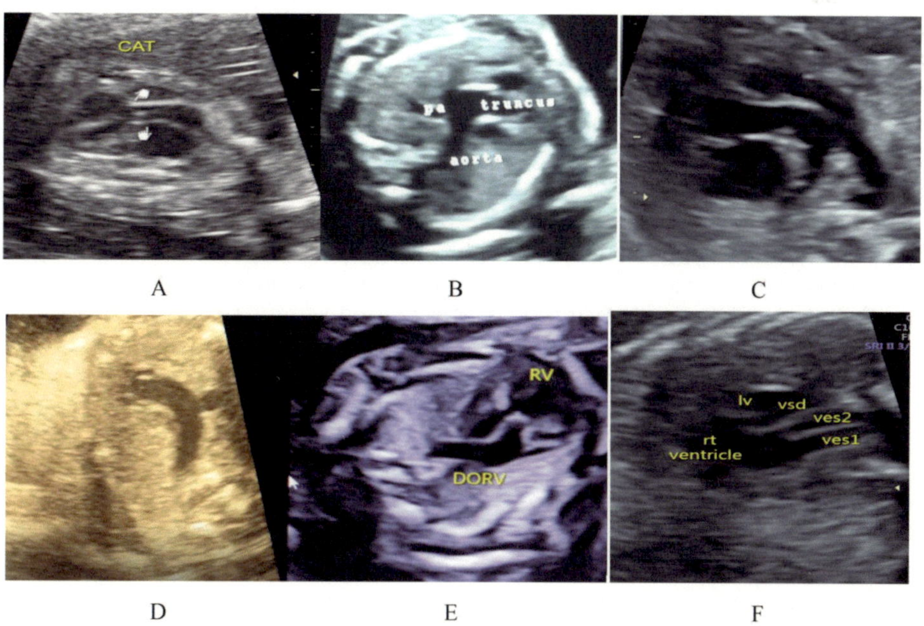

Figure 9.
(A) Five chamber view showing large overriding common arterial trunk. (B) Common arterial trunk with small pulmonary artery and large aorta. (C) Parallel origin of great vessels in DTGA. Aorta arising anteriorly from right ventricle and is right of the pulmonary artery which arises from left ventricle. (D) 3VT the aorta is seen as single large bent vessel as right convex shape i.e., I sign. (E, F) outflow tract view showing DORV.

of great vessels. Pulmonary artery atresia/stenosis is more common than aortic involvement. PS is most commonly associated with malformation in about 70% of cases [47] right sided aortic arch may be seen on 3VT view. The abnormal anatomic relation of great arteries can be better depicted on color Doppler. If atresia/stenosis of vessel is present, color Doppler helps to demonstrate a single large vessel on 3VT view. Cardiac malformations associated with DORV are mitral atresia, cleft in anterior mitral leaflet, ASD, AVSD, sub aortic stenosis, aortic coarctation, right aortic arch, persistent left svc and anomalous pulmonary venous return. DORV with AVSD may be noted in isomerism. DORV may also be noted with complex corrected transposition. In 12–40% of cases, chromosomal abnormalities including trisomies 18, 13 and 22q11 microdeletion are noted [48–50]. Poor prognostic signs associated with DORV are tubular or hypoplastic aorta, pulmonary atresia, hypoplastic left ventricle/single ventricle physiology, mitral atresia, AVSD and situs ambiguous.

Complete and congenitally corrected Transposition of great arteries: in complete transposition of great arteries (DTGA) atrioventricular concordance and ventriculoarterial discordance. Both great arteries display parallel course with aorta anterior and to right of pulmonary artery. It may present as simple or associate with other cardiac malformations (complex DTGA). VSD and PS are common association with DTGA and may be present alone or in combination in up to 30–40% of cases. Ultrasound findings are that five chamber view shows pulmonary artery arising from left ventricle and bifurcating shortly from its origin and aorta is arising from right ventricle in an anterior and parallel course to pulmonary artery. Transverse view in upper thorax demonstrates a single large anteriorly and superiorly placed vessel with SVC to its right. The single large vessel noted in 3VT view is Aorta and it assumes a right convex shape known as I sign (**Figure 9C** and **D**). On longitudinal view hockey stick appearance to aorta and candy cane appearance to pulmonary artery noted. Congenitally corrected transposition of great vessels (LTGA/ccTGA): characterized by atrioventricular and ventriculoarterial discordance. In ccTGA aorta is located anteriorly and left of the pulmonary artery. It has 2% recurrence risk in first degree relatives [51]. In some cases of ccTGA with dextrocardia or situs inversus, right atrium may be left sided and with double discordance of the ventricles and great vessels hemodynamically this condition resembles D-TGA. Situs inversus with ccTGA is noted in 5% of cases and dextro or mesocardia in 25% cases [52]. Sequential segmental analysis of fetal heart should be done to rule out situs abnormalities. Four chamber view assess ventricular morphology. Morphologic right ventricle in ccTGA is left posterior and is connected to left atrium. Morphology of right ventricle such as moderator band, apical attachment of AV valve, irregularity of the endocardial surface and a more triangle shape. Morphologic left ventricle is in right anterior and is connected to right atrium where it is characterized by smooth surface and elongated appearance with an Apex formation. Out flow tract shows pulmonary artery arising from right sided morphologic left ventricle and aorta from left sided right ventricle in parallel course with aorta anterior and left of the pulmonary artery. Here the PA arising from right sided ventricle has a course towards left side and aorta arising from left sided ventricle also courses towards left where as in DTGA aorta is coursing towards right side. Poor long-term prognosis is noted in ccTGA in association with Ebstein malformation of tricuspid valve, degree of TR, systemic right ventricular dysfunction and complete heart block. Survival rates exceeded 80% in prenatally diagnosed ccTGA when pregnancy was continued [53, 54].

Right aortic arch, double aortic arch and aberrant subclavian artery (ARSA):— Ultrasound findings in right aortic arch are: four chamber view shows descending aorta and is more centrally located. The detection and classification can be achieved in 3VT view where the aorta courses to right side of trachea. There are three subgroups: (1) right aortic arch with right ductus arteriosus (Rt V sign) here both the aorta and ductus arteriosus merges together on the right of trachea with a V configuration. There is mirror imaging branch pattern to normal left aortic arch noted. (2) Right aortic arch with left ductus arch (Usign): in this pattern, right-sided aorta with DA on to the left of trachea. Trachea is in between the DA and aorta (**Figure 10A** and **C**) in most of the cases it is associated with aberrant left subclavian artery. Arising from junction between ductus arteriosus and descending aorta called Kommerell diverticulum [55]. (3) Double aortic arch-aorta courses to right side of the trachea but bifurcates and one goes to left another one to right of trachea resembling Lambda configuration. Esophagus and trachea is entraped. Two vessels arise from each aortic arch.

Aberrant right subclavian artery (ARSA): in this, instead of three vessels, four vessels arises from left sided aortic arch from proximal to distal are right common carotid, left common carotid, left subclavian and ARSA. ARSA (**Figure 10B**) arises distally from aortic arch and courses towards left side of chest behind trachea and esophagus and to the right upper arm. This is also known as retrophayngeal right sub clavian artery or Lusorian artery. On 3VT ARSA is noted at the junction of aortic arch and ductus arteriosus with a course behind the trachea towards right shoulder. It may be isolated or commonly associated with conotruncal anomaly, 22q11microdeletion and trisomy 21.

Heterotaxy and situs inversus:-normal development and positioning of thoracic and abdominal organs is situs solitus. Situs inversus is mirror image arrangement of thoracic and abdominal viscera. Different arrangement of thoracic and abdominal viscera other than situs solitus and situs inversus is situs ambiguous or Heterotaxy syndrome or isomerism is characterized by an abnormal symmetry of the viscera that are normally dissimilar, which has different arrangement than situs solitus or situs inversus. This is due to abnormal lateralization of thoracic and abdominal viscera and is frequently associated with complex cardiac anomalies. Isomerism may be of right or left. Left isomerism (**Figure 11A**) the Ultrasound finding that strongly suggested in the presence of a combination of at least two of the following: (1) Viscerocardiac heterotaxy; (2) complete AVSD or other structural heart disease; (3) interruption of IVC with azygos continuation; (4) early fetal heart block; Right isomerism (**Figure 11B** and **C**) should be suspected in the presence of a combination of at least two of the following: (1) Viscerocardiac Heterotaxy, (2) structural heart disease, namely complete AVSD; (3) juxtaposition of IVC and descending aorta. If both interrupted IVC and complete heart block are observed, we can almost be sure that there is LAI. Left isomerism: bilateral left sidedness with maldevelopment of right-side structures. Morphologic left characteristics such as bilateral left bronchi, bilobed lungs, finger-like atrial appendages.

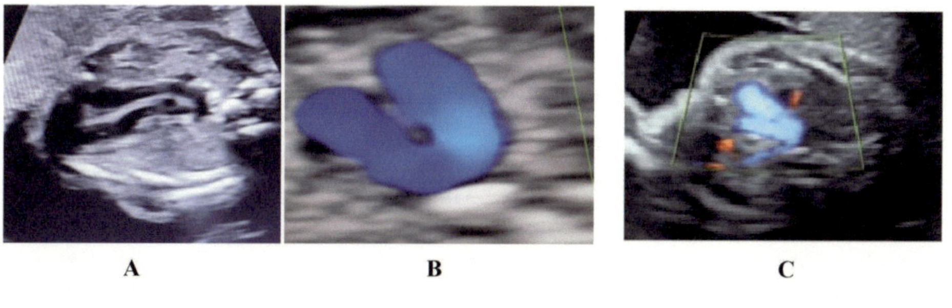

Figure 10.
(A) CCTGA with right aortic arch. (B) Right aortic arch with Usign. (C) ARSA coursing behind the trachea.

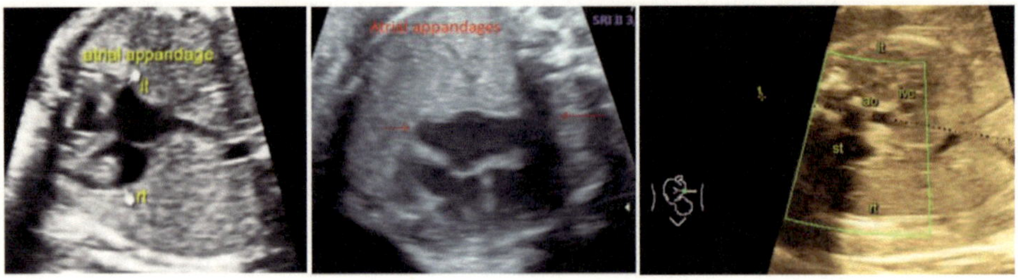

A B C

Figure 11.
(A) Left isomerism: finger like narrow bilateral symmetric left atrial appendages. (B) Broad pyramidal shaped symmetrical right atrial appendages in right isomerism. (C) Juxtaposition of aorta and IVC. Both on left side.

Inferior vena caval (IVC) interruption with azygous continuation, in which the hepatic segment of the inferior cava is absent, and the distal segment continues with the azygos or hemiazygos vein. A parasagittal view of abdomen and chest can demonstrate the azygose vein posterior to descending aorta. Color Doppler study shows opposite direction of flow in aorta and azygose vein noted. Right isomerism: bilateral structures with morphologic right characteristics, such as bilateral right atria, broad triangular atrial appendages, bilateral eparterial bronchi, and trilobed lungs. Ultrasound findings in right isomerism are Dextroversion is more common than left isomerism. More common cardiac anomaly associated are unbalanced AVSD and most of the times univentricular atrioventricular connection. TGA and DORV associated with pulmonary stenosis or atresia are associated commonly with right isomerism. Supracardiac TAPVC associated with right isomerism in 30%, infra diaphragmatic in 25% and cardiac in 30% and mixed in 15% observed. Visceral anomalies like malrotation and malfixation of the bowel, preduodenal portal vein, gastric volvulus, esophageal hiatal hernia, and biliary atresia are common in both left and right isomerism.

Situs inversus: in this, there will be mirror image arrangement of visceral organs in abdomen and thorax. Situs inversus associated cardiac anomalies are 0.3–5%in fetuses and newborn [56]. About 50% patients of Kartagener syndrome have situs inversus [57]. In situs inversus liver, IVC are on left side and spleen, stomach, heart and aorta are on right side.

Anomalies of systemic and pulmonary venous connections: they can occur as isolated or may be associated with simple cardiac anomalies like ASD and complex like Heterotaxy syndrome. Systemic venous malformation involves anomalies of IVC, SVC and coronary sinus. Persistent Left SVC (PLSVC) and interrupted IVC with azygos continuation are the most common systemic venous anomalies. The other rare venous malformation is abnormalities of ductus venosus, hepatic or umbilical veins.

PLSVC: it joins the coronary sinus on posterior left atrioventricular valve and drains to right atrium. On fetal echocardiography PLSVC (**Figure 12A**) appears as an extraneous vessel noted left to the ductal arch in three vessel trachea view. Very rarely PLSVC may be seen with absent right SVC (**Figure 12B**). Isolated PLSVC usually has no clinical significance. It is more commonly associated with other cardiac conditions (23% of PLSVC cases) They are Atrioventricular septal defect (AVSD), Double outlet right ventricle (DORV), Left out flow tract obstructive anomalies, Conotruncal anomalies and ventricular septal defect. The other Extra cardiac malformations including Heterotaxy syndrome (41–45%), Esophageal atresia, diaphragmatic hernia, IVC malformations, complex malformation syndromes

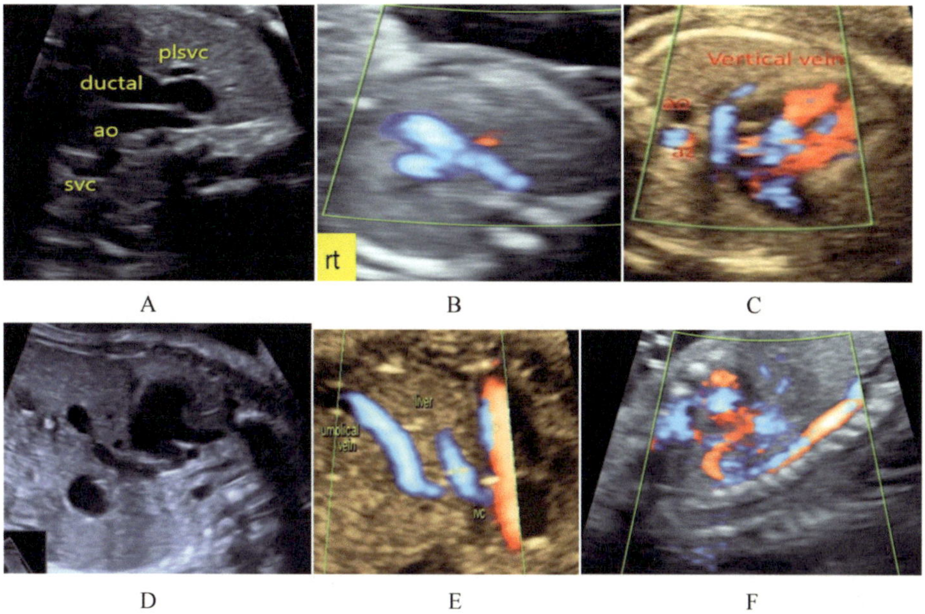

Figure 12.
(A) 3VTshowing 4vessels as in double SVC. (B) 3VT view showing 3 vessels in PLSVC with absent right SVC. (C) Supracardiac type of TAPVC. (D) Infra cardiac type of TAPVC with vertical vein coursing downwards. (E) Interrupted IVC-absent hepatic portion of IVC. (F) Azygos arch.

and chromosomal anomalies. Plane slightly inferior to four chamber view dilated coronary sinus can be noted. Normal diameter of coronary sinus is 1–3 mm; it courses perpendicular to inter atrial septum and opens into posterior wall of right atrium.

Interrupted IVC with azygos continuation: this is due to failure to form right subcardinal hepatic anastomosis results in absent hepatic segment of IVC (**Figure 12E** and **F**). The sonographic landmarks are dilated azygos vein alongside the Aorta in Abdominal circumference plane and four chamber view plane. In sagittal abdominal plane the descending Aorta and azygos vein run side by side with opposite direction of flow. Interrupted IVC has also been reported in isolated entity. In such cases it is clinically silent. It is more commonly associated about 80–90% with Left atrial isomerism.

Total Anomalous pulmonary connections (TAPVC) and partial anomalous connections (PAPVC): four pulmonary veins (PV) superior and inferior on both sides drains into posterior wall of left atrium. TAPVC involves all the pulmonary vein drains into right atrium directly or indirectly. Depending upon the anatomic site of anomalous connection four types of TAPVC noted 1supracardiac which is most common type, 2 cardiac, 3infra cardiac and mixed type [33]. Diagnosis is difficult prenatally. In a large series involving 424 cases with TAPVC only 8 were diagnosed prenatally. Ultrasound findings in four chamber view shows disproportion of right and left cardiac sizes with enlarged right sided chambers due to venous return. Area behind the heart in four chamber view plane shows increased distance between descending aorta and posterior wall of left atrium. There is no connection between pulmonary veins and left atrium. Which drains into the confluent vein or vertical vein. The confluent vein courses upward towards upper thorax drains into brachiocephalic vein in turn drains into Right atrium though SVC (**Figure 12C**). Vertical vein coursing downwards across the diaphragm in infra cardiac type (**Figure 12D**) or directly connects to right atrium or coronary sinus in cardiac type. In supra

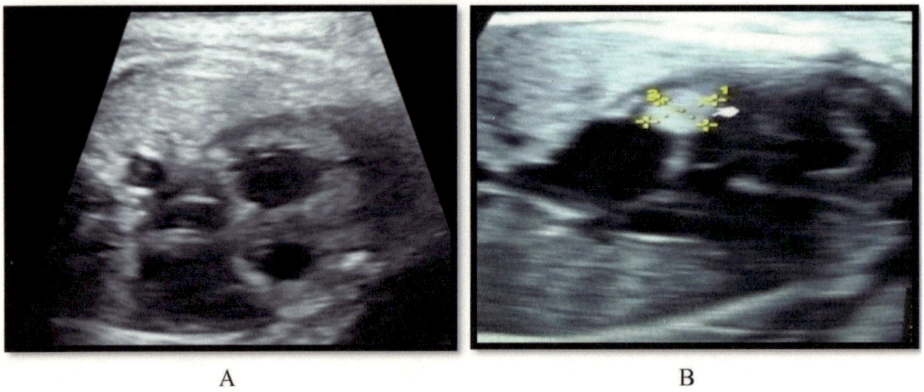

Figure 13.
(A) Hypertrophic cardiomyopathy. (B) Rhabdomyoma.

cardiac TAPVC at 3 vessel trachea view plane a fourth vessel i.e. vertical vein noted left of ductal arch. Blood flow in vertical vein in supra cardiac type flows superiorly towards upper thorax and there is dilated brachiocephalic vein noted. In cardiac type dilated coronary sinus in the absence of PLSVC should raise the suspicion of cardiac TAPVC. Infracardiac TAPVC the vertical vein formed behind the left ATRIA courses downwards along with esophagus through the diaphragm and drains into. portal veins. It is very difficult to see on routine gray scale ultrasound.in PAPVC difficult to detect and it is rarely reported prenatally. Scimitar syndrome: it is a combination of right lung hypoplasia, right pulmonary artery hypoplasia and PAPVC. In four chamber view, dextrocardia with right lung hypoplasia is noted. Right inferior pulmonary vein drains into IVC instead of left atrium.

Cardiomyopathies and fetal heart tumors: it is a disease of myocardium and is commonly associated with abnormal cardiac function. This can be manifested as dilated cardiomyopathy showing enlarged heart with dilated and decreased contractility or hypertrophic cardiomyopathy (**Figure 13A**) showing enlarged heart in association with ventricular wall hypertrophy. There may be reduced lumen of the effected ventricle. Mostly associated with diabetes mellitus. Pericardiac effusion is seen in cardiomyopathy. Heart tumors: 80–90% are rhabdomyomas (**Figure 13B**) but can also be teratoma, fibroma, myxoma, hamartoma, rhabdomyosarcoma and others. In Rhabdomyoma demonstrated in ultrasound as Ovale or circular well-defined echogenic mass. It may occur in the septum, wall or may be in the atrium and commonly associated with tuberous sclerosis.

Acknowledgements

The authors wish to express thanks to all parentages involved for giving permission to collect the presented data and also to Dr. Swapna Chouhan and Dr. D. Kamalakar Reddy, Shravya Diagnostics, for their contribution. Written informed consent was obtained from the pregnant women who participated in this study.

Author details

Madhavi Latha Routhu[1]* and Gudikandula Krishna[2]

1 Department of Radiology, MGM Hospital, Warangal, Telangana, India

2 Viral Research and Diagnostic Laboratory, Kakatiya Medical College, Warangal, Telangana, India

*Address all correspondence to: madhaviradiologist@gmail.com

References

[1] Hoffman JI, Christianson R. Congenital heart disease in a cohort of 19,502 births with long-term follow-up. The American Journal of Cardiology. 1978;**42**:641-647

[2] Benson DW. The genetics of congenital heart disease: A point in the revolution. Cardiology Clinics. 2002;**20**:385-394

[3] Fogel M, Copel JA, Cullen MT, et al. Congenital heart disease and fetal thoracoabdominal anomalies: Associations in utero and the importance of cytogenetic analysis. American Journal of Perinatology. 1991;**8**:411-416

[4] Friedman AH, Copel JA, Kleinman CS. Fetal echocardiography and fetal cardiology: Indications, diagnosis and management. Seminars in Perinatology. 1993;**17**:76-88

[5] Crawford DC, Chita SK, Allan LD. Prenatal detection of congenital heart disease: Factors affecting obstetric management and survival. American Journal of Obstetrics and Gynecology. 1988;**159**:352-356

[6] Bronshtein M, Gover A, Zimmer EZ. Sonographic definition of the fetal situs. Obstetrics and Gynecology. 2002;**99**:1129-1130

[7] Salomon LJ, Baumann C, Delezoide AL, et al. Abnormal abdominal situs: What and how should we look for? Prenatal Diagnosis. 2006;**26**:282-285

[8] Comstock CH. Normal fetal heart axis and position. Obstetrics and Gynecology. 1987;**70**:255-259

[9] Smith RS, Comstock CH, Kirk JS, et al. Ultrasonographic left cardiac axis deviation: A marker for fetal anomalies. Obstetrics and Gynecology. 1995;**85**:187-191

[10] Abuhamad AZ, Chaoui R. A Practical Guide to Fetal Echocardiography: Normal and Abnormal Hearts. Lippincott Williams & Wilkins; 2012

[11] Rubio AE, Lewin MB. Ventricular septal defects. In: Allen HD, Driscoll DJ, Shaddy RE, et al, editors. Moss and Adams' Heart Disease in Infants, Children, and Adolescents. 8th ed. Baltimore, MD: Williams & Wilkins; 2012. pp. 713-721

[12] Lincoln C, Jamieson S, Joseph M, et al. Transatrial repair of ventricular septal defects with reference to their anatomic classification. The Journal of Thoracic and Cardiovascular Surgery. 1977;**74**:183-190

[13] Soto B, Becker AE, Moulaert AJ, et al. Classification of ventricular septal defects. British Heart Journal. 1980;**43**:332-343

[14] Gomez O, Martinez JM, Olivella A, et al. Isolated ventricular septal defects in the era of advanced fetal echocardiography: Risk of chromosomal anomalies and spontaneous closure rate from diagnosis to age of 1 year. Ultrasound in Obstetrics & Gynecology. 2014;**43**:65-71

[15] Ferencz C, Rubin JD, Loffredo CA, et al. Epidemiology of congenital heart disease: The Baltimore-Washington infant study. In: Perspectives in Pediatric Cardiology. Mount Kisko, NY: Futura Publishing; 1981-1989. p. 1993

[16] Cetta F, Minich LL, Maleszewski JJ, et al. Atrioventricular septal defects. In: Allen HD, Driscoll DJ, Shaddy RE, et al, editors. Moss and Adams' Heart Disease in Infants, Children, and Adolescents.

8th ed. Baltimore, MD: Williams & Wilkins; 2012. pp. 691-712

[17] Allan LD, Sharland GK, Milburn A, et al. Prospective diagnosis of 1,006 consecutive cases of congenital heart disease in the fetus. Journal of the American College of Cardiology. 1994;**23**:1452-1458

[18] Machlitt A, Heling KS, Chaoui R. Increased cardiac atrial-to-ventricular length ratio in the fetal four-chamber view: A new marker for atrioventricular septal defects. Ultrasound in Obstetrics & Gynecology. 2004;**24**:618-622

[19] Delisle MF, Sandor GG, Tessier F, et al. Outcome of fetuses diagnosed with atrioventricular septal defect. Obstetrics and Gynecology. 1999;**94**:763-767

[20] Corsten-Janssen N, Kerstjens-Frederikse WS, du MarchieSarvaas GJ, et al. The cardiac phenotype in patients with a CHD7 mutation. Circulation. Cardiovascular Genetics. 2013;**6**:248-254

[21] Aubert S, Henaine R, Raisky O, et al. Atypical forms of isolated partial atrioventricular septal defect increase the risk of initial valve replacement and reoperation. European Journal of Cardio-Thoracic Surgery. 2005;**28**:223-228

[22] Studer M, Blackstone EH, Kirklin JW, et al. Determinants of early and late results of repair of atrioventricular septal (canal) defects. The Journal of Thoracic and Cardiovascular Surgery. 1982;**84**:523-542

[23] Allan LD, Crawford DC, Chita SK, et al. Familial recurrence of congenital heart disease in a prospective series of mothers referred for fetal echocardiography. The American Journal of Cardiology. 1986;**58**:334-337

[24] Nora JJ, Berg K, Nora AH. Cardiovascular Diseases: Genetics, Epidemiology, and Prevention. New York, NY: Oxford University Press; 1991

[25] Hornberger LK, Sahn DJ, Kleinman CS, et al. Antenatal diagnosis of coarctation of the aorta: A multicenter experience. Journal of the American College of Cardiology. 1994;**23**:417-423

[26] Paladini D, Volpe P, Russo MG, et al. Aortic coarctation: Prognostic indicators of survival in the fetus. Heart. 2004;**90**:1348-1349

[27] Brown DL, Durfee SM, Hornberger LK. Ventricular discrepancy as a sonographic sign of coarctation of the fetal aorta: How reliable is it? Journal of Ultrasound in Medicine. 1997;**16**:95-99

[28] Sharland GK, Chan KY, Allan LD. Coarctation of the aorta: Difficulties in prenatal diagnosis. British Heart Journal. 1994;**71**:70-75

[29] Chaoui R, Heling KS, Lopez AS, et al. The thymic-thoracic ratio in fetal heart defects: A simple way to identify fetuses at high risk for microdeletion 22q11. Ultrasound in Obstetrics & Gynecology. 2011;**37**:397-403

[30] Chaoui R, Kalache KD, Heling KS, et al. Absent or hypoplastic thymus on ultrasound: A marker for deletion 22q11.2 in fetal cardiac defects. Ultrasound in Obstetrics & Gynecology. 2002;**20**:546-552

[31] Volpe P, Marasini M, Caruso G, et al. Prenatal diagnosis of interruption of the aortic arch and its association with deletion of chromosome 22q11. Ultrasound in Obstetrics & Gynecology. 2002;**20**:327-331

[32] Van Mierop LH, Kutsche LM. Cardiovascular anomalies in DiGeorge

syndrome and importance of neural crest as a possible pathogenetic factor. The American Journal of Cardiology. 1986;**58**:133-137

[33] Uretzky G, Puga FJ, Danielson GK, et al. Complete atrioventricular canal associated with tetralogy of Fallot. Morphologic and surgical considerations. The Journal of Thoracic and Cardiovascular Surgery. 1984;**87**:756-766

[34] Rao BN, Anderson RC, Edwards JE. Anatomic variations in the tetralogy of Fallot. American Heart Journal. 1971;**81**:361-371

[35] Poon LC, Huggon IC, Zidere V, et al. Tetralogy of Fallot in the fetus in the current era. Ultrasound in Obstetrics & Gynecology. 2007;**29**:625-627

[36] Bharati S, Paul MH, Idriss FS, et al. The surgical anatomy of pulmonary atresia with ventricular septal defect: Pseudotruncus. The Journal of Thoracic and Cardiovascular Surgery. 1975;**69**:713-721

[37] Vesel S, Rollings S, Jones A, et al. Prenatally diagnosed pulmonary atresia with ventricular septal defect: Echocardiography, genetics, associated anomalies and outcome. Heart. 2006;**92**:1501-1505

[38] Boudjemline Y, Fermont L, Le Bidois J, et al. Prevalence of 22q11 deletion in fetuses with conotruncal cardiac defects: A 6-year prospective study. The Journal of Pediatrics. 2001;**138**:520-524

[39] Wertaschnigg D, Jaeggi M, Chitayat D, et al. Prenatal diagnosis and outcome of absent pulmonary valve syndrome: Contemporary single-center experience and review of the literature. Ultrasound in Obstetrics & Gynecology. 2013;**41**:162-167

[40] Sharland G. Common arterial trunk. In: Allan LD, Hornberger LK, Sharland GK, editors. Textbook of Fetal Cardiology. London, England: Greenwich Medical Media; 2000. pp. 288-303

[41] Volpe P, Paladini D, Marasini M, et al. Common arterial trunk in the fetus: Characteristics, associations, and outcome in a multicentre series of 23 cases. Heart. 2003;**89**:1437-1441

[42] Machlitt A, Tennstedt C, Korner H, et al. Prenatal diagnosis of 22q11 microdeletion in an early second-trimesterfetus with conotruncal anomaly presenting with increased nuchal translucency and bilateral intracardiac echogenic foci. Ultrasound in Obstetrics & Gynecology. 2002;**19**:510-513

[43] Sridaromont S, Feldt RH, Ritter DG, et al. Double outlet right ventricle: Hemodynamic and anatomic correlations. The American Journal of Cardiology. 1976;**38**:85-94

[44] Bradley TJ, Karamlou T, Kulik A, et al. Determinants of repair type, reintervention, and mortality in 393 children with double-outlet right ventricle. The Journal of Thoracic and Cardiovascular Surgery. 2007;**134** 967-973.e6

[45] Obler D, Juraszek AL, Smoot LB, et al. Double outlet right ventricle: Aetiologies and associations. Journal of Medical Genetics. 2008;**45**:481-497

[46] Chaoui R, Korner H, Bommer C, et al. Prenatal diagnosis of heart defects and associated chromosomal aberrations [in German]. Ultraschall in der Medizin. 1999;**20**:177-184

[47] Becker TA, Van Amber R, Moller JH, et al. Occurrence of cardiac malformations in relatives of children with transposition of the great arteries. American Journal of Medical Genetics. 1996;**66**:28-32

[48] Atallah J, Rutledge JM, Dyck JD. Congenitally corrected transposition of the great arteries (atrioventricular and ventriculoarterial discordance). In: Allen HD, Driscoll DJ, Shaddy RE, et al, editors. Moss and Adams' Heart Disease in Infants, Children, and Adolescents. 8th ed. Baltimore, MD: Williams & Wilkins; 2012. pp. 1147-1160

[49] Paladini D, Volpe P, Marasini M, et al. Diagnosis, characterization and outcome of congenitally corrected transposition of the great arteries in the fetus: A multicenter series of 30 cases. Ultrasound in Obstetrics & Gynecology. 2006;**27**:281-285

[50] Sharland G, Tingay R, Jones A, et al. Atrioventricular and ventriculoarterial discordance (congenitally corrected transposition of the great arteries): Echocardiographic features, associations, and outcome in 34 fetuses. Heart. 2005;**91**:1453-1458

[51] Chaoui R, Schneider MB, Kalache KD. Right aortic arch with vascular ring and aberrant left subclavian artery: Prenatal diagnosis assisted by three-dimensional power Doppler ultrasound. Ultrasound in Obstetrics & Gynecology. 2003;**22**:661-663

[52] DeVore GR, Sarti DA, Siassi B, et al. Prenatal diagnosis of cardiovascular malformations in the fetus with situs inversus viscerum during the second trimester of pregnancy. Journal of Clinical Ultrasound. 1986;**14**:454-457

[53] Bush A, Cole P, Hariri M, et al. Primary ciliary dyskinesia: Diagnosis and standards of care. The European Respiratory Journal. 1998;**12**:982-988

[54] Holzmann D, Ott PM, Felix H. Diagnostic approach to primary ciliary dyskinesia: A review. European Journal of Pediatrics. 2000;**159**:95-98

[55] Yoo SJ, Friedberg MK, Jaeggi E. Abnormal visceral and atrial situs and congenital heart disease. In: Yagel S, Gembruch U, Silverman N, editors. Fetal Cardiology: Embryology, Genetics, Physiology, Echocardiographic Evaluation, Diagnosis and Perinatal Management of Cardiac Diseases. New York, NY: Informa Healthcare; 2008. pp. 347-362

[56] Brown DW, Geva T. Anomalies of the pulmonary veins. In: Allen HD, Driscoll DJ, Shaddy RE, et al, editors. Moss and Adams' Heart Disease in Infants, Children, and Adolescents. 8th ed. Baltimore, MD: Williams & Wilkins; 2012. pp. 809-839

[57] Seale AN, Carvalho JS, Gardiner HM, et al. Total anomalous pulmonary venous connection: Impact of prenatal diagnosis. Ultrasound in Obstetrics & Gynecology. 2012;**40**:310-318

Chapter 7

Endocarditis and Cardiac Device Infections

Amparo Benedicto and Lourdes Domínguez

Abstract

The growing number of electronic intracardiac devices (pacemakers, resynchronizers and defibrillators) and non-electronic devices (percutaneous occluders) implanted, combined with certain common characteristics in the treated population (underlying heart disease, advanced age, kidney disease, multiple associated pathologies), have led to a change in the spectrum of presentation of endocarditis, with an increase in cases related to these devices. These infections pose diagnostic and therapeutic challenges due to the complexity of the patients, the microorganisms involved –who frequently generate the formation of biofilm- and the percutaneous or surgical techniques involved in the removal of material. All these circumstances require a multidisciplinary approach.

Keywords: endocarditis, cardiac implantable electronic device (CIED), infection, biofilm, prophylaxis

1. Introduction

Endocarditis is defined as the inflammation of the endothelium. The first case of endocarditis was described by Lazare Rivière in the seventeenth century. Since then, the clinical, etiological, epidemiological and therapeutic knowledge around it has expanded remarkably. Nevertheless, it is a complex disease in constant evolution that requires a multidisciplinary approach. Most endocarditis has an infectious cause of bacterial origin. Being a disease of the endocardium, it not only affects native structures -more frequently the valves or cardiac structures subjected to special hemodynamic conditions such as in congenital heart disease-, but also other endothelizable surfaces, such as valve prostheses, catheters, electrodes, or percutaneous devices.

In this chapter we will address endocarditis on Cardiac Implantable Electronic Devices (CIED).

2. Endocarditis and cardiac implantable electronic devices (CIED) with leads

2.1 Epidemiology

Infective endocarditis is a serious disease, whose incidence, despite therapeutic advances, remains relatively stable (although data regarding countries with low health resources are scarce). In developed countries, its incidence is estimated at 1 per 1000 hospital admissions and 1.5–9.6 cases per 100000 inhabitants [1, 2]. While in countries with limited resources it continues to be closely related to rheumatic valve disease, in developed countries it is fundamentally related to degenerative valve disease, valve prostheses and CIED. The use of implantable cardiac electronic devices (pacemakers [PM], implantable cardioverter-defibrillators [ICD], cardiac re-synchronized therapy [CRT]) has increased by 4.7% annually between 1993 and 2009 with a growth of 96% in the entire period. The number of implanted pacemakers increased by 55.6% (especially bicameral), while that of defibrillators did so by 504% [3, 4]. Such increase is due to a number of factors: the aging of the population, the complexity of their pathologies, the new indications and the advance in implantation techniques. However, the growth of infections associated with these devices has raised disproportionately and is estimated at 210% between 1993 and 2008 [4, 5].

2.2 Classification of CIED infections

- **Post-operative wound inflammation:** occurs within 30 days of implantation, with wound inflammation or 'stitch abscess', in the absence of definite evidence of infection and not necessarily requiring antimicrobial therapy (possible skin reaction to dressings, sutures or antiseptics) [6].

- **Uncomplicated generator infection:** cellulitis confined to the generator site, including purulent discharge, abscess, fistula or device erosion in the absence of systemic involvement, and negative blood cultures.

- **Complicated generator infection**: generator infection plus involvement of any part of the lead or development of systemic involvement (signs or symptoms or positive blood cultures).

- Lead infection.

    - Definite:

        a. Symptoms/signs of systemic infection, NO signs of generator pocket infection AND echocardiography consistent with vegetation(s) attached to lead(s) AND presence of major Duke microbiological criteria.

        b. Symptoms/signs of systemic infection, NO signs of generator pocket infection AND culture, histology or molecular evidence of infection on explanted lead.

    - Possible.

        a. Symptoms/signs of systemic infection AND echocardiography consistent with vegetation(s) attached to lead(s), BUT NO major Duke microbiological criteria present.

        b. Symptoms/signs of systemic infection AND major Duke microbiological criteria present, BUT NO echocardiographic evidence of lead vegetations.

        c. Pulmonary emboli are considered supportive evidence of lead infection in the absence of definite evidence of infection.

- CIED -associated native or prosthetic valve endocarditis.

Duke criteria for definite endocarditis satisfied, with echocardiographic evidence of valve involvement in a patient with an CIED in situ.

The last two forms are considered by the European Society of Cardiology (ESC) as endocarditis related to CIEDs, and we will now focus on them, not forgetting that they coexist with local infection of the generator pocket in up to 10–50% of cases (although in some recent series, the figure is closer to 10%, which suggests that causative microorganism reached PM leads by haematogenic way in a high proportion of case) [7].

Different epidemiological studies, with follow-up ranging from 6 weeks to 11 years, estimate the incidence of CDI-related infection at 2% [6, 8], although the figures are highly variable depending on the criteria used (0–6% and up to 19% if intra-abdominal devices are included) [9]. Between 10 and 23% of these infections meet the criteria for endocarditis [2, 7, 10].

A study in 7424 patients who underwent a pacemaker and/or ICD device implantation demonstrated an increasing incidence of IE in pacemakers [7]. It represented almost 10% with an increment from 1.25 to 9.32% of all IE between the period 1987–1993 compared to the period 2008–2013. Another prospective cohort study, using data from the International Collaboration on Endocarditis–Prospective Cohort Study (ICE-PCS), conducted from June 2000 through August 2006 in 61 centers in 28 countries, found that cardiac device infective endocarditis accounted for 6.4% of all cases of definite infective endocarditis [11].

2.3 Risk factors

Several studies have identified the following risk factors for the development of infection on CIED [2, 7, 8, 11–13]:

Factors associated with the patient: Several of them coexist in up to 50% of patients [7].

- Age, probably a confounding factor due to the higher number of comorbidities.
- Male sex.
- Diabetes Mellitus.
- Renal insufficiency.
- Other comorbidities such as heart failure or (chronic obstructive pulmonary disease (COPD).
- Neoplasia.
- Use of corticosteroids.
- States of immunosuppression.

Factors associated with the procedure

- Non-first implant: Infection is more frequent in replacement or update procedures (1–4%) than in first implantation (0.5–0.8%) The risk of CIED infection is much greater after generator change or device revision. It has been suggested that this is related to bacterial contamination of the avascular pocket that is formed around the generator, which may impede penetration of systemic antimicrobials and inflammatory cells during generator replacement. For this reason, some operators advocate the removal of the capsule in battery replacement.

- Shaving the skin with a blade (risk of disruption of the skin barrier).
- Poor preparation of the skin.
- Not using antibiotic prophylaxis.
- Fever in the previous 48 hours.
- Hematoma.
- Number of electrodes and complexity of the procedure.
- Duration of the procedure.
- Operator experience.

Factors related to other procedures and health care

- Previously carrying a transvenous transitory pacemaker.
- Invasive procedures related to health care (nosocomial and non-nosocomial) and or hospitalization, which may produce bacteremia leading to CIED infection, were identified in the previous 6 months in about 45–50% of the IE-ICED [7–11].

2.4 Physiopathology and etiology

According to estimates from the U.S Food and Drug Administration (FDA) and the European trade association representing the medical technology industries, (MedTech Europe), more than 500000 types of medical devices have currently entered the global market. Invasive medical devices, including indwelling and implantable devices, represent just a fraction of these [14, 15]. More than a million cardiovascular electronic devices are implanted worldwide each year [16]. Devices used in cardiovascular surgery and interventionism are inserted into the body tissues by breaching the skin or mucous membranes. No matter where the surgically invasive device is placed, it is a foreign body. Even a mild tissue response alters the local immune defenses, creating a "locus minoris resistentiae", which is vulnerable to bacterial attack. Especially the devices in contact with the bloodstream, can potentially cause sepsis.

CIED infection, can have a local or a distant origin.

2.4.1 Local origin

Human skin is very resistant to infection. This resistance is due to physical (thickness, exfoliation), chemical (pH, secretions) and immunological (cellular and humoral) factors.

The resident flora is also an important factor. This flora is made up of bacteria that live attached to the skin and under normal circumstances, they do not cause infection and prevent the proliferation of other strains as well. When the skin barrier is broken, the entry of microorganisms from the adjacent skin is facilitated. Most infections from these devices are caused by coagulase negative staphylococci

(CoNS), which are the most common microorganisms in the normal flora of the upper part of the skin of the thorax (especially *Staphylococcus epidermidis*). *Staphylococcus aureus* is not part of this resident flora, but it can become a persistent colonizer of the nasal mucosa, pharynx, and skin, especially in kidney patients, diabetics, some skin diseases, and hospital workers.

Phases of infection

- **Colonization** of the CIED pocket by microorganisms from the surgical equipment (air or personnel) or more frequently from the patient's own skin. Disinfection reduces the number of bacterial colonies, but in the presence of a foreign body, the inoculum to produce an infection is lower. The susceptibility of surgically invasive devices to bacterial colonization is due to reduced effectiveness of human immune defenses at the implant–tissue interface [12]. The longer the procedure, the higher the rate of colonization of the surgical sites.

However, colonization is not synonymous with infection, since it must occur: Adhesion and BIOFILM formation (**Figure 1**) [13, 14].
Biofilm formation occurs in five steps:

- *Initial reversible anchoring* of bacteria in "planktonic" or "free" form to surfaces by unspecific forces.

- *Irreversible anchorage*: Once anchored, a bacterial monolayer will begin to form and an extracellular protective matrix composed of extracellular polysaccharides, extracellular proteins, cellular debris and nucleic acids will begin to be produced. Both, along with the collagen and fibrinogen deposited in damaged tissues and on biomaterials, favors the anchorage of bacteria with specific receptors. The formation of hematomas facilitates this process.

- *Maturation:* the development of a biofilm favors the growth of the colonies, with a complex three-dimensional framework and a great resistance to antibiotics. Sometimes different bacterial species can coexist in the same biofilm. There are complex genetic interactions between the bacteria in these biolayers known as "quorum sensing".

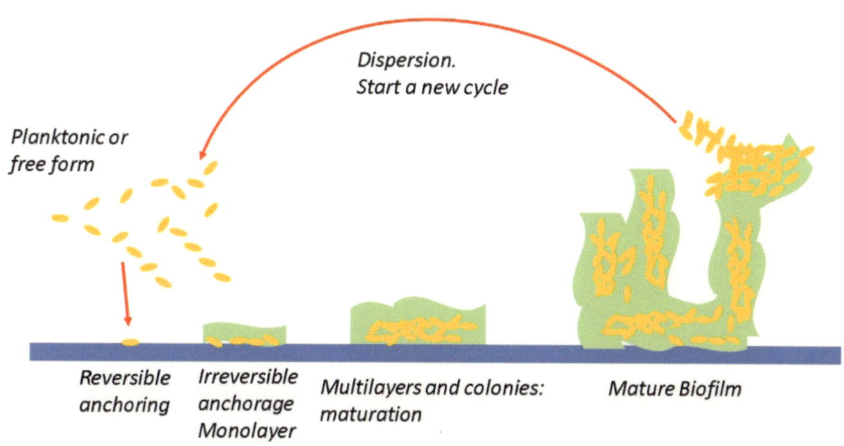

Figure 1.
BIOFILM formation.

- *Dispersion.* In the last step, some cells of the mature biofilm begin to dissociate and disperse again through the environment as planktonic cells to start a new cycle and thus the infection is dispersed.

2.4.2 Remote origin

During the early post-implant period, damage to the vascular wall and the formation of hematomas can favor the settlement of germs from the bloodstream in the implant area; thus, it is very important to avoid the development of bacteremia by removing unnecessary intravascular and urinary catheters.

The infection can spread to the endovascular structures, during the healing and resorption phases of hematomas, from the pacemaker pocket.

Conversely, and generally later, endovascular elements (electrodes) can present fibrin and platelet deposits on erosions produced by friction, deterioration or turbulent flows, on which bacterial colonies can settle and proliferate in a process similar to that of endocarditis, which can also spread to the adjacent endocardium.

Concomitant valve involvement is estimated in about 37.2% of cases, most frequently tricuspid valve [11], aortic or mitral valve vegetations are present in 10–15% of patients with CIED endocarditis and valve involvement in CIED infection is associated with higher in-hospital mortality.

As previously mentioned, between 40 and 50% of patients with CIED have a history of admission, manipulation or invasive procedure in the previous 6 months, potentially responsible for bacteremia. The risk is especially high when the bacteremia is due to *Staphylococcus aureus* (35–45%) [6].

In any case, given that many "presumed local" infections can progress to the intravascular components of the device and vice versa, the barrier between local and endovascular infection can be difficult to establish. Once the generator or proximal leads have eroded through the skin, a device should be considered infected, whatever the mechanism that caused the erosion.

2.5 Microbiology

Gram-positive bacteria are responsible for the vast majority of CIED infections (68–93%). Staphylococci, account for 60–80% of cases. Depending on the series, there is a predominance of infections caused by S Aureus or coagulase-negative staphylococcus (CoNS), although with few differences in their prevalence. Among the CoNS, *Staphylococcus epidermidis* and Staphylococcus Saprophyticus stand out. Methicillin resistance (MR) among Staphylococci varies among studies A high rate of MR in CoNS is associated with a healthcare environment source, reaching 50% in some series. For S aureus the rates of MR range between 2.6% (Germany) and 55% (USA). Gram-negative bacteria (GNB) are also identified in a percentage close to 15%. The higher proportion of GNB may be due to the large rate of different comorbidities, which is associated to more frequent invasive diagnosis or treatment measures. Polymicrobial infection sometimes involves more than one species of CoNS, (2–24% according to series). In a percentage between 8 and 15%, it was not possible to cultivate the responsible germ. Cases related to fungi are anecdotal [5, 6, 17–19].

2.6 Diagnosis

The diagnosis of IE-CEID, as in valve prostheses, is inconclusive in up to 30% of cases, according to the Duke criteria [20]. For this reason, in the guidelines published by the European Society of Cardiology in 2015, three additional criteria were proposed to increase sensitivity in diagnosis [19].

In any case, the IE-CEID diagnosis is based on three points [19, 21].

2.6.1 Clinical presentation

The clinical manifestations of IE-CIED can be variable, since it can combine signs and symptoms of local infection, with symptoms and signs of systemic infection.

When there is involvement of the pacemaker pocket, diagnosis can be easier since there will be typical signs of inflammation, such as pain, redness and increased temperature in the implantation area. In addition, there may be an increase in size, either due to the presence of hematoma related to the implant (which should alert to an increased risk of infection) or fluctuation due to the formation of pus, adhesion of the skin as well as spontaneous and sometimes intermittent pus drainage due to dehiscence of the suture or fistulization of the skin (**Figure 2**).

Any exteriorized device should be considered infected (although initial exteriorization was related to aseptic necrosis of the skin due to tension of the device in a small pocket).

Once the pocket is infected, the electrodes are frequently affected in its subcutaneous and extravascular portion, and affect the intravascular portion as well. When there is involvement of the intravascular components, that is, endocarditis of the leads and vascular part of the system, signs and symptoms of systemic infection will appear, with fever, chills, asthenia and anorexia. These data can appear larvae and in the absence of associated involvement of the pacemaker pocket, they can be more difficult to interpret. In a low percentage of patients, signs and symptom of frank sepsis will appear. In case of associated valvular involvement, data of valvular dysfunction and heart failure may also appear.

Clinical manifestations related to septic lung embolism may also appear from vegetations of the PM leads or tricuspid valve.

Among laboratory results data, the acute phase reactants (C-reactive protein, increased sedimentation rate, leukocytosis and procalcitonin) increase. Although these alterations point us towards a systemic infection, acute phase reactants can also appear in local infections.

Regarding the chronology of infections, several aspects must be taken into account:

- In the first 30 days, skin or exudate or superficial erythema may appear in relation to infection of the suture or allergic reaction,
- Depending on the responsible germ, the temporary clinical course may vary. In the case of S Aureus infections, parturition is usually earlier and

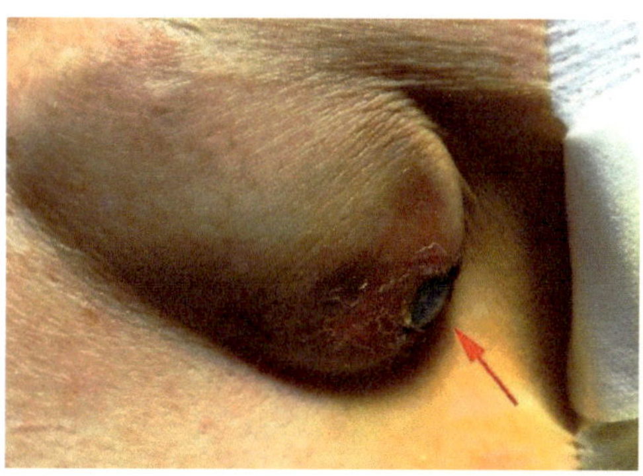

Figure 2.
Exteriorized device.

the progression to systemic disease faster than in the case of germs such as S Epidermidis or *Propionibacterium acnes*, in which it can be latent and even reactivate late with delayed handling.

2.6.2 Microbiological evidence

We have already discussed the main agents involved, now we will address how and when microbiological samples should be collected and processed. Appropriate microbiological samples include: culture of blood, lead fragments (ideally distal and proximal), lead vegetation (proximal and distal tips), generator pocket tissue and pus from a generator pocket wound.

Blood sample extraction [6, 21].

- Should be collected as soon as possible, and whenever possible before starting antibiotic treatment.

- Collection of multiple samples increases diagnostic sensitivity: three sets of aseptically collected, optimally filled blood cultures should be taken from peripheral sites with ≥6 h between them, especially in patients with non-acute presentation.

- To avoid an undesirable delay in patients with suspected IE-CIED and severe sepsis or septic shock at the time of presentation, two sets of optimally filled blood cultures should ideally be taken at different times within 1 h and prior to the start of empirical antimicrobial therapy.

- Follow -up blood cultures should be obtained 48 to 72 h after antimicrobial therapy is begun, and every 48–72 hours until clearance of bacteremia is documented.

- Blood cultures should be taken 48–72 h after removal of an infected CIED.

Regarding blood culture, the following considerations must be taken into account:

- In a variable percentage, around 10%, it will not be possible to grow any microorganism.

- The interpretation of a single positive culture for an organism, common contaminant of the skin flora, should not be interpreted systematically as bacteremia and should be evaluated within the overall clinical context.

- In case of bacteremia originated at a clear distant infectious focus (abdominal, urinary, respiratory) and due to germs that do not frequently cause endocarditis on devices (enterobacteria, pneumococci), affectation of the device should not be assumed unless proven otherwise.

- All cultured samples must be processed in different culture media and in specific media for slow-growing organisms.

- When interpreting the results of the cultured electrodes, it should be considered their potential contamination when extracted through the explant area.

- To the contrary, in the presence of remote bacteremia by S Aureus, the risk of device infection is very high (35–45%).

2.6.3 Imaging

Different imaging techniques are used for the diagnosis of IE – CIED and, therefore, we will speak of Multimodal imaging when referring to them [21, 22].

First line technique, due to its availability and safety, is echocardiography. Initially, an echocardiogram should be performed in all patients with CIED infection, either local or systemic. Transthoracic echocardiogram (TTE) will allow us to globally assess all the structures of the heart as well as their function (**Figure 3**). Despite the advantage of the proximity of the right cavities to the thoracic wall, the presence of metallic electrodes generates artifacts that make it difficult to assess associated vegetations. Occasionally, images compatible with vegetations can be identified, associated with the electrodes, the valves or the endocardium; although their absence does not exclude the diagnosis, since sensitivity is low.

Regardless of the result of the TTE, a Transesophageal echocardiography (TOE) should be performed in all patients with CIED infection suspected of systemic involvement, and probably in carriers of intracardiac devices in the presence of S Aureus bacteremia (**Figure 4**). Even though the sensitivity is higher than in ETT, it is still less than 100% in the case of devices. The reasons for the low sensitivity include: the small part visualized of the cava, the difficulty to assess electrodes in the coronary sinus, or the lesser proximity to the transducer. Three-dimensional (3D) echo, if available, can provide information about vegetation's morphology and size (**Figure 5**). On the other hand, there are images that are difficult to interpret as they may correspond to fibrin strands or small thrombi adhering to the surface of the leads, more frequent in the right cavities due to a slower flow.

In some centers, intracardiac echo (ICE) is also used for the diagnosis of vegetations based on electrodes, with greater sensitivity for the detection of vegetations in the case of high suspicion without diagnostic images. As drawbacks, it is an invasive and expensive technique [23].

In the case of uncertain diagnosis and high suspicion of endocarditis in the absence of diagnostic criteria or doubts about the extent of a local infection,

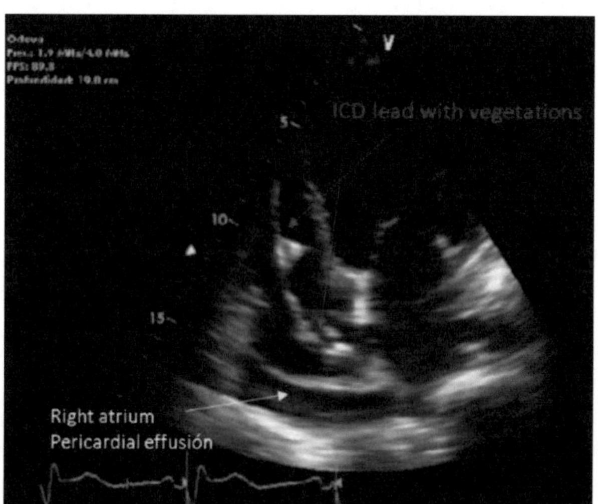

Figure 3.
Lead vegetation TTE.

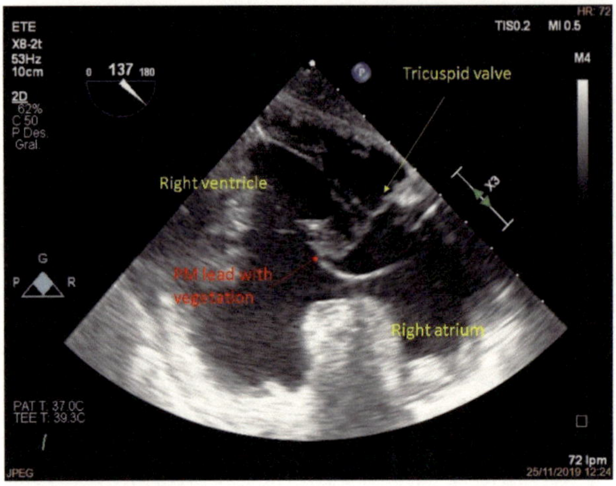

Figure 4.
Lead vegetation TOE.

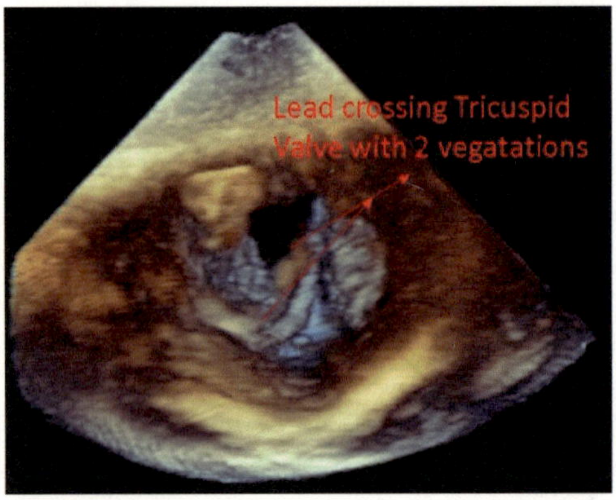

Figure 5.
Lead vegetation 3D echo.

Nuclear Medicine or hybrid technique can be used, based on the detection of metabolic or inflammatory activity.

Positron Emission Tomography-CT (PET-CT) is generally performed using a single acquisition (generally at 1 h) after administration of 18F-FDG, which is actively incorporated in vivo by activated leucocytes, monocytes, macrophages and CD4+ T-lymphocytes accumulating at the sites of infection. Its limitations are the low resolution for foci smaller than 5 mm, its price, the high radiation and the early post-implant or post-surgery period, since the isotope uptake can occur in any inflamed tissue or with metabolic activity, including thrombi and tumors. Sensibility of this test it is estimated around 87% and its specificity around 94% (**Figures 6** and 7).

Scintigraphy (SPECT) with labeled leukocytes can be combined with CT. Compared to PET-CT, it has the disadvantages of a lower availability, a longer duration -since it requires 2 separate acquisitions (2 and 24 hours)- and the use of blood products. On the other hand, it is cheaper, has greater utility in the post-implantation/postoperative period, exposes less radiation and a greater specificity is reported, close to 100% (except for non-pyogenic agents such as Candida or Coxiella, rarely implicated in CIED infection) [24, 25].

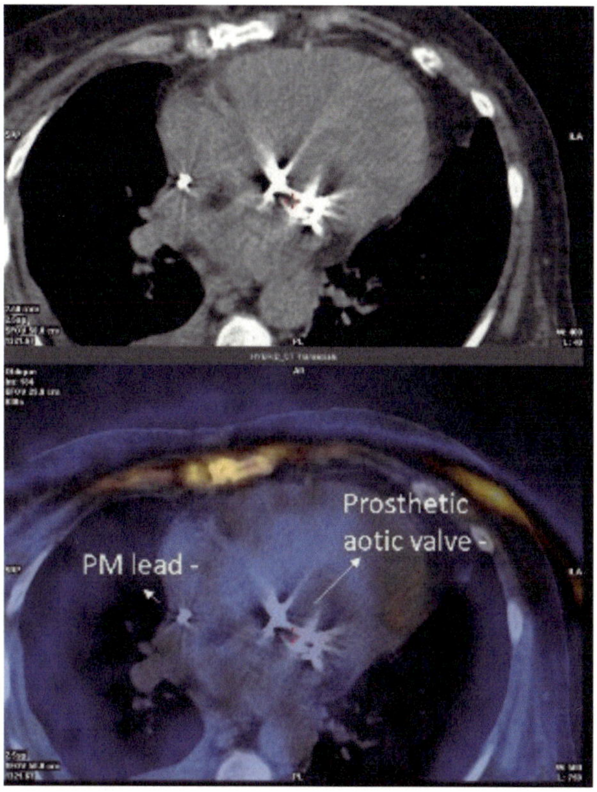

Figure 6.
PET-TAC-.

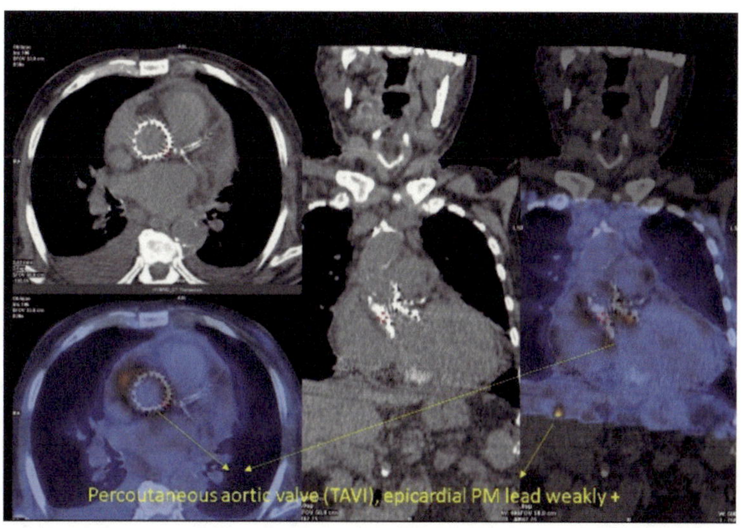

Figure 7.
PET-TAC+.

Beyond imaging techniques focused on evaluating of vegetations and inflammatory activity, a chest radiograph in 2 projections or even a CT should be performed to assess the type of device (sometimes unknown), the presence of breakage, torsion or dislocation of the electrodes or the generator displacement, and to assess the pulmonary parenchyma as there may be images suggestive of septic embolism or infectious pulmonary involvement (**Figure 8**).

2.7 Prevention and prophylaxis

Before addressing the treatment of IE-CIED we will discuss how to prevent infectious complications.

2.7.1 General measures

Any implant procedure must be performed following the usual aseptic surgical standards. Additionally, it is recommended to adhere to the following guidelines:

- Carry out the procedure in an appropriate place, with adequate ventilation. The air requirements specified for cardiac catheterization laboratories (15 air changes/hour) are less than the 25 air changes/hour recommended for the operating room [6].

- Do not shave the skin with blades. When trimming hair, shave with a single-use electric head or with depilatory cream, before the procedure and outside the implant room [6, 30].

- Prepare the skin with an alcoholic solution of chlorhexidine (minimum 2%) or as an alternative for allergic individuals, use povidone iodine in alcohol [6, 18, 27–29].

- Avoid unnecessarily long procedures, best if performed by a first operator or an experienced supervisor [6, 11, 26, 30].

- Carry out a correct hemostasis to avoid the formation of hematoma. In the case of anticoagulated patients in whom anticoagulation should not be interrupted, do not use bridging therapy with heparin and look for an INR close to 2. Individualize treatment in the rest of antiplatelet or anticoagulated patients. Local thrombin solutions can be considered to facilitate hemostasis [18, 26].

- Do not perform procedures in patients with suspected active infection or fever in the past 48 hours [6, 11, 18].

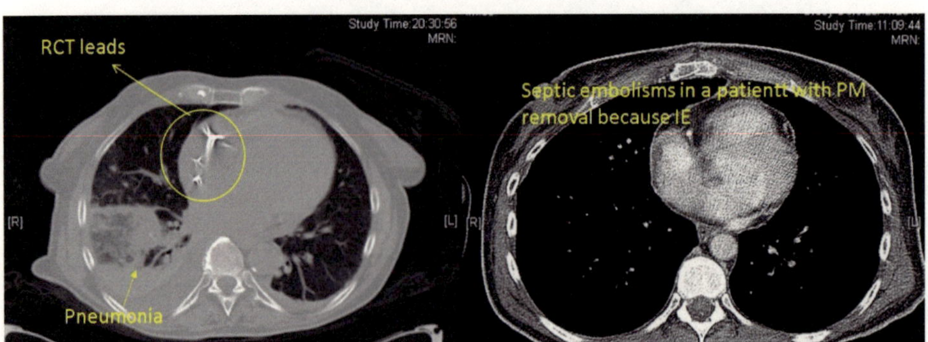

Figure 8.
Pulmonary infectious involvement in IE-CIED. TC.

- Consider the subpectoral implantation in malnourished or very thin patients [18, 26, 30].

2.7.2 Antibiotic prophylaxis

Antimicrobial prophylaxis should be administered on time to ensure, at the time of incision and throughout the procedure, that the tissue and plasma concentrations exceed the MIC for the microorganisms commonly associated with infection. This would normally be within 1 h for intravenous drugs given as a bolus or short infusion, but for some longer infusions that are given over 30 minutes or more, they may need to be started earlier to ensure that the infusion is completed at least 20 minutes before incision (e.g. vancomycin and fluoroquinolones) [6, 18, 19, 26–30].

Currently, the use of a dose of cefazolin (2 gr) or another first-generation cephalosporin or flucloxacillin (1–2 g) is recommended, one hour prior to the procedure. In patients allergic to Beta lactams or when the local incidence of MR Staphylococci is very high, vancomycin is recommended (vancomycin requires a mg/kg iv slower rate of infusion to prevent systemic vasodilatation and erythema within 2 hours before incision) or teicoplanin as an alternative regimen. If a glycopeptide is to be used, teicoplanin has some practical advantages over vancomycin in terms of administration as it can be given as a bolus (400 mg iv 5 minutes) rather than a long infusion. Teicoplanin resistance is more frequent than vancomycin resistance among Staphylococci (including CoNS), but both are uncommon. In case of allergy to both, assess linezolid/daptomycin.

In very prolonged procedures or in case of heavy bleeding, a second dose of intraprocedural antibiotic can be considered [12].

For elective procedures, *S. aureus* colonization can be detected by nasal swabs. Nasal treatment with mupirocin and chlorhexidine skin washing can reduce colonization and has been shown in some surgical studies to reduce the risk of infection, but there are no studies relating specifically to CIED interventions [6, 18, 30].

Antibiotic doses after wound closure are not recommended [6, 30]. The use of local antibiotic delivery is not recommended [6, 21, 30] as well.

Antimicrobial 'envelopes' have been developed to deliver antimicrobial agents locally into the generator pocket at the time of implantation or generator replacement. A product that delivers rifampicin and minocycline locally was tested in a randomized, controlled clinical trial WRAP-IT to assess its safety and efficacy in a population of patients who were at increased risk for CIED pocket infection. The envelope was significantly more effective at preventing infection than standard protocols. There is no formal recommendation for the use of these covers but it could be considered in high-risk patients [29, 30].

Antimicrobial prophylaxis is not recommended for dental or other invasive procedures not directly related to device manipulation to prevent CIED infection, except in case of infected tissue manipulation [26].

2.8 IE-CIED treatment

Treatment is based on two pillars: the removal of the device and antimicrobial therapy.

2.8.1 The removal of the device

Complete removal of the device, electrodes, or abandoned remains, is indicated in patients with any CIED infection, with the exception of superficial infections related to the incision and provided that they do not occur with exteriorization of the device or erosion of the skin [24, 30–32].

Explantation is indicated in case of:

- local pocket infections without data of systemic involvement (negative blood cultures).
- infections of the pocket with systemic involvement, without vegetations on the electrodes or valves.
- infections of the pocket with systemic involvement, with evidence of vegetations in electrodes and/or valves and/or embolisms.

The device should also be removed in CIED carriers in case of [21, 30]:

- bacteremia or fungaemia caused by S Aureus, CoNS, Cutibacterium spp. and Candida spp.
- bacteremia with Alpha- or Beta-Hemolytic Streptococcus spp. and Enterococcus spp. as first-line treatment or as a second step in case of recurrent/continued bacteremia despite appropriate antibiotic therapy.
- bacteremia with non-Pseudomonal/Serratia Gram-negative bacteria or Pneumococci in case of recurrent/continued bacteremia, in spite of appropriate antibiotic therapy when no other identifiable source for recurrence or continued infection is found.
- patients with infective valve endocarditis without definite involvement of the CIED system.

The device must be completely removed as early as possible. Percutaneous removal is indicated as first choice when possible. Surgical approach is indicated when there is an indication for surgery associated with endocarditis in another location or after incomplete percutaneous removal. For large vegetations, greater than 20 mm, surgery may be considered the first option from the outset, due to a hypothetical higher risk of pulmonary embolism, although this cut-off point is arbitrary. The aspiration of large vegetations is reported before the percutaneous extraction of the electrodes. Removal of the system percutaneously is usually relatively simple when it is performed early after implantation, since there is less fibrosis around the device elements and implies more difficulty and risk of complications the longer the period after implantation and the complexity of the device.

The extraction should be done in expert centers by interventional cardiologists, electrophysiologists or cardiac surgeons. The percentage of complete removal of the device is high>90% with the techniques and materials currently available (specific stylets, mechanical dissection sheaths, with radiofrequency or laser, ties, etc.) (**Figure 9**). Implant removal requires centers with availability of urgent cardiac surgery, given that, although the percentage of complications is low, they can be serious and lead to vital compromise. The risk of serious complications is 2–4%, the most severe being cardiac avulsion or tear (CA / T) with tamponade and vascular avulsion or tear (VA/T). In the case of surgical extraction, (**Figure 10**) the percentage of complications observed is higher and it seems related to a greater severity of the patients [30–32].

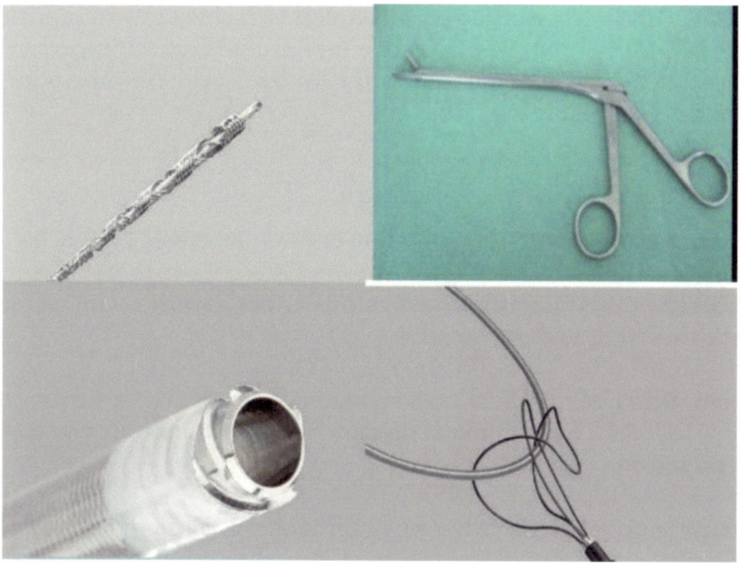

Figure 9.
Materials for percutaneous.

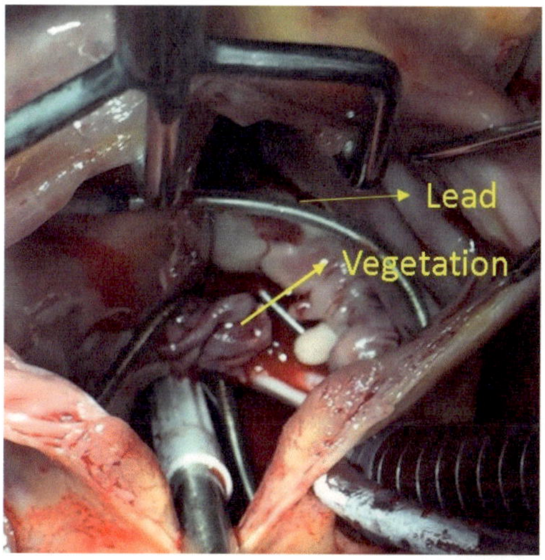

Figure 10.
Lead with big vegetation, surgical removal.

In 3–15% of patients with an indication of removal of the device, this will not be carried out for various reasons, especially a very high surgical risk or the patient's own refusal [6, 10].

2.8.2 The antimicrobial therapy

Intravenous (iv) antimicrobial therapy should be guided whenever possible by microbiological documentation and antibiogram; this is the reason why the correct collection and sample processing is so important.

The empirical antibiotic regimens recommended by a consensus of various scientific societies, European Heart Rhythm Association (EHRA), Heart Rhythm Society (HRS), Asia Pacific Heart Rhythm Society (APHRS), Latin American Heart Rhythm Society (LAHRS), International Society for Cardiovascular Infectious

Diseases (ISCVID), European Society of Clinical Microbiology and Infectious Diseases (ESCMID), European Association for Cardio-Thoracic Surgery (EACTS)] [30] are listed in **Table 1**. The duration of the treatment will continue once the device is removed as follows:

- Isolated pocket infection (negative blood culture): 10–14 days.
- Systemic infection without vegetation on leads or valves +/– pocket infection:
  4 weeks (2 weeks if negative blood culture after extraction with total treatment duration not shorter than 4 weeks).
- Systemic infection: IE-CIED with vegetation on leads and/or valves + embolism: 4–6 weeks + oral antibiotic therapy follow-up if indicated by secondary infectious focus.

Long-term suppressive therapy with iv antibiotic, according to the recommendations in prosthetic valve endocarditis for 4–6 weeks, is reasonable for patients in whom the device cannot be totally or partially removed, due to the high rates of failure, relapse or reinfection [33].

2.9 New device implant

After the removal of a CIED, the indication for a new implant must be reconsidered. This must be done critically and individually [19, 26, 30].

It is estimated that, in about 30% of patients, implantation of a new device is not indicated. The reason may be that there is no longer any indication, that the explanted device was not correctly indicated, or that the patient himself rejects a new implant. In the case of a new reimplantation, it will be necessary to assess whether a similar device is indicated, or whether it should be different, generally of less complexity or "downgrade" [31, 34].

If the indication for a new implant is confirmed, it should be deferred until the infection is controlled, if possible after obtaining negative blood cultures for at least 72 hours after the explant. In patients dependent on cardiac stimulation, who require temporary stimulation, an electrode ipsilateral to the explant will be used, through a venous access different from that used by the previous one. To prevent manipulations due to instability of the electrode, with a greater risk of contamination, the use of an active fixation electrode connected to an external battery and fixed to the skin is recommended, until it is safe to implant the definitive device [6, 34].

If a device with electrodes (RTC, bicameral pacing) is indicated, it should be implanted initially on the contralateral side. If not, implantation of an epicardial pacemaker or a MicraTM Transcatheter Pacing System (TPS; Medtronic, Minneapolis, MN, USA) femoral leadless pacemaker may be considered. The lead-free pacemaker avoids the possibility of a primary infection of the generator pocket and thanks to its smaller overall surface area and the progressive encapsulation once implanted (**Figure 11**), it would theoretically present less risk of secondary infection in the presence of systemic infection [35].

In the case of patients with an indication for defibrillator reimplantation, without the need for permanent pacing, resynchronization or anti-tachycardia therapy, the implantation of a subcutaneous defibrillator should be considered (the infection rate requiring removal of the device is 2.4% after 3 years of follow up) (**Figure 12**) [36].

Isolated pocket infection	10–14 days post-extraction
-Systemic symptoms	
Empirical treatment/ - blood cultures	-Vancomycin: 30–60 mg/kg/d iv in 2–3 doses
Directed at MR * CoNS and S Aureus	-Alternative: Daptomycin 8–10 mg/kg iv od
+ Systemic symptoms	+/–
(Empirical treatment/ - blood cultures)	-Cephalosporin: standard dose
For additional Gram- coverage	-Alternative: Gentamicin** 5–7 mg/kg iv od
After culture result	Flucloxacillin: 8 g/d iv in 4 doses
If sensitive Staphylococcus	Alternative: 1st generation cephalosporin standard dose
	Partial oral treatment often used
Systemic infections without vegetation on leads or valves +/-pocket infection	
	4 weeks post-extraction_(consider 2w if -blood_cultures)
Empirical treatment/ - blood cultures	Vancomycin: 30–60 mg/kg/d iv in 2–3 doses
Directed at MR Staphylococci and Gram- bacteria	Alternative: Daptomycin 8–10 mg/kg od
	+
	Cephalosporin: standard dose iv
	Alternative: Gentamicin 5–7 mg/kg iv o d
After culture result	Flucloxacillin: 8 g/d iv in 4 doses
If sensitive Staphylococcus	Alternative: 1st generation cephalosporin standard dose
Systemic infections with vegetation on leads or valves +/-pocket infection	
	Lead vegetation: 2 weeks post-extraction (total 4w except S Aureus)
	Native valve vegetation: 4 weeks post-extraction
	Prosthetic valve vegetation: (4-) 6 weeks post-extraction
Empirical treatment/ - blood cultures	Vancomycin:30–60 mg/kg/d iv in 2–3 doses
	Alternative: Daptomycin 8–10 mg/kg od
	+
	Cephalosporin: standard dose
	Alternative: Gentamicin 5–7 mg/kg iv od
Adjust to culture result according to ESC endocarditis guidelines 2015	
If prosthetic valve and staphylococcal infection:	Add Rifampicin after 5–7 days: 900–1200 mg/day orally (or iv) in 2 doses
*adapt to local resistance	
**adjust according to kidney function	od: once day

Table 1.
IE-CIED Empirical antibiotic regimens recommended.

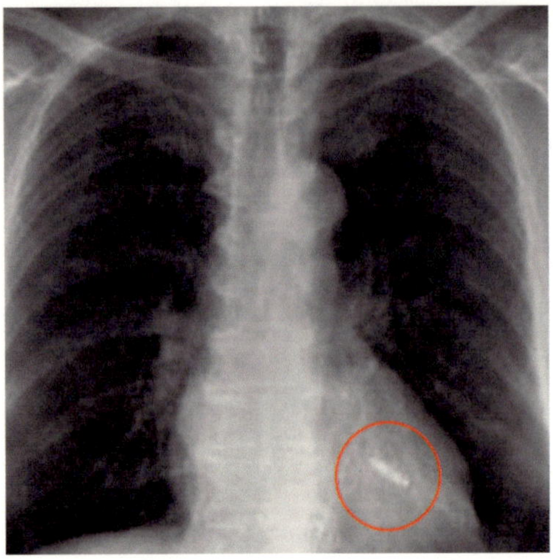

Figure 11.
MICRA.

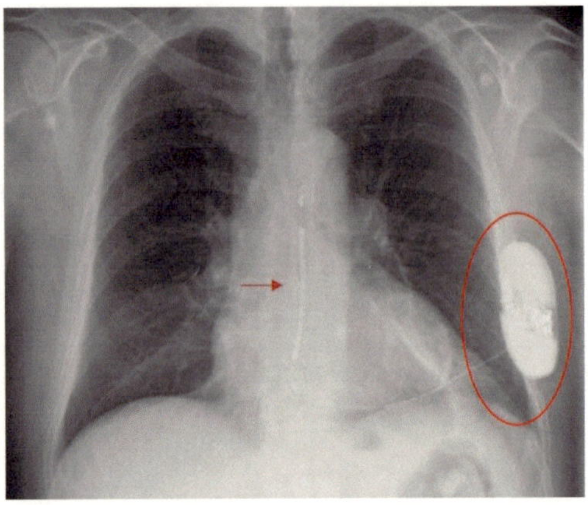

Figure 12.
Subcutaneous defibrillator.

2.10 Prognosis

CIED infection is a serious pathology with a 30-day hospital mortality estimated between 4.6–11% (despite the heterogeneity of the studies) [37]. Studies that included only patients with CIED -IE reported high mortality: 24.5–29% with follow-up periods of up to a year and explant rates of 80–100% [6]. It is associated with systemic infection and sepsis, complications derived from extraction and reimplantation and the own comorbidities of the patients. Long-term mortality is between 1.5 and 2.4 times higher than in CIED carriers without infectious complications. Mortality is high during the first year following CIED infection, but many deaths are not infection related. Abnormal renal function is the most consistently identified risk factor for mortality. Failure to remove an infected device is associated with relapse and mortality. CIED-IE has a higher mortality than localized generator pocket infection.

For all these reasons, infections in patients with CIED and especially those with suspected or confirmed systemic involvement should be considered a medical emergency, that must receive a multidisciplinary approach by a team made up of specialists in infectious diseases and microbiology, interventional cardiologists, electrophysiologists, clinicians and experts in multimodal imaging, surgeons and experts in other imaging techniques such as radiologists and nuclear medicine [38].

3. Conclusions

Infective endocarditis is a prevalent pathology in developed countries. Its spectrum is changing and its association with intracardiac devices has increased disproportionately in recent decades. Affected patients are especially vulnerable to complications due to both their cardiac and extra-cardiac pathologies and their frequent contact with health-related procedures. Most of these infections are caused by S Aureus and CoNS, many times carriers of antibiotic resistance and must be treated early and aggressively by multidisciplinary teams. We must be careful in the indication and choice of devices and exquisite in the prevention of infections since once established, therapeutic failure entails high morbidity and mortality.

Acknowledgements

All the staff of the Cardiology Imaging Department of the Hospital de la Princesa for the work we share daily.

The Infectious Diseases Service of Hospital de la Princesa, for their intense dedication to infective endocarditis.

Marta and Carmen Terrón for supervising the translation.

Conflict of interest

The author declares no conflict of interest.

Author details

Amparo Benedicto* and Lourdes Domínguez
Cardiology Imaging Department, Hospital Universitario de La Princesa, Madrid, Spain

*Address all correspondence to: ambebe2000@yahoo.es

References

[1] Bin Abdulhak AA, Baddour LM, Erwin PJ, Hoen B, Chu VH, Mensah GA, Tleyjeh IM. Global and regional burden of infective endocarditis, 1990-2010: A systematic review of the literature. Glob Heart. 2014 Mar;9(1):131-143. doi: 10.1016/j.gheart.2014.01.002. PMID: 25432123.

[2] Ambrosioni J, Hernandez-Meneses M, Téllez A, Pericàs J, Falces C, Tolosana JM, Vidal B, Almela M, Quintana E, Llopis J, Moreno A, Miro JM; Hospital Clinic Infective Endocarditis Investigators. The Changing Epidemiology of Infective Endocarditis in the Twenty-First Century. Curr Infect Dis Rep. 2017 May;19(5):21. doi: 10.1007/s11908-017-0574-9.PMID:28401448.

[3] Greenspon AJ, Patel JD, Lau E, Ochoa JA, Frisch DR, Ho RT, Pavri BB, Kurtz SM. 16-year trends in the infection burden for pacemakers and implantable cardioverter-defibrillators in the United States 1993 to 2008. J Am Coll Cardiol. 2011 Aug 30;58(10):1001-1006. doi: 10.1016/j.jacc.2011.04.033. PMID: 21867833.

[4] Mond HG, Proclemer A. The 11th world survey of cardiac pacing and implantable cardioverter-defibrillators: Calendar year 2009--a world Society of Arrhythmia's project. Pacing Clin Electrophysiol. 2011 Aug;34(8):1013-1027. doi: 10.1111/j.1540-8159.2011.03150.x. Epub 2011 Jun 27. PMID: 21707667.

[5] Mateos Gaitán R, Boix-Palop L, Muñoz García P, Mestres CA, Marín Arriaza M, Pedraz Prieto Á, de Alarcón Gonzalez A, Gutiérrez Carretero E, Hernández Meneses M, Goenaga Sánchez MÁ, Cobo Belaustegui M, Oteo Revuelta JA, Gainzarain Arana JC, García Vázquez E, Martínez-Sellés M. Infective endocarditis in patients with cardiac implantable electronic devices: A nationwide study. Europace. 2020 Jul 1;22(7):1062-1070. doi: 10.1093/europace/euaa076. PMID: 32390046

[6] Sandoe JA, Barlow G, Chambers JB, Gammage M, Guleri A, Howard P, Olson E, Perry JD, Prendergast BD, Spry MJ, Steeds RP, Tayebjee MH, Watkin R; British Society for Antimicrobial Chemotherapy; British Heart Rhythm Society; British Cardiovascular Society; British Heart Valve Society; British Society for Echocardiography. Guidelines for the diagnosis, prevention and management of implantable cardiac electronic device infection. Report of a joint Working Party project on behalf of the British Society for Antimicrobial Chemotherapy (BSAC, host organization), British Heart Rhythm Society (BHRS), British Cardiovascular Society (BCS), British Heart Valve Society (BHVS) and British Society for Echocardiography (BSE). J Antimicrob Chemother. 2015 Feb;70(2):325-59. doi: 10.1093/jac/dku383. Epub 2014 Oct 29. PMID: 25355810.

[7] Fournier PE, Casalta JP, Habib G, Messana T, Raoult D. Modification of the diagnostic criteria proposed by the Duke endocarditis service to permit improved diagnosis of Q fever endocarditis. Am J Med. 1996 Jun;100(6):629-633. doi: 10.1016/s0002-9343(96)00040-x. PMID: 8678083

[8] Hercé B, Nazeyrollas P, Lesaffre F, Sandras R, Chabert JP, Martin A, Tassan-Mangina S, Bui HT, Metz D. Risk factors for infection of implantable cardiac devices: Data from a registry of 2496 patients. Europace. 2013 Jan;15(1):66-70. doi: 10.1093/europace/eus284. Epub 2012 Oct 24. PMID: 23097224.

[9] Mela T, McGovern BA, Garan H, Vlahakes GJ, Torchiana DF, Ruskin J,

Galvin JM. Long-term infection rates associated with the pectoral versus abdominal approach to cardioverter-defibrillator implants. Am J Cardiol. 2001 Oct 1;88(7):750-753. doi: 10.1016/s0002-9149(01)01845-8. PMID: 11589841.

[10] Klug D, Balde M, Pavin D, Hidden-Lucet F, Clementy J, Sadoul N, Rey JL, Lande G, Lazarus A, Victor J, Barnay C, Grandbastien B, Kacet S; PEOPLE Study Group. Risk factors related to infections of implanted pacemakers and cardioverter-defibrillators: Results of a large prospective study. Circulation. 2007 Sep 18;116(12):1349-1355. doi: 10.1161/CIRCULATIONAHA.106.678664. Epub 2007 Aug 27. PMID: 17724263.

[11] Athan E, Chu VH, Tattevin P, Selton-Suty C, Jones P, Naber C, Miró JM, Ninot S, Fernández-Hidalgo N, Durante-Mangoni E, Spelman D, Hoen B, Lejko-Zupanc T, Cecchi E, Thuny F, Hannan MM, Pappas P, Henry M, Fowler VG Jr, Crowley AL, Wang a; ICE-PCS investigators. Clinical characteristics and outcome of infective endocarditis involving implantable cardiac devices. JAMA. 2012 Apr 25;307(16):1727-1735. doi: 10.1001/jama.2012.497. PMID: 22535857.

[12] Fernando Arribas, María López-Gil, Rafael Salguero y Javier Chimeno Unidad de Arritmias. Servicio de Cardiología. Hospital Universitario 12 de Octubre. Madrid. España. Algunos aspectos relacionados con la implantación del desfibrilador automático implantable Rev Esp Cardiol Supl. 2008;8:51A-64a

[13] Anderson DJ, Podgorny K, Berríos-Torres SI, Bratzler DW, Dellinger EP, Greene L, Nyquist AC, Saiman L, Yokoe DS, Maragakis LL, Kaye KS. Strategies to prevent surgical site infections in acute care hospitals: 2014 update. Infect Control Hosp Epidemiol. 2014 Jun;35(6):605-27. doi: 10.1086/676022. PMID: 24799638; PMCID: PMC4267723.

[14] Arciola CR, Campoccia D, Montanaro L. Implant infections: Adhesion, biofilm formation and immune evasion. Nat Rev Microbiol. 2018 Jul;16(7):397-409. doi: 10.1038/s41579-018-0019-y. PMID: 29720707.

[15] www.immunology.org/es/public-information/bitesized-immunology / pathogens-and-disease/ Biofilms and their role in pathogenesis Birte Hollmann, Mark Perkins, Centro de Ciencias Biomoleculares Dean Walsh, Universidad de Nottingham

[16] McIntyre WF, Healey JS. Cardiac implantable electronic device infections: From recognizing risk to prevention. Heart Rhythm. 2017 Jun;14(6):846-847. doi: 10.1016/j.hrthm.2017.03.027. Epub 2017 Mar 23. PMID: 28343911.

[17] Bongiorni MG, Tascini C, Tagliaferri E, Di Cori A, Soldati E, Leonildi A, Zucchelli G, Ciullo I, Menichetti F. Microbiology of cardiac implantable electronic device infections. Europace. 2012 Sep;14(9):1334-1339. doi: 10.1093/europace/eus044. Epub 2012 Mar 7. PMID: 22399202.

[18] Padfield GJ, Steinberg C, Bennett MT, Chakrabarti S, Deyell MW, Bashir J, Krahn AD. Preventing cardiac implantable electronic device infections. Heart Rhythm. 2015 Nov;12(11):2344-2356. doi: 10.1016/j.hrthm.2015.06.043. Epub 2015 Jun 30. PMID: 26142295.

[19] Habib G, Lancellotti P, Antunes MJ, Bongiorni MG, Casalta JP, Del Zotti F, Dulgheru R, El Khoury G, Erba PA, Iung B, Miro JM, Mulder BJ, Plonska-Gosciniak E, Price S, Roos-Hesselink J, Snygg-Martin U, Thuny F, Tornos Mas P, Vilacosta I, Zamorano JL; ESC Scientific Document Group. 2015 ESC guidelines for the management of infective endocarditis: The task force for the Management of

Infective Endocarditis of the European Society of Cardiology (ESC). Endorsed by: European Association for Cardio-Thoracic Surgery (EACTS), the European Association of Nuclear Medicine (EANM). Eur heart J. 2015 Nov 21;36(44):3075-3128. doi: 10.1093/eurheartj/ehv319. Epub 2015 Aug 29. PMID: 26320109.

[20] Li JS, Sexton DJ, Mick N, Nettles R, Fowler VG Jr, Ryan T, Bashore T, Corey GR. Proposed modifications to the Duke criteria for the diagnosis of infective endocarditis. Clin Infect Dis. 2000 Apr;30(4):633-638. doi: 10.1086/313753. Epub 2000 Apr 3. PMID: 10770721

[21] UPTODATE Infections involving cardiac implantable electronic devices: Epidemiology, microbiology, clinical manifestations, and diagnosis authors: Adolf W Karchmer, MDVivian H Chu, MD, MHS www.uptodate.com

[22] Uslan DZ, Dowsley TF, Sohail MR, Hayes DL, Friedman PA, Wilson WR, Steckelberg JM, Baddour LM. Cardiovascular implantable electronic device infection in patients with Staphylococcus aureus bacteremia. Pacing Clin Electrophysiol. 2010 Apr;33(4):407-413. doi: 10.1111/j.1540-8159.2009.02565.x. Epub 2009 Sep 30. PMID: 19793360.

[23] Narducci ML, Pelargonio G, Russo E, Marinaccio L, Di Monaco A, Perna F, Bencardino G, Casella M, Di Biase L, Santangeli P, Palmieri R, Lauria C, Al Mohani G, Di Clemente F, Tondo C, Pennestri F, Ierardi C, Rebuzzi AG, Crea F, Bellocci F, Natale A, Dello Russo A. Usefulness of intracardiac echocardiography for the diagnosis of cardiovascular implantable electronic device-related endocarditis. J Am Coll Cardiol. 2013 Apr 2;61(13):1398-1405. doi: 10.1016/j.jacc.2012.12.041. PMID: 23500279.

[24] Horgan SJ, Mediratta A, Gillam LD. Cardiovascular imaging in infective endocarditis: A multimodality approach. Circ Cardiovasc Imaging. 2020 Jul;13(7):e008956. doi: 10.1161/CIRCIMAGING.120.008956. Epub 2020 Jul 20. PMID: 32683888

[25] Patricia Muñoz, HUGM Novedades en el diagnóstico y tratamiento de la endocarditis Avances en el diagnóstico, nuevos criterios VII CONGRESO SEICAV 2018 . Oral presentation

[26] Baddour LM, Epstein AE, Erickson CC, Knight BP, Levison ME, Lockhart PB, Masoudi FA, Okum EJ, Wilson WR, Beerman LB, Bolger AF, Estes NA 3rd, Gewitz M, Newburger JW, Schron EB, Taubert KA; American Heart Association Rheumatic Fever, Endocarditis, and Kawasaki Disease Committee; Council on Cardiovascular Disease in Young; Council on Cardiovascular Surgery and Anesthesia; Council on Cardiovascular Nursing; Council on Clinical Cardiology; Interdisciplinary Council on Quality of Care; American Heart Association. Update on cardiovascular implantable electronic device infections and their management: a scientific statement from the American Heart Association. Circulation. 2010 Jan 26;121(3):458-77. doi: 10.1161/CIRCULATIONAHA.109.192665. Epub 2010 Jan 4. PMID: 20048212.

[27] Darouiche R, Mosier M, Voigt J. Antibiotics and antiseptics to prevent infection in cardiac rhythm management device implantation surgery. Pacing Clin Electrophysiol. 2012 Nov;35(11):1348-1360. doi: 10.1111/j.1540-8159.2012.03506.x. Epub 2012 Sep 4. PMID: 22946683.

[28] Darouiche RO, Wall MJ Jr, Itani KM, Otterson MF, Webb AL, Carrick MM, Miller HJ, Awad SS, Crosby CT, Mosier MC, Alsharif A, Berger DH. Chlorhexidine-alcohol versus povidone-iodine for surgical-site antisepsis. N Engl J Med. 2010 Jan 7;362(1):18-26. doi: 10.1056/NEJMoa0810988. PMID: 20054046.

[29] Tarakji KG, Mittal S, Kennergren C, Corey R, Poole JE, Schloss E, Gallastegui J, Pickett RA, Evonich R, Philippon F, McComb JM, Roark SF, Sorrentino D, Sholevar D, Cronin E, Berman B, Riggio D, Biffi M, Khan H, Silver MT, Collier J, Eldadah Z, Wright DJ, Lande JD, Lexcen DR, Cheng A, Wilkoff BL; WRAP-IT investigators. Antibacterial envelope to prevent cardiac implantable device infection. N Engl J Med. 2019 May 16;380(20):1895-1905. doi: 10.1056/NEJMoa1901111. Epub 2019 Mar 17. PMID: 30883056.

[30] Blomström-Lundqvist C, Traykov V, Erba PA, Burri H, Nielsen JC, Bongiorni MG, Poole J, Boriani G, Costa R, Deharo JC, Epstein LM, Saghy L, Snygg-Martin U, Starck C, Tascini C, Strathmore N; ESC Scientific Document Group. European Heart Rhythm Association (EHRA) international consensus document on how to prevent, diagnose, and treat cardiac implantable electronic device infections-endorsed by the Heart Rhythm Society (HRS), the Asia Pacific Heart Rhythm Society (APHRS), the Latin American Heart Rhythm Society (LAHRS), International Society for Cardiovascular Infectious Diseases (ISCVID) and the European Society of Clinical Microbiology and Infectious Diseases (ESCMID) in collaboration with the European Association for Cardio-Thoracic Surgery (EACTS). Europace. 2020 Apr 1;22(4):515-549. doi: 10.1093/europace/euz246. PMID: 31702000; PMCID: PMC7132545

[31] Patel D, Khan F, Shah H, Bhattacharya S, Adelstein E, Saba S. Cardiac implantable electronic device lead extraction in patients with underlying infection using open thoracotomy or percutaneous techniques. Cardiol J. 2015;22(1):68-74. doi: 10.5603/CJ.a2014.0038. Epub 2014 May 20. PMID: 24846514

[32] Zucchelli G, Di Cori A, Segreti L, Laroche C, Blomstrom-Lundqvist C, Kutarski A, Regoli F, Butter C, Defaye P, Pasquié JL, Auricchio A, Maggioni AP, Bongiorni MG; ELECTRa Investigators. Major cardiac and vascular complications after transvenous lead extraction: Acute outcome and predictive factors from the ESC-EHRA ELECTRa (European Lead extraction ConTRolled) registry. Europace. 2019 May 1;21(5):771-780. doi: 10.1093/europace/euy300. PMID: 30590520

[33] Tan EM, DeSimone DC, Sohail MR, Baddour LM, Wilson WR, Steckelberg JM, Virk A. Outcomes in patients with cardiovascular implantable electronic device infection managed with chronic antibiotic suppression. Clin Infect Dis. 2017 Jun 1;64(11):1516-1521. doi: 10.1093/cid/cix181. PMID: 28329125.

[34] Döring M, Hienzsch L, Ebert M, Lucas J, Dagres N, Kühl M, Hindricks G, Knopp H, Richter S. Extraction of infected cardiac implantable electronic devices and the need for subsequent re-implantation. Int J Cardiol. 2020 Jun 15;309:84-91. doi: 10.1016/j.ijcard.2019.12.044. Epub 2019 Dec 27. PMID: 31973885

[35] El-Chami MF, Soejima K, Piccini JP, Reynolds D, Ritter P, Okabe T, Friedman PA, Cha YM, Stromberg K, Holbrook R, Fagan DH, Roberts PR. Incidence and outcomes of systemic infections in patients with leadless pacemakers: Data from the Micra IDE study. Pacing Clin Electrophysiol. 2019 Aug;42(8):1105-1110. doi: 10.1111/pace.13752. Epub 2019 Jul 2. PMID: 31232461

[36] Boersma L, Barr C, Knops R, Theuns D, Eckardt L, Neuzil P, Scholten M, Hood M, Kuschyk J, Jones P, Duffy E, Husby M, Stein K, Lambiase PD; EFFORTLESS Investigator Group. Implant and midterm outcomes of the subcutaneous implantable cardioverter-defibrillator registry: The EFFORTLESS study. J Am Coll Cardiol. 2017 Aug

15;70(7):830-841. doi: 10.1016/j.jacc.2017.06.040. PMID: 28797351.

[37] Sohail MR, Henrikson CA, Braid-Forbes MJ, Forbes KF, Lerner DJ. Mortality and cost associated with cardiovascular implantable electronic device infections. Arch Intern Med. 2011 Nov 14;171(20):1821-1828. doi: 10.1001/archinternmed.2011.441. Epub 2011 Sep 12. PMID: 21911623

[38] Holte E, Dweck MR, Marsan NA, D'Andrea A, Manka R, Stankovic I, Haugaa KH. EACVI survey on the evaluation of infective endocarditis. Eur Heart J Cardiovasc Imaging. 2020 Aug 1;21(8):828-832. doi: 10.1093/ehjci/jeaa066. PMID: 32361725; PMCID: PMC7369685.

Chapter 8

Contemporary and Evolving Treatment of Tricuspid Endocarditis

Vira I. Ayzenbart and Mark Joseph

Abstract

The current treatment paradigm for right sided infective endocarditis is rapidly evolving. The existing recommendations for right sided infective endocarditis include medical therapy with surgical therapy used in certain situations. Surgical therapy is based on the size of the vegetation, presence of infective complications and certain causative organisms as well the retention of intracardiac devices. Unfortunately, medical therapy alone is usually not enough to clear the infection, especially when intravenous drug use is associated as the etiology. Intravenous drug use is associated with a high rate of recidivism in tricuspid valve endocarditis. Even with indications for surgery, these patients present an ethical dilemma as most of these patients will re-infect their valves post-surgery. This often provides little option than for the surgeon to re-operate in a setting with a higher risk of mortality and morbidity. We present an evolving technique of percutaneous extirpation of vegetation, allowing for rapid clearance of endocarditis, less chance of failure of medical therapy with a lower risk profile for complication.

Keywords: tricuspid endocarditis, percutaneous treatment, cardiac implantable device endocarditis, CIDE, extirpation

1. Introduction

Endocarditis is defined as inflammation of the inner layer of the endocardium, usually involving the heart valves and or chambers of the heart, the valves being more commonly affected than the heart chambers [1]. Endocarditis is further categorized into non-bacterial thrombotic endocarditis (NBTE) or noninfectious endocarditis, and infectious endocarditis (IE) [2]. NBTE is rare and associated with malignancy and chronic inflammatory states such as systemic lupus erythematosus, rheumatoid arthritis, ANCA-vasculitis, burns, and sepsis [2, 3]. Conversely, IE is more common, with annual incidence of 3–10 cases per 100,000 people [4, 5]. It occurs due to bacterial and less commonly due to fungal infections [1, 4, 5]. *Staphylococcus aureus* is now the leading cause of IE, accounting for about 26.6% of all cases [4]. Staphylococci, streptococci (including the viridans group) and enterococci comprise about 80–90% of all cases of IE [4, 5]. The other 10–20% of cases are due culture negative endocarditis and fastidious organisms such bartonella species, brucella species, *Coxiella burnetii*, haemophilus species, *Aggregatibacter actinomycetenomitans*, *Cardiobacterium hominis*, *Eikenella corrodens*, *Kingella kingae* and *Tropheryma whipplei* [5]. Endocarditis is characterized by lesions, known as vegetations. These vegetations follow endocardial injury where platelets and fibrin form a nidus which becomes secondarily infected by microorganisms circulating in the blood. (1) Endocarditis can involve both the right and left side of the heart and often can have differing causative organisms and etiologies. Left sided endocarditis can involve the aortic valve, mitral valve and in severe cases can involve the aorto-mitral curtain causing damage to the electrical structures of the heart. Right sided endocarditis typically involves the valvular structures on the right side of the heart most commonly the tricuspid valve and less often the pulmonary valve. In addition, the right sided endocarditis may also involve foreign bodies that are typically found transversing the right atrium such as pacemaker leads, central lines.

2. Right sided infective endocarditis

Right sided Infective Endocarditis (RSIE) accounts for about 10% of all IE cases [6]. Typically, these patients are younger with fewer medical comorbidities and less underlying valve disease as compared to patients with left-sided IE [6]. RSIE involves both tricuspid valve endocarditis (TVE) and cardiac implantable device endocarditis (CIDE). RSIE is most frequently seen with intravenous drug use (IVDU). Other predisposing risk factors include use of central venous catheters, cardiovascular implanted electronic devices, congenital heart disease, prosthetic heart valves, and end-stage renal disease on hemodialysis [5, 6]. Mortality rate of RSIE is typically 5–15% [6]. The risk factors and independent predictors of death are age, *Staphylococcus aureus* infection, heart failure, embolic events and health care-associated IE [5].

2.1 Tricuspid valve endocarditis

2.1.1 Epidemiology

Ninety percent of RSIE involves the tricuspid valve, of which infection resulting from intravenous drug use (IVDU) constitutes approximately 30–40% of all tricuspid valve endocarditis cases. The incidence of tricuspid lesions in IVDU is approximately 50–65%, with a prevalence of about 2–5% per year [6]. With ongoing IVDU, IE reoccurs in about 28% of cases due to prior damage or replacement of the valve [6]. *Staphylococcus aureus* is the predominant causative organism in TVIE, just as in all types on of IE [4, 6]. The opioid epidemic over the last several years has seen an increase in patients with IVDU as subsequently an increase in TVE. Heroin abuse has more than doubled over the past decade along with TVE during the same period. A study by Wallen et al. showed a fivefold increase in surgical volume for tricuspid endocarditis from 2011 to 2017. In addition, the average age of patients seemed to decrease from 52.85 +/−19.6 years to 39.2 +/−12.9 over the same five-year period [7]. In addition, multiple other studies have reported an increase in tricuspid-related IE corresponding to an increase in IVDU during the same period [8–10].

2.1.2 Treatment and prognosis

As a whole, RSIE carries a good prognosis. TVIE clears in 70–85% of cases with antibiotic treatment alone. Non-operatively treated TVIE carries an in-hospital mortality of 7–11% [6]. Non operative treatment typically consists of 4–6 weeks of intravenous antibiotics. However, approximately 5–16% cases of RSIE will require surgical intervention [6]. Indications and timing for surgery are less clear for RSIE than for left-sided infectious endocarditis (LSIE). According to the most recent AHA/ACC guidelines, surgery for native RSIE is indicated for patients with antibiotic failure, multi-drug-resistant organisms, tricuspid vegetations greater than 2 cm, embolic complications, or right-sided heart failure with poor response to diuretics [11, 12]. Most patients with infected prosthetic TV will require surgery, except in patients with unacceptable intra-operative mortality risk [6]. Surgery is less often performed for TV regurgitation due to IE, as it is more amendable to medical management and unlike aortic or mitral valve regurgitation, most patients can tolerate TV regurgitation up to a certain period [6]. Patients with isolated TVIE have an operative mortality between 0 and 15% and excellent survival. The post-surgical in-hospital mortality for TVIE is less than 10% and long term post-surgical mortality for TVIE is less than 15%, but increased in the presence of additional risk factors such as continued intravenous drug abuse, hemodialysis, valve replacement, *S. aureus*, and vegetation greater than 20 mm [6].

2.1.3 Current surgical options

Over the years, various surgical options have been used in TVIE. Surgical options range from valve repair or replacement to the removal of the tricuspid valve leaflets and chordae tendinae without replacement (valvectomy). Valvectomy, essentially commits the patient to require surgical repair, but has been used with success to temporize a patient while fighting ongoing systemic infection [6]. According to a systematic review by Luc et al., the post-operative 30-day mortality, right heart failure, and recurrent endocarditis was the same with valvectomy compared to surgical valve replacement for endocarditis but with a slightly higher non-significant trend towards higher postoperative right heart failure and 30-day mortality [13]. Tricuspid reoperation rate, however, was higher in valvectomy (56%) versus valve replacement (14%) in addition to an increased likelihood of prolonged ventilation (40% vs. 26%) in the valvectomy group [13].

Tricuspid valvectomy can be a feasible option in patients with active ongoing IVDU, normal pulmonary pressure, normal biventricular heart function, high degree of valvular destruction and high risk of reoperation, recidivism and recurrence for infection [13, 14]. Valvectomy with valve replacement as a staged procedure can allow patients to self-select in terms of their ability to maintain adequate follow-up, undergo detoxification and drug rehabilitation, optimize their social and financial situation, and demonstrate abstinence from IVDU prior to tricuspid valve replacement. However, valvectomy is largely falling out of favor due to the potential of severe right heart failure and the ventricularization of right atrial pressures [13, 15]. In patients with normal heart function pre valvectomy, severe right heart failure with symptoms of peripheral edema and ascites can occur within 6–9 months post valvectomy [6]. Therefore, patient with elevated pulmonary artery pressure are therefore not candidates for complete valvectomy [6].

The preferred surgical procedure is that of repair, particularly because it adheres to the basic principles cited for the successful surgical treatment of infective endocarditis. These include aggressive and extensive debridement of vegetations; correction of defects that have developed; use of autologous tissue to avoid implantation of artificial material [13, 16]. Most centers will prioritize valve repair prior to valve replacement or valvectomy [13].

2.1.4 Valve choice with replacement

Both bioprosthetic valves and mechanical valves have been used for valve replacement in TVIE. The gold standard anticoagulation after mechanical valve replacement is warfarin. Warfarin is can be difficult to manage as levels are dependent on patients' variable vitamin K intake and requires frequent monitoring. Furthermore, problems with compliance with monitoring and anticoagulation therapy is more frequently seen in patients with IVDU and this population is also the most common to present with recurrent right-sided endocarditis and require surgery for valve replacement. With bioprosthetic valve replacement, only first three months of anticoagulation after replacement are required to prevent thrombosis, although this practice itself can be variable [17, 18]. This time frame allows for reendothelialization to the suture zone [17]. Due to decreased duration of anticoagulation, bioprosthetic valves are associated with lower rates of bleeding complications [19].

Another advantage of bioprosthetic valve replacement compared to mechanical valve, is the thrombosis risk. Obstruction of the tricuspid mechanical prosthesis due to thrombosis is 20 times more frequent than left-sided prosthetic valve thrombosis [17]. This is likely due to low flow state of the right heart compared to the left. Lastly, Patients with bioprosthetic valve replacement are still candidates for pacemaker and ICD placement as compared to mechanical valves [6]. Similarly, embolic events are more common with mechanical valves [19]. Ergo, prosthetic valve replacement may be a better option from this perspective. Mechanical tricuspid valve replacement may be beneficial from the durability perspective as they last longer than bioprosthetic valves [6, 19]. Previously average failure time for tricuspid bioprosthetic valve was 7 years [19]. However, the durability of new bioprosthetic valves have improved over the years as recent data suggest no difference in long term data between bioprosthetic and mechanical valves at 15 years [20]. Additionally, mitral homografts have been used in the tricuspid space but with limited experience and long-term data [21].

2.1.5 Percutaneous options for valve replacement

Percutaneous tricuspid valve replacement (PTVR) creates unique challenges as compared to the left side. One, the tricuspid annulus is large is size compared to the mitral annulus and can be further increased with right ventricular dilation. For large valve replacement, large caliber sheaths and large bore venous access must be obtained [22]. Only jugular and femoral veins can accommodate such large bores of up to 45 French [22]. Trans-atrial approach has been used in the past; however, this requires surgical expertise. Two, tricuspid valves are more difficult to anchor percutaneously as there is limited calcification and the structure itself is dynamic (changes in diameter in systole and diastole). Three, PTVR carries an increased risk post-procedural conduction defects just as with surgical repair [6, 21]. Frequently with percutaneous replacement the tricuspid annulus becomes stretched. This can cause a complete atrio-ventricular (AV) block, requiring pacemaker placement, due to proximity of the AV node and the bundle of His to the tricuspid valve. Similarly, proximity of the tricuspid valve to the right coronary artery, coronary sinus, vena cava create additional challenges with percutaneous placement and valve design [22]. Furthermore, patients with pacemaker or ICD devices are not great candidates for percutaneous tricuspid valve replacement as placement of a valve may dislodge leads. Lastly, there is very limited data on the percutaneously placed tricuspid valve replacement durability and more studies are necessary. Unlike, for surgical tricuspid valve replacement there are no guidelines regarding timing of percutaneous valve aortic valve replacement after infective endocarditis. Without surgical debridement or percutaneous debulking and with antibiotics use alone, there is a high theoretical reinfection risk of the new tricuspid valve placed using a percutaneous approach after endocarditis.

2.2 Cardiac implantable device endocarditis

Cardiac implantable device endocarditis (CIDE) involves cardiovascular implantable electronic devices (CIED) which include permanent pacemakers (PPM), implantable cardiac defibrillators (ICD), and cardiac resynchronization systems (CRT). CIDE is diagnosed based on the presence of the following four criteria:

- Presence of a cardiac device;
- No other source of infection;
- A positive culture for typical causative agents from the pocket of the device or its leads; and
- Echocardiographic findings of vegetation on the tricuspid valve or at the end of the electrical lead [23].

Specifically, for CIDE diagnosis, the Duke criteria should be used. Patient presentation can be variable and can involve all or just a few symptom including fevers, rigors, anorexia, fatigue, local tissue inflammation. In addition, there may be possible purulent discharge, device exposure, focal pain that may help localize the primary site of infection. Other symptoms could be neurologic or cardiac consistent with embolic stroke, or symptoms of volume overload [23].

2.2.1 Epidemiology

Intracardiac device infections constitute approximately 10% of all endocarditis cases [24]. CIEDs have been implanted in patient as early as 1960s, but over the last two decades had significant increase in incidence. According to American Heart Association update, between 1997 and 2004, PPM placement increased by 19% and ICD placement increased by 60% [25]. Other studies quote an even higher increase of 30% for PPM and over 500% for ICDs [26]. In the United States greater than 500,000 PPMs and ICDs are implanted per year with over 4 million implanted between 1993 and 2008 [27]. Notably, more patients who are elderly and those with many comorbidities have been receiving these devices [25]. In developed countries 20–35% of CIEDs were placed in patients older than 80 years of age [25].

Over the years, changing the implantation site of ICD from abdomen (associated with 3.2% infection rate) to pectoral site (associated with 0.5% infection rate) initially decreased the incidence of device related infections [25]. Despite the innovation in PPM and ICD technology together with better surgical technique, the rate of infections associated with cardiac devices has increased by 124–210% [25, 26]. About 1.8–31.1 cases of CIED infection per 1000 device years has been reported for PPM and ICD devices and overall higher rates of infection with ICDs and CRTs [27]. This change is likely due to increased rate of CIED implantation in people over the age of 65 and presences of major comorbidities such as renal failure, respiratory failure, heart failure and diabetes [26]. CIED infections are associated with up to 18% of morbidity and mortality and increase by 47% per decade hospital charges [26].

Early infection typically arises from device implantation [27]. With first time implantation the rate of CIED related infection is 0.5–1% and 1–5% with device replacement or upgrade [27]. CIED related infection can involve the bloodstream, the generator pocket, the leads, or endocardial structures [26, 27]. Late infection typically arises from patient poor health or other clinically significant processes.

Almqvist et al., further divides the spectrum of CIED infections into six different categories: early post-implantation inflammation, uncomplicated pocket infection, complicated pocket infection, definite CIED lead infection, possible CIED lead infection, CIED-associated endocarditis, and probable CIED infection [26].

2.2.2 CIED infection risk factors

Patients with chronic kidney disease, long-term corticosteroid use, presence of more than 2 pacing leads, diabetes mellitus, heart failure and oral anticoagulation are at higher risk for CIED infection [25, 26]. Use of preprocedural temporary pacing, fever within 24 hours prior to implantation, blood stream infections, and early reintervention were also associated with higher risk of CIED infection [25]. Lower rates of CIED infection was associated with antibiotic perioperative prophylaxis new device placement, use of pectoral approach rather than abdominal or transthoracic approach, and device placement by a high-volume physician [25].

2.2.3 Pathogenesis and microbiology

Source of microorganisms often originate from the skin during the implantation of the electrical agent in the subcutaneous tissue, from the pocket in which the electrical agent is placed, the tunnel that forms around the lead before its point of entry into the blood vessel or from bacteria unrelated to the CIED, which may be present in the form of a foreign body placed on or in contact with the endocardial tissue, or that applies pressure to the endocardial tissue and tricuspid valve [23, 27]. Alternatively, contamination of the CIED can occur at different stages or from various causes. This includes but is not limited to manufacturing or packaging, infection prior to or during implantation, secondary to surgical site infection or via hematogenous seeding from a distant site or after erosion through the skin [24, 25, 27].

Physical and chemical properties such as electrostatic charge, surface tension and hydrophobicity of each device plays an important role in the interaction with bacteria and development of bacterial attachment and biofilm formation [23]. More hydrophobic surfaces such as polyvinyl chloride, polyethylene, silicone, latex and stainless steel are associated with higher microbial adherence [24]. Pathogens are more likely to adhere to irregular surfaces and may also adhere to the patient's matrix proteins (fibrinogen, fibronectin and collagen) that coat the surface of an implanted device [25]. CIED infections are more likely to occur due to gram positive bacteremia than gram negative bacteremia [25]. Staphylococci species, especially coagulase negative staph, have a knack for adhesion to CIEDs via host matrix proteins and to each other thus forming biofilms [24, 25]. Coagulase negative staphylococci comprise 42% of all PPM and ICD infections, followed by oxacillin sensitive *S. aureus* (25%), oxacillin resistant *S. aureus* (4%), with the remaining causative organisms being other gram positive cocci (4%), gram negative bacilli (9%), fungal (2%), polymicrobial (7%), and unidentified/culture negative (7%) [28].

2.2.4 The role of biofilm

Biofilm is a group of one or more microbial species firmly attached to a device surface and each other and covered by extracellular polymeric matrix [24, 25]. This matrix provides a protective barrier and results in antibiotic resistance and extreme difficult of bacterial irradiation that frequently requires device explanation [24, 25]. Some bacteria are more adept to adhering to non-biological materials such as staphylococci.

2.2.5 Treatment and prognosis

Antibiotics are generally empirically initiated after obtaining at least three sets of blood cultures. These usually consists of broad-spectrum intravenous antibiotics covering both gram-positive and gram-negative bacteria, including methicillin/oxacillin-resistant *Staphylococcus aureus* [29]. Antibiotic therapy alone without device removal, however, is associated with a 7 times increase in 30-day mortality [28]. Treatment of CIDE as recommended per the 2017 HRS Consensus Document include complete device and lead removal in addition to antibiotics [29]. Immediate system removal is associated with a 3 times decrease in 1-year mortality as compared to preliminary antibiotic treatment and delayed system removal [30]. Mortality rates in patients with endocarditis who had systems removed and antimicrobial therapy are 18% or less compared with up to 66% on antibiotic therapy alone [27]. Multiple clinical studies have now demonstrated a 97.7% clinical success rate with hardware removal in addition to antibiotic therapy [30].

2.2.6 Duration of treatment

The start of antibiotic therapy duration is counted from the first day of negative blood cultures, therefore it is reasonable to obtain blood cultures every 24 to 48 hours until they are negative [31]. If the patient requires surgery and the surgical cultures are negative, then the duration of therapy is still counted from the first day of negative blood cultures [31]. If surgical cultures are positive, then the start of antibiotic therapy duration occurs the next day, after the achievement of source control [31]. This applies to post device removal as well as some authors recommend obtaining new blood cultures 48–72 hours post device removal [26]. If the need for CIED remains in patients treated for bacteremia, negative blood cultures should be documented at least 72 hours prior to new device implantation [29]. Duration of treatment usually consists of 4–6 weeks of IV antibiotics, in addition to removal of CIED [29].

3. Evolving percutaneous options for treatment

Given that 10–15% of patients fail medical therapy, percutaneous treatment options as an adjunct to medical therapy have now started to become mainstream. Specifically, the use of AngioVac device (AngioDynamics, Latham, New York) has begun to get traction because of its ease of use, low risk profile and ability to debulk the vegetation and prevent septic pulmonary emboli. The AngioVac system is a veno-venous extracorporeal system. The most common configuration is as a bilateral femoral venous platform or via the right internal jugular and femoral platform. The system mainly consists of a cannula and a circuit along with a trap, which captures the undesirable material. AngioVac is currently used in the setting of thromboembolic disease, particularly in the vena cava or the right atrium. Both the cannula and circuit are indicated for use in procedures requiring extracorporeal circulatory support for periods up to six hours for removal of fresh, soft thrombi or emboli. The cannula and circuit are designed to be used with off shelf pump, filter and reinfusion cannula. The device itself leverages the use of blood flow through a centrifugal pump to create negative pressure in order to extirpate undesirable intravascular material, such as thrombus, emboli or vegetation.

3.1 Cannula

The current iteration of the cannula is in its third generation. It is available in either a 180- or 20-degree angled tip (**Figure 1**). The cannula itself is radiopaque with a self-expanding nitinol tip which allows for visualization under fluoroscopic imaging. The tip is funnel shaped which allows for greater contact surface area of the unwanted material and the cannula shaft supported by a flat stainless-steel coiled wire within the catheter body to support greater pushability, kink resistance, and column strength. The cannula is further supported by a slide over sheath (**Figure 2**), which allows the user to maintain the desired angle needed to engage the unwanted material.

3.2 Circuit

The circuit consists of ½ inch tubing typically used for extracorporeal circulation with the use of quick connectors which allow for greater efficiency and ease of use. The quick connector are rotating adapters that allows for rotation of the cannula independently without twisting or kinking the circuit tubing. In addition, the circuit has a built in Y-Adapter with touhy insert allowing for over-the-wire capability through a working side port (**Figure 3**). This allows the user to use up to a 17 French adjunctive device alongside the cannula if needed.

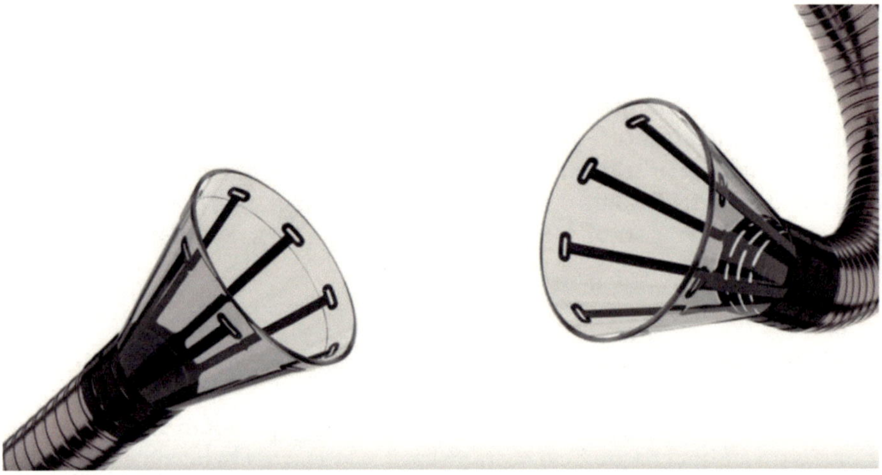

Figure 1.
AngioVac cannula.

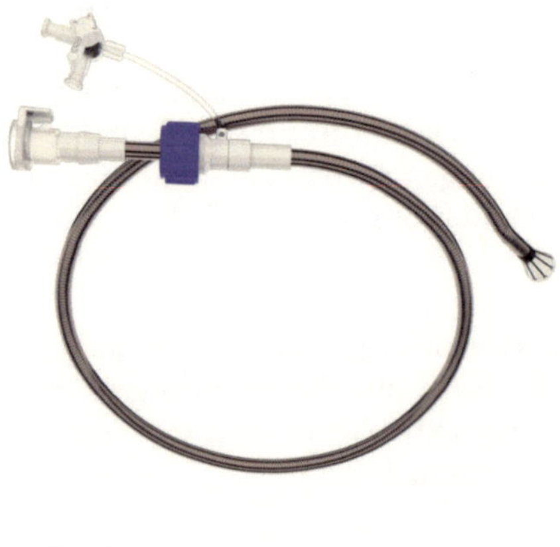

Figure 2.
AngioVac cannula with slide over sheath.

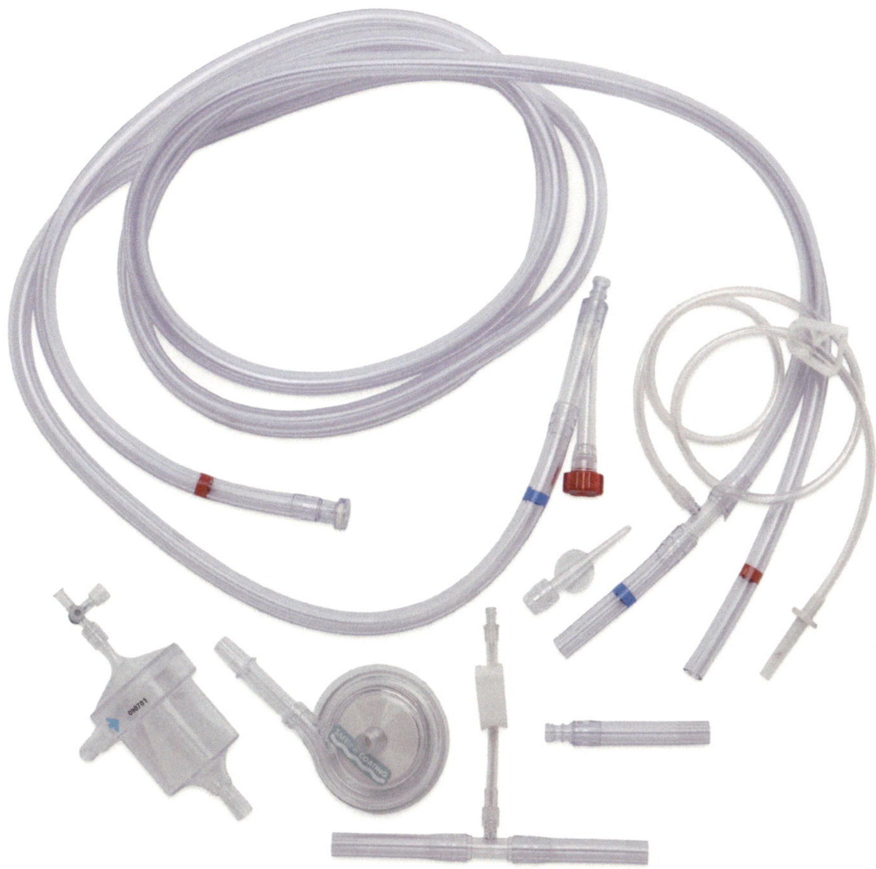

Figure 3.
AngioVac circuit.

3.3 Pump

The pump used with this system can be any off the shelf centrifugal pump. The centrifugal pump leverages negative pressure with increase in flow rates to extirpate undesirable material into the trap. Typical flow rates are around 3-4 Liters/minute. Once the material is engaged, flows will almost always come down to zero, but the negative pressure of the pump circulating allows the material to be suctioned up into the cannula and subsequently into the circuit and trap. Cavitation can occasionally occur but is well tolerated on the right side especially if the patient does not have a patent foramen ovale. When cavitation occurs, clamping the inflow and outflow and deairing the circuit is made simple due to the quick connectors.

3.4 Placement

As mentioned earlier, the AngioVac cannula can be used in the vena cava as well as the right atrium. It is not indicated for use in the pulmonary artery, but centers have used it in the right ventricle on occasion to extirpate vegetation or clot underneath the tricuspid valve. As centers have gained more experience with thromboembolism mainly in the right atrium, more centers are now using AngioVac for vegetations particularly on the tricuspid valve [32–34]. Access is obtained usually percutaneously in both femoral veins or through the right internal jugular vein and a femoral vein for a veno-venous configuration (**Figure 4**).

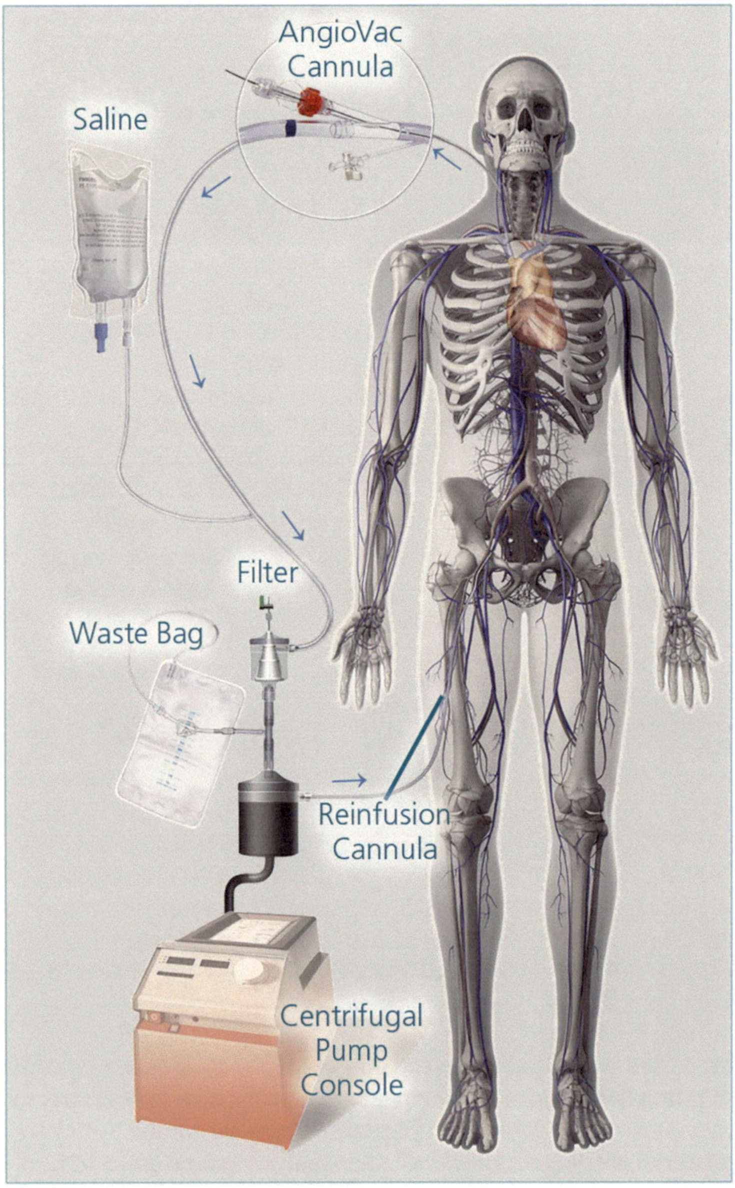

Figure 4.
AngioVac placement and configuration.

3.5 Indications

The surgical indications for TVE are less clear than that of endocarditis involving the left side of the heart. Current indications for surgery include vegetations >2 cm, evidence of septic pulmonary emboli, methicillin resistant organism, fungal infections and structural deterioration causing severe tricuspid valve regurgitation and heart failure [21]. However, given the repeat IVDU in these patients a surgical treatment is less likely to last for long due to repeat episodes of TVE. More concerning is the potential of prosthetic valve endocarditis which almost always necessitates a reoperation. Surgeons often find themselves in an ethical dilemma when patients represent needing a reoperation, especially when they have failed a second or third time. The risk of reoperation steadily increases and at some point, the risks outweigh the benefits.

However, a percutaneous option is more appealing due to its less invasive nature and the fact that it can be done multiple times without increasing the risk for the patient.

4. Current data

4.1 Percutaneous valve debulking in tricuspid valve endocarditis

Although vast data for the use of percutaneous valve debulking (PTVD) is rare, there are some retrospective data available. George et al., look at a review of 33 consecutive patients over 40 months who were declined traditional surgical management for TVE. Procedural success was defined as the removal of >1 cm of particulate and/or the ability to removal additional particulate. Patients were young with a vast majority being positive for IVDU (73%) with staphylococcal species being the most common causative agent. (75%). The average size of the tricuspid vegetation was 2.1 + 0.7 cm. More than 75% of patients had clearance of bacteremia within 48 hours of the procedure. Roughly 43.5% of patients however had worsening of their tricuspid regurgitation [32]. The same group also compared PTVD to valve replacement in a retrospective study which showed that the 1-year mortality was unchanged between the two cohorts, with the PTVD cohort having a shorter hospital length of stay [33].

A recent multicenter retrospective review showed at in 89 patients, 70% of patients had complete clearance of bacteremia within 48 hours of the procedure with only one patient requiring surgery for severe TR and heart failure. Surprisingly, the TR was unchanged in most patients (60%) and improved in 20% and worsened in 20%. The group of patient who had worsening of their TR were those who was on the borderline of mild–moderate and moderate–severe TR [34].

4.2 AngioVac in CIDE

Recent data from Starck et al. in 101 patients undergoing lead extraction with vegetation showed low risk and possible survival benefit when PTVD was combined with lead extraction [35]. Extraction was performed with either mechanical, laser or traction alone in the setting of a femoral to femoral venous configuration of AngioVac. This resulted in a theoretical reduction of septic pulmonary emboli with low intraprocedural complication rate. Overall, thirty-day mortality was 3% which was due to severe sepsis.

5. Conclusion

RSIE is increasing particularly due to the incidence of patients with CIEDs and IVDU particularly due to the opioid epidemic (7–10). Medical management alone is these groups of patients leads to medical failure and can lead to further complications such as septic pulmonary emboli. Surgical intervention in TVE is associated with higher risk of recurrent infection, thromboembolic and bleeding complications and reoperation with valve replacement [6]. In addition, contemporary series have shown that valve repair is preferred over replacement especially in IVDUs [6, 36, 37]. In addition to current recommendations, the use of percutaneous aspirational techniques provide a unique and effective way to treat these patients. These techniques are evolving and may become standard of care involving a multidisciplinary approach and avoid the need for surgical intervention at the time of presentation and potentially allow for a greater chance of needing of having a repair rather than a replacement in patients with structural deterioration of their valve.

Conflict of interest

Dr. Mark Joseph is a consultant for AngioDynamcis.

Author details

Vira I. Ayzenbart and Mark Joseph*
Virginia Tech Carilion School of Medicine, Roaonke, Virginia, USA

*Address all correspondence to: mjoseph@carilionclinic.org

References

[1] Chu VH, Sexton DJ. Pathogenesis of vegetation formation in infective endocarditis. Up to Date Web site. Available from : https://www.uptodate.com/contents/pathogenesis-of-vegetation-formation-in-infective-endocarditis. [Accessed: 2020-11-18]

[2] Ferraz de Campos FP, Takayasu V, Kim EIM, Benvenuti LA. Non-infectious thrombotic endocarditis. Autops Case Rep. 2018 Apr 18;8(2):e2018020. doi: 10.4322/acr.2018.020.

[3] Muñoz-Grajales C, Chavarriaga JC, Márquez JD, Pinto LF. Noninfective endocarditis in microscopic polyangiitis: Report of a case with a successful response to immunosuppressive therapy. Reumatol Clin. 2019 Sep-Oct;15(5):e21-e23. English, Spanish. doi: 10.1016/j.reuma.2017.07.005. Epub 2017 Aug 16.

[4] Rajani R, Klein JL. Infective endocarditis: A contemporary update. Clin Med (Lond). 2020 Jan;20(1):31-35. doi: 10.7861/clinmed.cme.20.1.1.

[5] NEJM IE article -- cite

[6] Hussain ST, Witten J, Shrestha NK, Blackstone EH, Pettersson GB. Tricuspid valve endocarditis. Ann Cardiothorac Surg, 2017; 6(3): 255-261.

[7] Wallen TJ, Szeto W, Williams M, Atluri P, Arnaoutakis G, Fults M, Sultan I, Desai N, Acker M, Vallabhajosyula PJ. Card Surg. 2018 May; 33(5):260-264. DOI:10.111/jocs.13600.

[8] Hartman L, Barnes E, Bachmann L, et al.: Opiate injection-associated infective endocarditis in the Southeastern United States. Am J Med Sci 352:603-608, 2016.

[9] Wurcel AG, Anderson JE, Chui KKH, et al.: Increasing infectious endocarditis admissions among young people who inject drugs. Open Forum Infect Dis 3:157, 2016.

[10] Hoen B, Duval X. Infective Endocarditis. N Engl J Med 2012; 268:1425-33.

[11] Nishimura RA, Otto CM, Bonow RO, et al.: 2017 AHA/ACC Focused Update of the 2014 AHA/ACC guideline for the management of patients with valvular heart disease: A report of the American College of Cardiology/American Heart Association task force on clinical practice guidelines. Circlation 2017.

[12] Edelstein S, Yahalom M. Cardiac device-related endocarditis: Epidemiology, pathogenesis, diagnosis and treatment – a review. Int J Angiol. 2009 Winter; 18(4): 167-172.

[13] Luc JGY, Choi JH, Kodia K, Weber MP, Horan DP, Maynes EJ, Carlson LA, Massey HT, Entwistle JW, Morris RJ, Tchantchaleishvili V. Valvectomy versus replacement for the surgical treatment of infective tricuspid valve endocarditis: a systematic review and meta-analysis. Ann Cardiothorac Surg. 2019 Nov;8(6):610-620.

[14] Munro AI, Jamieson WR, Tyers GF, et al. Tricuspid valve replacement: porcine bioprostheses and mechanical prostheses. Ann Thorac Surg 1995;60:S470-3; discussion S473-4.

[15] Yanagawa B, Elbatarny M, Verma S, et al. Surgical Management of Tricuspid Valve Infective Endocarditis: A Systematic Review and Meta-Analysis. Ann Thorac Surg 2018;106:708-14.

[16] Musci M, Siniawski H, Pasic M, et al. Surgical treatment of right-sided active infective endocarditis with or without involvement of the left heart: 20-year single center experience. Eur J Cardiothorac Surg 2007;32:118-25.

[17] Roudaut R, Serri K, Lafitte S. Thrombosis of prosthetic heart valves: diagnosis and therapeutic considerations. Heart. 2007;93(1):137-142. doi:10.1136/hrt.2005.071183.

[18] Beller JP, Krebs ED, Hawkins RB, Mehaffey JH, Quader MA, Speir AM, Kiser AC, Joseph M, Yarboro LT, Teman NR, Ailawadi G. Non-vitamin K oral anticoagulant use after cardiac surgery is rapidly increasing. J Thorac Cardiovasc Surg. 2020 Nov;160(5):1222-1231. doi: 10.1016/j.jtcvs.2019.09.064

[19] Altaani HA, Jaber S. Tricuspid Valve Replacement, Mechnical vs. Biological Valve, Which Is Better?. Int Cardiovasc Res J. 2013;7(2):71-74.

[20] Kang Y, Hwang HY, Sohn SH, Choi JW, Kim KH, Kim KB. Fifteen-Year Outcomes After Bioprosthetic and Mechanical Tricuspid Valve Replacement. Ann Thorac Surg. 2020 Nov;110(5):1564-1571. DOI:10.1016/j.athoracsur.2020.02.040.

[21] Couetil J-PA, Argyriadis PG, Shafy A, et al. Partial replacement of the tricuspid valve by mitral homografts in acute endocarditis. Ann Thorac Surg 2002;73:1808-12. 10.1016/S0003-4975(02)03574-9

[22] Demir OM, Regazzoli D, Mangieri A, et al. Transcatheter Tricuspid Valve Replacement: Principles and Design. Front Cardiovasc Med. 2018;5:129. Published 2018 Sep 19. doi:10.3389/fcvm.2018.00129.

[23] Sandoe JAT, Barlow G, Chambers JB. Guidelines for the diagnosis, prevention and management of implantable cardiac electronic device infection. J Antimicrob Chemother. 2015; 70: 325-359.

[24] Greenspon AJ, Patel JD, Lau E, Ochoa JA, Frisch DR, Ho RT, Pavri BB, Kurtz SM. 16-year trends in the infection burden for pacemakers and implantable cardioverter-defibrillators in the United States 1993 to 2008. J Am Coll Cardiol. 2011 Aug 30;58(10):1001-6. doi: 10.1016/j.jacc.2011.04.033.

[25] Lambert CT, Tarakji KG. Cardiac implantable electronic device infection. Cleveland Clinic Journal of Medicine. 2017 December;84(suppl 3):47-53.

[26] Almqvist M, Mattson G, Razmi R, Magnusson P. Cardiac Implantable Electronic Device-Related Infections. June 17th 2019 .DOI: 10.5772/intechopen.86395

[27] Sohail MR, Uslan DZ, Khan AH, Friedman PA, Hayes DL, Wilson WR, Steckelberg JM, Stoner S, Baddour LM. Management and outcome of permanent and implantable cardioverter-defibrillator infections. J Am Coll Cardiol. 2007;49:1851-1859.

[28] Le KY, Sohail MR, Friedman PA, et al. Impact of timing of device removal on mortality in patients with cardiovascular implantable electronic device infections. Heart Rhythm 2011;8:1678-85.

[29] Kusumoto FM, Schoenfeld MH, Wilkoff BL, et al. 2017 HRS expert consensus statement on cardiovascular implantable electronic device lead management and extraction. 2017; 14(12): e503-e551.

[30] Wazni O, Epstein LM, Carillo RG, et. al. Lead Extraction in the Contemporary Setting: The LExICon Study: A Multicenter Observational Retrospective Study of Consecutive Laser Lead Extractions. J Am Coll Cardiol. 2010;55:579-586.

[31] Baddour LM, Epstein AE, Erickson CC, et al. Update on cardiovascular implantable electronic device infections and their management: A scientific statement from the American Heart Association. Circulation. 2010;121: 458-477.

[32] George B, Voelkel A, Kotter J, et al. A novel approach to percutaneous removal of large tricuspid valve vegetations using suction filtration and veno-venous bypass: A single center experience. Catheter Cardiovasc Interv. 2017;9:1009-1015.

[33] George BJ, Santos P, Donaldson K, Musa, et al. A retrospective comparison of tricuspid valve surgery to tricuspid valve vegetation debulking with AngioVac for isolated tricuspid endocarditis. Published abstract. JACC 2019. March 12;73 (9).

[34] Joseph M, Reddy VS. Percutaneous Treatment Option for Treating Tricuspid Valve Endocarditis. (submitted for publication)

[35] Starck CT, Schaerf RHM, Breitenstein A, Najibi S, Conrad J, Berendt J, Esmailian F, Eulert-Grehn J, Dreizler T, Falk V. Transcather aspiration of large pacemaker and implantable cardioverter-defibrillator lead vegetations facilitating safe transvenous lead extraction. Europace. 2020 Jan 1;22 (1):133-138. DOI: 10.1093/europace/euz283.

[36] Dawood MY, Cheema FH, Ghoreishi M, et al.: Contemporary outcomes of operations for tricuspid valve infective endocarditis. Ann Thorac Surg 99:539-546, 201.

[37] Witten JC, Hussain ST, Shrestha NK, et al.: Surgical treatment of right-sided infective endocarditis. J Thorac Cardiovasc Surg 157:1418-1427, 2019.e14.

Chapter 9

Surgery for Tricuspid Valve Endocarditis in the Current Era

Sameh M. Said

Abstract

Tricuspid valve endocarditis (TVE) continues to be on the rise and has been mostly attributed to the growing epidemic of intravenous drug abuse (IVDA). Other risk factors include long-term indwelling central venous catheters and implantable cardiac devices. While medical management continues to be the first line therapy, surgery is indicated when medical management fails, and in the presence of hemodynamic deterioration, recurrent septic pulmonary embolization and/or persistent sepsis. Tricuspid valve (TV) excision once was the main surgical strategy, but other options include TV repair/reconstruction and replacement. Remaining challenges include management of drug-induced endocarditis and the best strategy for recurrent infection.

Keywords: endocarditis, tricuspid valve endocarditis, intravenous drug abuse, implantable cardiac devices

1. Introduction

Infective endocarditis remains a serious disease that is associated with significant morbidity and mortality. The overall incidence is relatively low, about 5/100,000 person-years [1]. In the current era, aggressive medical therapy and earlier surgical interventions with few exceptional circumstances have been the goal. Recent literature shows relatively stable mortality rates, despite the improvement in diagnostic and therapeutic tools including medical therapy and surgical techniques [2]. Isolated TVE overall is less common in comparison to left sided endocarditis. In a study of 801 adult patients with endocarditis, tricuspid or multivalvular involvement was present in 31.2% and this was a significant risk factor of early mortality on multivariate analysis [3]. The incidence of TVE is increasing, mostly related to the growing epidemic of drug abuse. In the report by Seratnahaei et al., the incidence of tricuspid endocarditis increased from 6% between 1999 and 2000 to 36% between 2009 and 2010 [4].

2. Epidemiology

Right-sided endocarditis occurs at lower incidence in comparison to left-sided infection due to the less common pathology that involves the right heart in addition to the lower pressures and decrease oxygen content in comparison to the left side of the heart [5].

Right-sided endocarditis represents 5–10% of infective endocarditis cases [6], and TVE constitutes the majority of these cases. Of all surgeries for endocarditis in North America, 4.1% involves TVE [7].

IntechOpen

3. Natural history

Isolated TVE has been reported to have a favorable prognosis and good response to medical therapy with few exceptions. Ginzton and colleagues studied 16 patients (12 had history of IVDA) with TVE to define echocardiographic criteria to help identifying those at risk for complications or need for TV surgery [8]. The authors concluded that TV vegetations tend to resolve with time, however, those with persistent infection, cardiomegaly and right heart failure are at increased risk, and no M mode or two-dimensional echocardiographic feature is a predictor of outcome.

This tendency for TV vegetations to resolve overtime is different from left-sided endocarditis which tend to persist. This could be related to bacteriological cure or silent embolization to the lung overtime.

4. Risk factors

- *Intravenous Drug Abuse (IVDA)*

    - This is the most common predisposing factor for right sided endocarditis and it ranges between 2 and 5% per year.

    - Approximately 15 opioid overdose deaths and 5 heroin overdose death per 100,000 population reported in 2016, in comparison to 6 opioid overdose deaths and one heroin overdose death per 100,000 population in 2010, according to the Centers for Disease Control data [9]. This growing epidemic of drug abuse constitutes a major risk factor for TVE. In an analysis of the Society of Thoracic Surgeons national database, isolated TV operations were performed in 1613 patients with intravenous drug-associated TV endocarditis between 2011 to 2016 [10].

    - Structural abnormalities of the TV have been noticed in those with chronic use of injected drugs. These abnormalities have been visualized by echocardiography and include leaflet thickening, and/or prolapse with or without regurgitation [11].

- *Long-term Indwelling Catheters*

    - One of the most common complications of long-term indwelling central venous catheters that are used for long-term hemodialysis or long-term delivery of medications such as chemotherapy has been infection [12]. The incidence of this type of infection is increasing and is parallel to the increase use of indwelling central venous catheters. In the United Sates, it is estimated that about 35,000 cases of catheter-related *Staphylococcus aureus* infection are reported each year with 6% of them developing into endocarditis [13].

- *Implantable Cardiac Devices*

    - This is a severe type of infection that is seen in patients with permanent pacemakers and defibrillators, and its incidence has been on the rise due to the increase use of these devices. In a prospective study of 2760 patients by Athan et al. [14], the incidence of cardiac device-related infection was 6.4%. Coexisting valvular involvement was present in 37.3%, of which 24.3% was TVE.

 - ○ The risk of infection after pacemaker implantation is 0.5–1% in the first year after implantation and with the increase complexity of the implanted device, and the need for device replacement or revision procedures, it increases further [15].

- *Congenital Heart Defects*

 - ○ Patients with ventricular septal defect (VSD) and left-to-right shunts are at risk of endocarditis. TV involvement occurs secondary to the jet lesion against the anterior or the septal leaflets of the TV. Current guidelines do not recommend endocarditis prophylaxis anymore in those with acyanotic heart defects due to the low risk of its occurrence in this population [16].

 - ○ Endocarditis in the presence of atrial septal defects is extremely rare due to the slow velocity of the shunt flow, and only few reported cases exist in the literature. An explanation of such occurrence could be related to the development of tricuspid regurgitation secondary to right ventricular volume overload which increases the risk of TV involvement [17].

5. Microbiology

The most predominant organism is *Staphylococcus aureus* (60–90%). In IVDA, there has been an increase in methicillin-resistance and polymicrobial infection [18]. Coagulase-negative Staphylococcus infection occurs more frequently in the presence of prosthetic valves and indwelling central catheters. Although infection with Streptococci can occur (<10%), it remains higher in left-sided endocarditis [19]. There is also increase in infection with Pseudomonas and other gram-negative bacteria. Fungal infection is not uncommon and has been associated with high mortality especially in immunocompromised patients and those with intracardiac devices [20].

6. Clinical presentations

Clinical presentation may vary depending on degree of involvement/destruction of the tricuspid valve and presence or absence of complications. The most common presentation has been persistent fever, chills, anorexia, fatigue, cough, dyspnea, dizziness, cardiac murmur, and varying degrees of heart failure. Septic shock may occur in severe cases.

7. Complications of tricuspid endocarditis

The most common complications are related to valvular destruction with subsequent varying degrees of tricuspid regurgitation. Large vegetations can lead to valvular obstruction or recurrent septic pulmonary embolization (**Figure 1(A)**) and hemoptysis or pulmonary abscesses (**Figure 1(B)**). This repeat pulmonary embolization can result in elevation of the right-sided pressures, which in the presence of atrial level shunting, can lead to systemic embolization as well [21]. In severe cases, abscess formation is not uncommon [22], so as varying degrees of atrioventricular block. Acute diffuse glomerulonephritis secondary to immune complex formation and complement C3 deposition in the renal glomeruli resulting in acute renal failure

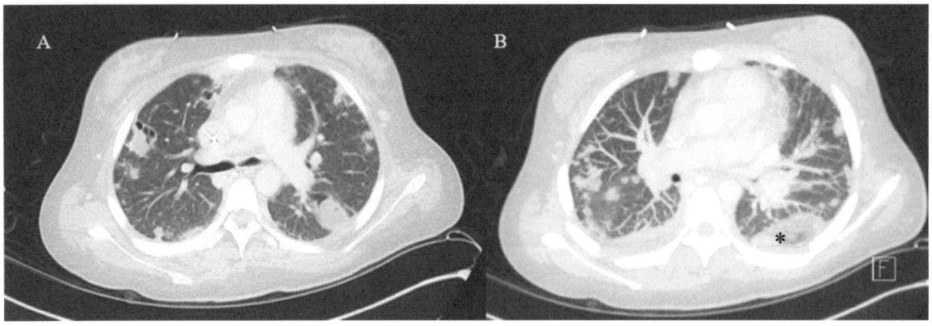

Figure 1.
(A and B). Preoperative computed tomography scan in a patient with isolated tricuspid valve endocarditis secondary to intravenous drug use showing: (A) multiple bilateral septic pulmonary emboli with cavitation. Notice in (B), the development of necrotic changes with possible abscess (asterisk) formation in the left lung.

has been reported with *Staphylococcus aureus* [23]. When sepsis is uncontrolled, this can lead to right heart failure, septic shock, and multiorgan failure.

Acquired VSD can occur after an episode of endocarditis. Gerbode described in 1958 [24] an acquired form of left ventricular-to-right atrial shunting with successful repair. Acquired Gerbode defect is a type of paramembranous VSD that is associated with left ventricular-to-right atrial shunting which can occur above (Type I), below (Type II) or both sides (Type III) of the septal leaflet of the TV [25].

8. Diagnosis

Diagnosis depends on high index of suspicion and by identifying the patient's risk factors and the occurrence of the usual manifestation of infection such as persistent fever and other signs of bacteremia. Echocardiography remains the most appropriate initial test in these patients. Both transthoracic and transesophageal modalities are important to confirm the diagnosis, identify the presence of vegetations (**Figure 2**; **Video 1**—https://bit.ly/3mDCQxK), evaluate the degree of TV destruction/regurgitation (**Video 2**—https://bit.ly/3mDCQxK), rule out any intra-cardiac shunts and evaluate the left side of the heart for any evidence of multivalvular involvement.

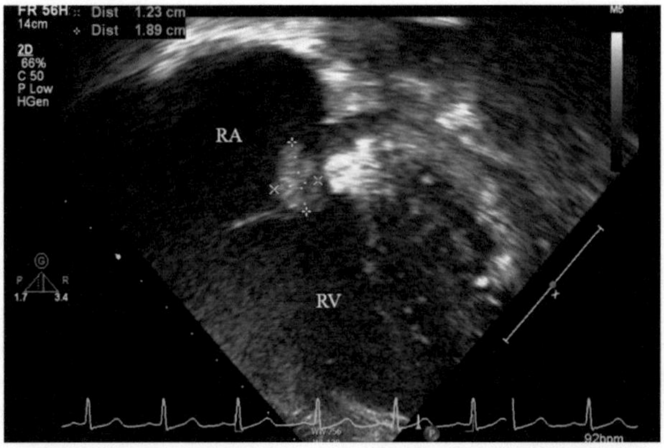

Figure 2.
A large tricuspid valve vegetation (1.9 × 1.2 mm) is shown on preoperative transthoracic echocardiography. RA: Right atrium; RV: Right ventricle.

Computed tomography (CT) scan is indicated to evaluate the lung parenchyma and vasculature. Due to the difficulty in diagnosing septic pulmonary emboli, we obtain chest CT scan routinely as this may change the timing of intervention. Other relevant tests depend on presence of other systemic manifestations of infection/embolization may include other cross-sectional imaging, brain imaging etc.

It is important to know that it is difficult to apply the Duke's criteria [26] to diagnose TVE due to: (1) the unique anatomy of the structures in the right side of the heart which could simulate vegetations, (2) embolization if occurred is pulmonary rather than systemic which is difficult to diagnose until it evolves into pulmonary infarcts or abscesses, and (3) many of the radiologic findings can be mistaken for pneumonia.

9. Treatment

- *Medical Treatment*

  In general, right-sided endocarditis resolves with medical treatment in the majority of cases (70–85%).

- *Surgical Treatment*

  Although antibiotics remained the first line treatment for TVE, several patients may fail this line of therapy and require surgical interventions. In addition, those who have residual TV regurgitation will need either early or late reconstruction or replacement of the TV.

  ○ Indications for Surgical Intervention

The following constitutes reasonable indications for surgical intervention [27]:

1. Right heart failure secondary to severe tricuspid regurgitation with poor response to medical therapy.

2. Persistent bacteremia/sepsis (> 7 days) with poor response to antibiotics which sometimes occurs in the presence of a highly virulent bacteria (*Staphylococcus aureus*, and Pseudomonas bacteremia), and infection with organisms that are difficult to eradicate such as fungi.

3. Recurrent septic pulmonary embolism with or without right heart failure.

4. Large TV vegetations (>20 mm) with or without right heart failure.

5. Abscess (more common in the presence of a prosthesis)

  ○ Timing of Surgery

While the exact timing of surgery remains unclear in many of these scenarios, it should be a team approach in decision with input from the cardiologist, cardiac surgeon, and the infectious disease specialist. In absence of urgent/emergent surgical indications (persistent sepsis, recurrent septic embolization, and heart failure), surgery is usually done on elective basis after a good duration of antibiotic therapy and appearance of negative blood cultures. This increases the chance of successful valve repair and minimize risk of recurrent infection. Decision is a bit more complicated in IVDA and in those with recurrent endocarditis.

Other factors that may affect the timing include: (1) the presence of infected intracardiac devices, (2) the causative organism (fungal may not respond to medical therapy), and (3) the presence of concomitant left-sided infection.

◦ **Surgical Options**

The principles of surgical treatment for isolated TVE follows the same principles in endocarditis cases which include thorough debridement, vegetation removal (**Figure 3**), and excision of all infected non-viable tissues. The preference after that will be to minimize the use of prosthetic materials especially in patients with history of IVDA and to attempt TV repair if possible.

◦ *Tricuspid Valvectomy*

Excision of the TV has been proposed for those with massive valvular destruction and concerns with compliance to therapy, continued IVDA, and increased risk with repeat operations for infected prosthetic TV [28]. In the presence of low-normal pulmonary vascular resistance, this option may work as a temporary measure till sepsis is controlled.

The downside of this approach is right heart failure with development of ascites, peripheral edema and low cardiac output and this should be considered as a bridge for valve replacement once infection is cleared.

◦ *Tricuspid Valve Repair*

TV repair should be strongly considered especially in IVDA cases to minimize the use of prosthetic materials and prosthesis that can lead to recurrent infection. The technique of valve reconstruction depends on the degree of valvular destruction:

1. **Direct Suturing:** suitable for small defects that is limited to one or two leaflets.

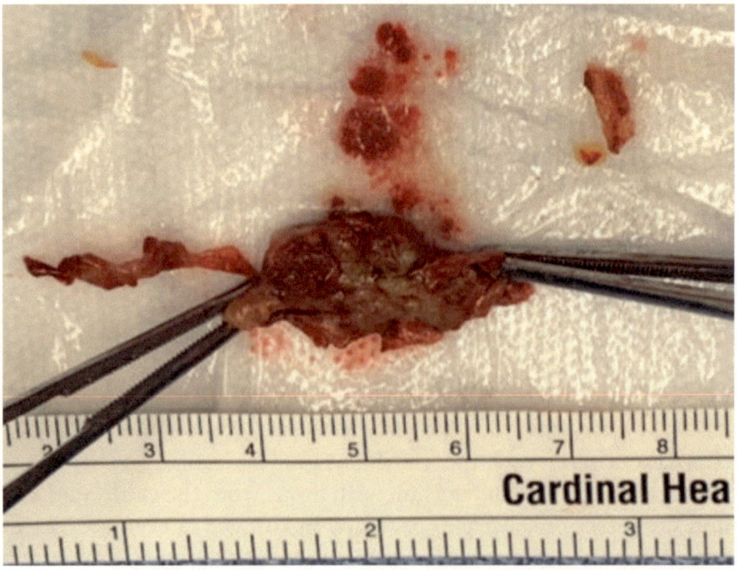

Figure 3.
Intraoperative photo showing a large, excised vegetation from the posterior leaflet of the tricuspid valve. This was performed in a 16-year-old who presented with isolated tricuspid valve endocarditis secondary to intravenous drug abuse and underwent successful tricuspid valve repair after excision of the vegetations.

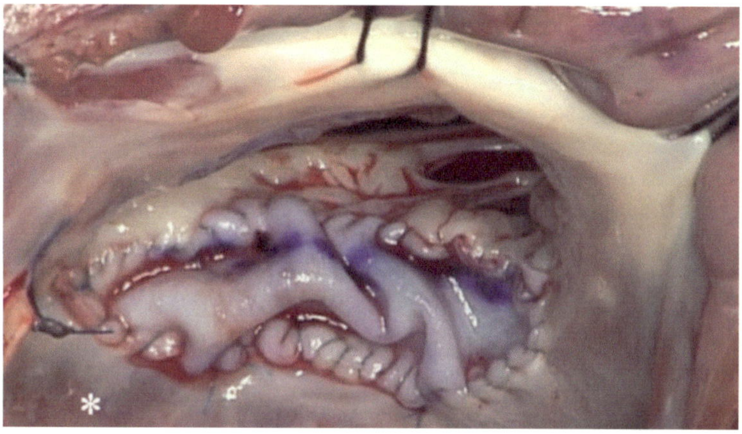

Figure 4.
Intraoperative photo showing a bovine pericardial patch that is used to augment the septal leaflet of the tricuspid valve and improve coaptation in a patient who presented with severe tricuspid valve regurgitation and history of endocarditis. Notice that augmentation should be done in the belly of the leaflet and not at the free leading edge. Also notice the area of the atrioventricular node (asterisk).

2. **Patch Repair** (**Figure 4**): our preference has been to use autologous pericardium or bovine pericardium to repair larger defects in the leaflet after excision of the vegetation and debridement of infected tissues.

3. **Leaflet Replacement:** a complete replacement of one leaflet can be performed using a variety of materials such as autologous or bovine pericardium. Multiple artificial chordae (neo-chordae) may be needed to join the newly formed leaflet with the papillary muscles of the TV and prevent prolapse.

4. **Bicuspidization of the TV:** this is suitable more when infection is localized to the posterior leaflet which can be excised, and both the anterior and septal leaflets are mobilized to form a bicuspid valve.

5. **Annuloplasty:** annuloplasty maneuvers are needed when the tricuspid annulus is dilated to support the repair and minimize recurrence of regurgitation. This varies from suture annuloplasty (Kay's or De Vega's) to a ring annuloplasty (**Figure 5(A)** and **(B)**). Several studies reported that ring annuloplasty is superior to suture annuloplasty in terms of recurrence of regurgitation [29].

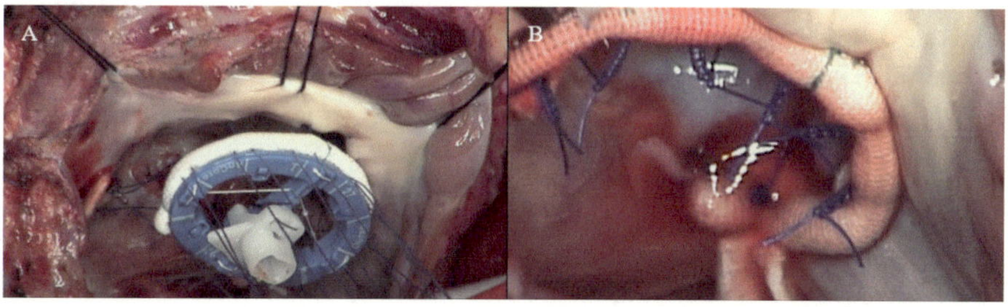

Figure 5.
(A and B). Intraoperative photos showing the technique of tricuspid valve ring annuloplasty. We prefer to use non-pledgeted prolene sutures in a horizontal mattress fashion (A) to secure the ring due to the fragility of the right atrioventricular junction. It is important to secure the ring from the anteroseptal to posteroseptal commissures. The last stitch (pledgeted) is placed within the mouth of the coronary sinus which is critical to reduce the length of the inferior annulus as most of the recurrence of regurgitation occurs due to re-dilation of the tricuspid annulus in this area.

○ *Tricuspid Valve Replacement*

While TV repair is preferred, TV replacement remains the most commonly performed procedure [30]. Bioprostheses have been the first choice but mechanical prostheses have been also used in these cases. In a study by Cho et al., there was no difference in long-term valve-related complications such as thromboembolic or bleeding events between mechanical and biological prostheses [31].

Total autologous reconstruction of the TV using autologous/bovine pericardium or extracellular matrix reconstruct has been reported in some case reports to avoid the use of the prosthetic materials in the setting of infection [32]. We do not know the long-term outcome of such maneuvers.

- *Special Circumstances*

○ **Isolated TV Vegetations without Valvular Destruction**

In some unique scenarios, large vegetations have been identified on the tricuspid valve without any evidence of valvular destruction or in some patients where the risk of surgery is quite high. Percutaneous aspiration of these large vegetations has been performed as an alternative to surgery [33]. The AngioVac system (AngioDynamics, Latham, NY) was approved in 2014 by the US Food and Drug Administration for removal of intravascular materials such as thrombi and emboli.

This system consists of two percutaneous venous cannulae (reinfusing/drainage) that are connected to an extracorporeal circuit pump head and bubble trap. Thrombotic materials/vegetations are aspirated when the pump is started and then the blood is circulated through a filter prior to returning to the patient. In a study by George et al., the authors reported the outcomes of percutaneous aspiration in 33 patients with large vegetations. Most of these patients (91%) were discharged home with reduced vegetations size in two-thirds [34]. This seems to be a reasonable option especially in those with prohibitive risk of surgery and in those with recurrent infection especially IVDA.

The obvious risks associated with percutaneous aspiration includes pulmonary embolization and vascular access complications.

○ **Prosthetic Tricuspid Valve Endocarditis**

In the presence of TV prosthesis, infection will be difficult to eradicate without removal of the prosthesis. This subgroup of patients may require early and aggressive surgical eradication of infection to minimize in-hospital mortality and morbidities. There is a higher risk of heart block in this subgroup of patients.

○ **Management of Implantable Cardiac Devices/Indwelling Catheters**

All infected leads and devices have to be removed. Hospital mortality is less when infected devices are identified earlier and removed promptly. Extraction of these devices by interventional cardiologist/electrophysiologist is preferred if possible, over the surgical extraction due to higher success and lower complication rates. One option, in less severe cases, is to remove these infected leads/devices, use temporary leads for pacemaker-dependent patients and continue antibiotic therapy and reevaluate the TV later, if repair or replacement is needed.

In severe cases that require urgent surgery, TV repair/replacement with concomitant extraction of the infected leads/devices is a better approach. Temporary pacemaker leads can be used with subsequent endovenous implantation of a new permanent system once infection is cleared is a reasonable approach.

Other options for pacemaker-dependent patients is to use leadless pacemakers or trans-coronary sinus approach to avoid placing the lead through a freshly repaired TV or replaced tricuspid prosthesis. We have used epicardial permanent pacemaker system as well in some of these complex cases with limited vascular access.

This is a team decision that should be discussed thoroughly between the electrophysiologist, cardiologists, cardiac surgeon, and the patient.

- **Concomitant Left Sided Disease (Multi-valvular Endocarditis)**

Those with left sided involvement have worse outcomes in comparison with isolated TVE. These patients will require early surgical intervention to decrease mortality and improve outcomes. In a study by Musci and colleagues, 30-day survival was 96.2% for isolated right sided involvement in comparison to 72% for combined right and left-sided endocarditis [35].

- **Mycotic Aneurysms**

Mycotic aneurysms involving the pulmonary vasculature are less common and small number of cases have been reported in the literature [36]. Staphylococcus and streptococcus species are the most common organisms involved in developing these aneurysms, but it can also occur in the settings of mycobacterial or fungal infections. Clinical manifestations are usually related to the underlying endocarditis and manifestations specific to these mycotic aneurysms are rare except when rupture occurs which can lead to catastrophic hemoptysis.

Computed tomography scan is the most reliable for detection of these aneurysms. Due to the high mortality associated with rupture of these aneurysms, transcatheter embolization is recommended, although successful antibiotic therapy have been documented in those with small aneurysms that are stable [37].

- **Concomitant Pulmonary Emboli**

In patients with TV endocarditis and large vegetations, the search for evidence of pulmonary embolization is necessary especially in the presence of hemodynamic instability or acute new pulmonary manifestations. Concomitant pulmonary embolectomy at the time of TV surgery may be considered in patients with large bilateral/unilateral emboli especially if they are accessible. We have performed a retrograde pulmonary embolectomy in a recent case of TVE in an IVDA with CT evidence of bilateral pulmonary septic emboli. This technique is valuable in the presence of emboli in the distal pulmonary arterial bed that may not be accessible with the traditional pulmonary embolectomy technique [38].

- **Recurrent Endocarditis**

The highest risk of recurrence occurs among those with IVDA [39]. In a study by Huang and colleagues, the authors followed 87 patients who survived their first episode of endocarditis and up to 25% of these patients experienced recurrence of infection within a year of the first episode [40]. Outcomes of repeat operation in this population has been poor with increased mortality. In another study by Jeganathan and colleagues, 68 patients underwent repeat TV operations with early mortality of 13.2% and higher incidence of postoperative bleeding, low cardiac output syndrome, renal failure, and stroke [41]. A debate continues regarding offering IVDA patients and those who are noncompliant, repeat surgery when infection recurs.

10. Prognosis

The majority of TVE respond to medical therapy but is associated with higher risk of recurrence, specifically in IVDA.

The overall prognosis of isolated TV endocarditis is better than left-sided and multivalvular infection. This may be due to younger age of patients, less occurrence of systemic embolization or development of drug-resistance, in addition to the fewer significant hemodynamic derangements that may occur from tricuspid regurgitation in contrast to aortic and/or mitral involvement.

The following have been associated with poor prognosis according to several reports: (1) persistent sepsis with failure to respond to medical therapy, (2) development of right heart failure, (3) fungal infection, (4) recurrent pulmonary embolization, (5) septic shock, and (6) multivalvular involvement.

11. Surgical outcomes

The estimated operative mortality for surgery for TVE is between 6 and 10% [42]. Excision of the TV has been associated with high morbidity due to right heart failure [43], and TV replacement has been associated with increased risk of recurrent infection and need for permanent pacemaker.

Yanagawa and colleagues reported the outcome sin 1165 patients who underwent surgery for TVE. The indications were recurrent pulmonary embolization, right heart failure, persistent sepsis and concomitant left-sided infection. TV repair was possible in 2/3 of these patients and the majority underwent TV replacement with a bioprosthesis. The authors concluded that both TV repair and replacement have good long-term survival, but repair is associated with less risk of need for pacemaker, recurrence of infection and reoperation [44].

Di Mauro et al. reported the surgical outcomes of isolated TVE in 157 patients (IVDA was present in 38%) of a multicenter registry. Repair was performed in 49%, while replacement with a bioprosthesis was the main procedure in 46% and a mechanical prosthesis was used in 5%. Early mortality was 11% with no difference between repair or replacement. The authors identified the following factors as predictors of poor outcomes: older age, IVDA, fungal endocarditis, repeat operation, the use of a prosthesis, and the presence of intracardiac devices [45].

In a recent systemic review and metanalysis of 752 patients with TVE by Luc and colleagues, tricuspid valvectomy was performed in 14%, while 86% underwent TV replacement. There was more prolonged duration of mechanical ventilation in the valvectomy group, but there was no significant difference in early mortality, right heart failure and recurrence of endocarditis between the two groups. The authors concluded that tricuspid valvectomy is an acceptable initial therapy in those with IVDA to help identify those who will self-select as candidates for later valve replacement [46].

12. Conclusions

TVE has several features that are unique in comparison to left-sided infection. These include the different population demographics, etiology of infection, response to medical therapy and prognosis. High index of suspicion and use of appropriate imaging modalities facilitate early diagnosis and early initiation of appropriate therapy. Surgery remains indicated in those with failure to respond to medical therapy and in the presence of complications. The same principle of surgery for endocarditis apply which are adequate and thorough debridement of all infected materials and excision of all vegetations. Extraction of all associated infected cardiac devices is critical to ensure complete eradication of all sources of infection. Excision of the TV is associated with higher morbidity due to ongoing right heart failure, and TV repair is preferred over replacement if feasible. Debate remains ongoing in regard to offering surgery for those with recurrent infection and specifically IVDA.

Author details

Sameh M. Said
Division of Pediatric Cardiovascular Surgery, Masonic Children's Hospital, Department of Surgery, University of Minnesota, Minneapolis, Minnesota, USA

*Address all correspondence to: ssaid@umn.edu

References

[1] Tleyjeh IM, Steckelberg JM, Murad HS, Anavekar NS, Ghomrawi HM, Mirzoyev Z, et al. Temporal trends in infective endocarditis: a population-based study in Olmsted County, Minnesota. JAMA 2005; 293: 3022-3028

[2] Mylonakis E, Calderwood SB, Medical P. Infective endocarditis in adults. The New England Journal of Medicine 2001; 345: 1318-1330

[3] Said SM, Abdelsattar ZM, Schaff HV, Greason KL, Daly RC, Pochettino A, et al. Outcomes of surgery for infective endocarditis: a single-center experience of 801 patients. European Journal of Cardio-Thoracic Surgery 2018 Feb 1;53(2):435-439

[4] Seratnahaei A, Leung SW, Charnigo RJ, Cummings MS, Sorrell VL, Smith MD. The changing "face" of endocarditis in Kentucky: An increase in tricuspid cases. American Journal of Medicine. 2014; 127, 04: 786.e1, 009-786.e6

[5] Goud A, Abdelqader A, Dahagam C, Padmanabhan S. Isolated pulmonic valve endocarditis presenting as neck pain. J Community Hosp Intern Med Perspect. 2015; 5:29647

[6] Murdoch DR, Corey GR, Hoen B, Miró JM, Fowler VG Jr, Bayer AS, et al. Clinical presentation, etiology, and outcome of infective endocarditis in the 21st century: The International Collaboration on Endocarditis-Prospective Cohort Study. Archives of Internal Medicine 2009; 169: 463-473

[7] Gaca JG, Sheng S, Daneshmand M, Rankin JS, Williams ML, O'Brien SM, Gammie JS. Current outcomes for tricuspid valve infective endocarditis surgery in North America. The Annals of Thoracic Surgery 2013; 961374-961381

[8] Ginzton LE, Siegel RJ, Criley JM. Natural history of tricuspid valve endocarditis: a two-dimensional echocardiographic study. The American Journal of Cardiology 1982; 49(8): 1853-1859

[9] Center for Disease Control and Prevention. Drug Overdose Death Data. Available at: https://www.cdc.gov/drugoverdose/data/statedeaths.html. Accessed June 26, 2018

[10] Slaughter MS, Badhwar V, Ising M, Ganzel B, Sell-Dottin K, Jawitz OK, et al. Optimum surgical treatment for tricuspid valve infective endocarditis: an analysis of the society of thoracic surgeons national database. J Thorac Cardiovasc Surg 2019 *(Article in press)*

[11] Pons-Llado G, Carreras F, Borras X, Cadafalch J, Fuster M, Guardia J, Casas M. Findings on Doppler echocardiography in asymptomatic intravenous heroin users. The American Journal of Cardiology 1992; 69: 238-241

[12] Bassi KK, Girl AK, Pattanayak M, Abraham SW, Pandey KK. Totally implantable venous access ports: Retrospective review of long-term complications in 81 patients. Ind J Can 2012; 49:114-118

[13] Yamashita S, Noma K, Kuwata G, Miyoshi K, Honaga K. Infective endocarditis at the tricuspid valve following central venous catheterization. Journal of Anesthesia 2005; 19:84-87

[14] Athan E, Chu VH, Tattevin P, Selton-Suty C, Jones P, Naber C, et al. Clinical characteristics and outcome of infective endocarditis involving implantable cardiac devices. JAMA 2012; 307: 1727-1735

[15] Doring M, Richter S, Hindricks G. The diagnosis and treatment of

pacemaker-associated infection. Deutsches Ärzteblatt International 2018; 115: 445-452

[16] Wilson W, Taubert KA, Gewitz M, Lockhart PB, Baddour LM, Levison M, et al. Prevention of infective endocarditis: guidelines from the American Heart Association: a guideline from the American Heart Association Rheumatic Fever, Endocarditis, and Kawasaki Disease Committee, Council on Cardiovascular Disease in the Young, and the Council on Clinical Cardiology, Council on Cardiovascular Surgery and Anesthesia, and the Quality of Care and Outcomes Research Interdisciplinary Working Group. Circulation. 2007; 116: 1736-54

[17] Shimbo M, Watanabe H, Abe T, Sato T, Koyama T, Yamamoto H, Ito H. Isolated Atrial Septal Defect Complicated by Tricuspid Valve Infective Endocarditis. Intern Med. 2015;54(19):2463-5

[18] Habib G, Lancellotti P, Antunes MJ, Bongiorni MG, Casalta JP, Del Zotti F, et al. 2015 ESC guidelines for the management of infective endocarditis: the task force for the management of infective endocarditis of the European Society of Cardiology (ESC). Endorsed by: European Association for Cardio-Thoracic Surgery (EACTS), the European Association of Nuclear Medicine (EANM). European Heart Journal 2015; 36: 3075-3128

[19] Akinosoglou K, Apostolakis E, Marangos M, Pasvol G. Native valve right sided infective endocarditis. European Journal of Internal Medicine 2013; 24:510-519

[20] Siciliano RF, Gualandro DM, Sejas ONE, Ignoto BG, Caramelli B, Mansur AJ, et al. Outcomes in patients with fungal endocarditis: a multicenter observational cohort study. International Journal of Infectious Diseases 2018; 77: 48-52

[21] Farrant O, Scozzi G, Hughes R. Systemic septic emboli in tricuspid endocarditis due to an atrial communication with a right-to-left shunt. BML Case Reports 2020 Feb 20;13(2):e233477

[22] Yuan SM. Right-sided infective endocarditis: recent epidemiologic changes. International Journal of Clinical and Experimental Medicine 2014; 7: 199-218

[23] Boils CL. Endocarditis-associated glomerulonephritis. In: Satoskar AA, Nadasdy T, editors. Bacterial infections and the kidney. Cham: Springer; 2017. p. 87-116

[24] Gerbode F, Hultgren H, Melrose D, Osborn J. Syndrome of left ventricular right atrial shunt; successful surgical repair of defect in five cases, with observation of bradycardia on closure. Annals of Surgery 1958; 148: 433-446

[25] Perry EL, Burchell HB, Edwards JE. Congenital communication between the left ventricle and the right atrium; co-existing ventricular septal defect and double tricuspid orifice. Proc Staf Meet Mayo Clin. 1949; 24: 198-206

[26] Li JS, Sexton DJ, Mick N, Nettles R, Fowler Jr VG, Ryan T, et al. Proposed modifications to the Duke criteria for the diagnosis of infective endocarditis. Clinical Infectious Diseases 2000; 30: 633-638

[27] Shmueli H, Thomas F, Flint N, Setia G, Janjic A, Siegel R. Right -sided infective endocarditis 2020: Challenges and updates in diagnosis and treatment. Journal of the American Heart Association 2020 Aug 4; 9(15): e017293

[28] Hussain ST, Witten J, Shrestha NK, Gordon SM, Houghtaling PL, Bakaeen FG, et al. Tricuspid valve endocarditis. Ann Cardiothorac Surg 2017; 6: 255-261

[29] Matsuyama K, Matsumoto M, Sugita T, Nishizawa J, Tokuda Y, Matsuo T, Ueda Y. De Vega annuloplasty and Carpentier-Edwards ring annuloplasty for secondary tricuspid regurgitation. The Journal of Heart Valve Disease 2001; 10: 520-524

[30] Protos AN, Trivedi JR, Whited WM, Rogers MP, Owolabi U, Grubb KJ, et al. Valvectomy versus replacement for the surgical treatment of tricuspid endocarditis. The Annals of Thoracic Surgery 2018; 106: 664-669

[31] Cho WC, Park CB, Kim JB, Jung SH, Chung CH, Choo SJ, Lee JW. Mechanical valve replacement versus bioprosthetic valve replacement in the tricuspid valve position. Journal of Cardiac Surgery. 2013; 28: 212-217

[32] Gerdisch MW, Boyd WD, Harlan JL, Richardson JB Jr, Flack JE 3rd, Palafox BA, et al. Early experience treating tricuspid valve endocarditis with a novel extracellular matrix cylinder reconstruction. The Journal of Thoracic and Cardiovascular Surgery 2014 Dec;148(6):3042-3048

[33] Divekar AA, Scholz T, Fernandez JD. Novel percutaneous transcatheter intervention for refractory active endocarditis as a bridge to surgery-AngioVac aspiration system. Catheterization and Cardiovascular Interventions 2013; 81: 1008-1012

[34] George B, Voelkel A, Kotter J, Leventhal A, Gurley J. A novel approach to percutaneous removal of large tricuspid valve vegetations using suction filtration and veno-venous bypass: a single center experience. Catheterization and Cardiovascular Interventions 2017; 90: 1009-1015

[35] Musci M, Siniawski H, Pasic M, Amiri A, Stein J, Siniawski H, et al. Surgical treatment of right-sided active infective endocarditis with or without involvement of the left heart: 20-year single center experience. European Journal of Cardio-Thoracic Surgery 2007;32: 118-125

[36] Knowles KA, Alvin M, Dunn E. Mycotic pulmonary artery aneurysm secondary to septic emboli. BMJ Case Rep 2017 Dec 13bcr2017223439

[37] Wilson TN, Tew K, Taranath A. Multiple mycotic aneurysms of the pulmonary arteries resolving with conservative management: multislice CT examination findings. Journal of Thoracic Imaging 2008; 23: 197-201

[38] Hussain ST, Bartholomew JR, Leacche M, Tong MZY. Retrograde pulmonary embolectomy for acute pulmonary embolism: A simplified technique. The Annals of Thoracic Surgery 2017; 103: e473–e474

[39] Alagna L, Park LP, Nicholson BP, Keiger AJ, Strahilevitz J, Morris A, et al. Repeat endocarditis: analysis of risk factors based on the International Collaboration on Endocarditis - Prospective Cohort Study. Clinical Microbiology and Infection 2014; 20:566-575

[40] Huang G, Barnes EW, Peacock JE. Repeat infective endocarditis in persons who inject drugs: "take another little piece of my heart". Open Forum Infect Dis. 2018 Nov 16;5(12): ofy304

[41] Jeganathan R, Armstrong S, Al-Alao B, David T. The risk and outcomes of reoperative tricuspid valve surgery. The Annals of Thoracic Surgery 2013; 95: 119-124

[42] Kamalakannan D, Pai RM, Johnson LB, Gardin JM, Saravolatz LD. Epidemiology and clinical outcomes of infective endocarditis in hemodialysis patients. The Annals of Thoracic Surgery 2007; 83: 2081-2086

[43] Arbulu A, Holmes RJ, Asfaw I. Surgical treatment of intractable right

sided infective endocarditis in drug addicts: 25 years' experience. The Journal of Heart Valve Disease 1993; 2: 129-137; discussion 138-29

[44] Yanagawa B, Elbatarny M, Verma S, Hill S, Mazine A, Puskas JD, Friedrich JO. Surgical management of tricuspid valve infective endocarditis: a systematic review and meta-analysis. The Annals of Thoracic Surgery 2018; 106: 708-714

[45] Di Mauro M, Foschi M, Dato GMA, Centofanti P, Barili F, Corte AD, et al. Surgical treatment of isolated tricuspid valve infective endocarditis: 25-year results from a multicenter registry. International Journal of Cardiology 2019; 292: 62-67

[46] Luc JGY, Choi JH, Kodia K, Weber MP, Horan DP, Maynes EJ, et al. Valvectomy versus replacement for the surgical treatment of infective tricuspid valve endocarditis: a systematic review and meta-analysis. Ann Cardiothorac Surg. 2019 Nov;8(6):610-620